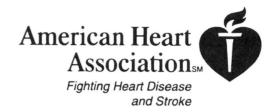

American Heart
Association℠

*Fighting Heart Disease
and Stroke*

Monograph Series

VENTRICULAR FIBRILLATION:
A PEDIATRIC PROBLEM

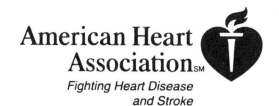

American Heart Association℠

Fighting Heart Disease and Stroke

Monograph Series

Venetricular Fibrillation
A Pediatric Problem

Edited by

Linda Quan, MD

Associate Professor of Pediatrics
University of Washington School of Medicine
Seattle, Washington

and

Wayne H. Franklin, MD

Nemours Cardiac Center
Division of Pediatric Cardiology
Alfred I. duPont Hospital for Children
Wilmington, DE

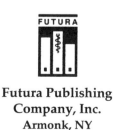

Futura Publishing
Company, Inc.
Armonk, NY

Preface

This monograph constitutes a unique compendium of the multi-faceted issues surrounding ventricular fibrillation (VF) in the pediatric patient. This single arrhythmia in the pediatric patient is a fascinating, complex phenomenon; understanding it in its different settings, the infant with congenital heart disease to the previously normal drowning child, to the adolescent with QT abnormalities, would reveal the secrets of the developing myocardium in a changing milieu. While it is the focus of attention in adult cardiac research, VF has received little attention in research of pediatric cardiac resuscitation. The number of children at risk is increasing. Advances in cardiac surgery, improved recognition of predisposing factors, ability to diagnose and treat VF by out-of-hospital personnel as well as nonmedical people, and improved treatment regimens have all served to make pediatric VF an emerging field.

This book represents a cross-fertilization among those studying VF from differing perspectives with a variety of tools. It attempts to define the current knowledge about VF in the pediatric patient from the epidemiological, physiological, and clinical perspectives. It brings together examinations of the developmental factors at the molecular, cellular, and pathophysiological level associated with VF, and identifies questions about the research and treatment of this condition that must be answered in order to save children's lives. We would like to thank Dianne L. Atkins, MD, Lisa Carlson, RN, Richard Kerber, MD, Vinay Nadkarni, MD, and Richard Robinson, PhD, for their help during the planning phase. We are also indebted to the many other outstanding scientists and clinicians who contributed to the book.

Linda Quan, MD
Wayne H. Franklin, MD

Contributors

Dianne L. Atkins, MD Associate Professor, Department of Pediatrics, University of Iowa, Iowa City, IA

Robert A. Berg, MD Professor of Pediatrics, Department of Pediatrics, Pediatric Critical Care Medicine, University of Arizona Health Sciences Center, Tucson, AZ

Charles I. Berul, MD Associate in Cardiology, Pediatric Cardiology, Children's Hospital, Harvard Medical School, Boston, MA

Thomas J. Callahan, PhD Director, OCRND, Food and Drug Administration, Rockville, MD

Carole C. Carey, MD Electrical Engineer, Food and Drug Administration, Rockville, MD

Leon Chameides, MD Clinical Professor of Pediatrics, Pediatric Cardiology, Hartford Hospital, University of Connecticut, Hartford, CT

Howard M. Corneli, MD Associate Professor of Pediatrics, Primary Children's Medical Center, University of Utah, Salt Lake City, UT

Robert Delagi, MA, NREMT-P Chief, Prehospital Medical Operations, Suffolk County Emergency Medical Services, Yaphank, NY

David J. Driscoll, MD Professor of Pediatrics, Section of Pediatric Cardiology, Mayo Clinic, Rochester, MN

Wayne H. Franklin, MD Nemours Cardiac Center, Alfred I. duPont Hospital for Children, Wilmington, DE

Richard A. Friedman, MD Pediatric Cardiology, Texas Children's Hospital, Baylor College of Medicine, Houston, TX

Arthur Garson, Jr., MD, MPH Texas Children's Hospital, Houston, TX

Joanne S. Ingwall, PhD Professor of Medicine (Physiology), Brigham and Women's Hospital, Boston, MA

Richard E. Kerber MD   Professor of Medicine, Division of Cardiology, University of Iowa, Iowa City, IA

Jack Kron, MD   Professor, Division of Cardiology, Oregon Health Sciences University, Portland, OR

John H. McAnulty, MD   Professor and Chief, Division of Cardiology, School of Medicine, Oregon Health Sciences University, Portland, OR

Vinay Nadkarni, MD   Director, Pediatric Intensive Care, Alfred I. duPont Institute, Wilmington, DE

James C. Perry, MD   Director of Cardiology, Electrophysiology, and Pacing, Children's Heart Institute, San Diego Children's Hospital, San Diego, CA

Linda Quan, MD   Associate Professor, University of Washington School of Medicine, Seattle, WA

Richard B. Robinson, PhD   Professor of Pharmacology, Department of Pharmacology, Columbia University, New York, NY

Michael R. Rosen, MD   Professor of Pediatrics, Department of Pharmacology, College of Physicians & Surgeons of Columbia University, New York, NY

Michael J. Silka, MD   Professor and Chief, Division of Pediatric Cardiology, Children's Hospital, Los Angeles, University of Southern California, Los Angeles, CA

Ronald E. Stickney   Senior Research Engineer, Medtronic Physio-Control Corporation, Redmond, WA

Jeffrey A. Towbin, MD   Associate Professor of Pediatrics (Cardiology), Baylor College of Medicine, Texas Children's Hospital, Houston, TX

George F. Van Hare, MD   Associate Professor of Pediatrics, Department of Pediatric Cardiology, Stanford University, Palo Alto, CA

Glenn T. Wetzel, MD   Associate Professor of Pediatrics, University of California Los Angeles School of Medicine, Los Angeles, CA

Arno L. Zaritsky, MD   Department of Pediatrics, Children's Hospital of the King's Daughters, Norfolk, VA

Contents

SECTION VII
Pharmacologic Treatment

SECTION VIII
Outcomes

SECTION IX
Prevention

SECTION X
Summary: Where Do We Go From Here?

Sudden Death in the Pediatric Patient with an Ostensibly Normal Heart

Developmental Changes in Normal Substrate for Lethal Arrhythmias

Chapter 1

Energetics of the Developing Heart:
Implications for Understanding Ion Movement

Joanne S. Ingwall, PhD

The following hypothesis is considered in this chapter: ventricular fibrillation (VF) causes and is caused by disturbances in energy metabolism and ion homeostasis. All processes in the heart either directly or indirectly depend on chemical energy in the form of adenosine triphosphate (ATP). Supporting the importance of energetics for normal heart function, this chapter includes a discussion about the fundamentals of the chemistry of ATP in the heart, and includes examples of how the chemistry of ATP in the developing heart differs from that in the adult heart as well as an example of the metabolic consequences and predictability of VF in the adult heart. The chapter concludes with some recommendations for future studies.

The Chemistry of ATP in the Heart

Mammalian ventricular tissue contains ~5 μmol of ATP per gram wet weight, which corresponds to a concentration of 8 to 10 mmol/L of intracellular water or 30 to 35 μmol per gram of cardiac protein. The concentration of ATP ([ATP]) is essentially constant throughout maturation of the heart, and is highly regulated. Chemical energy is stored in the phosphoryl bonds of ATP (Figure 1). Cleavage of the terminal phosphoryl bond of ATP by ATPases releases chemical energy, which is converted into the work of contraction and relaxation, ion movements, and macromolecular synthesis. The reaction is:

Supported by NIH grants HL-26215, HL43170, and HL52350.

From: Quan L, Franklin WH (eds). Ventricular Fibrillation: A Pediatric Problem. Armonk, NY: Futura Publishing Company, Inc.; ©2000.

$$ATP + H_2O \rightarrow ADP + Pi + H^+ \tag{1}$$

Chemical energy that can be used to do work in this way is called the free energy of ATP hydrolysis, ΔG.

Kinetics

The amount of ATP in the heart, $\sim$0.6 g for a 250-g heart, is sufficient to maintain pump function for less than 50 beats. Thus, the cell must continually resynthesize ATP to maintain normal myocardial pump function and cellular viability. Using a conservative value for the rate of ATP synthesis (and use) of $\sim$1 mmol/L s^{-1}, it can be calculated that we use $\sim$7 kg of ATP in a day! The distinction between the concentration of ATP versus its turnover rate is central to our understanding of bioenergetics. In the normal heart, [ATP] remains high and con-

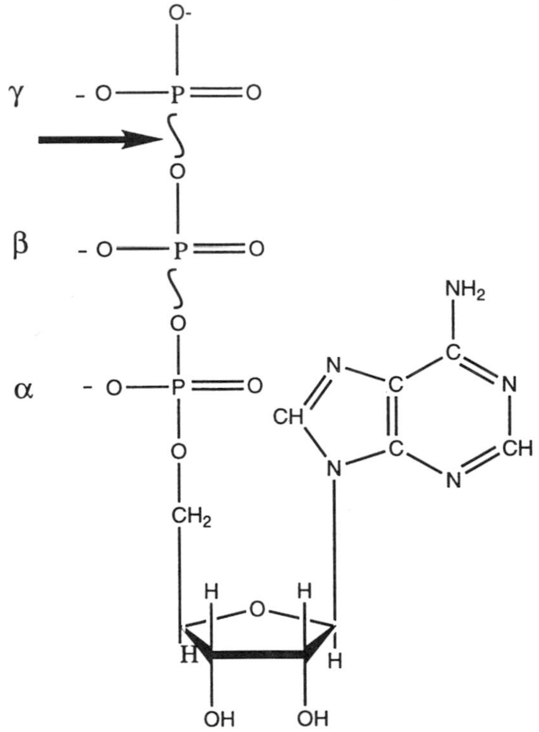

ATP

Figure 1. Structure of adenosine triphosphate.

stant but its rate of synthesis and degradation (turnover rate) varies. The energetics of increasing cardiac work illustrate this principle. As the workload of the heart increases, oxygen consumption (a good index of ATP synthesis rate in the mitochondria) proportionately increases; yet ATP content is essentially unchanged. Thus, the rate at which ATP is made and used (turnover rate), but not its concentration, increases as work increases. This example also illustrates the important principle that ATP synthesis rate matches ATP utilization rate.

Given the critical need to maintain a constant and high level of ATP, it is not surprising that the cell uses many reactions and pathways to synthesize ATP. In order of decreasing velocity (measured for the intact rat heart), the major ATP synthesizing pathways (see Figure 2) are the creatine kinase (CK) reaction ($\sim$10 mmol/L s^{-1}), oxidative phosphorylation ($\sim$1 mmol/L s^{-1}), and glycolysis ($\sim$0.03 mmol/L s^{-1}). [ATP] is maintained essentially constant by the integration of these multiple pathways for ATP synthesis. Normally, ATP production by oxidative phosphorylation is sufficient to meet the constantly changing demands for energy. Under some conditions, the CK reaction uses the energy stored in the phosphoryl bond of phosphocreatine (PCr) (present in heart in concentrations twice that of ATP) to replete the ATP pool.

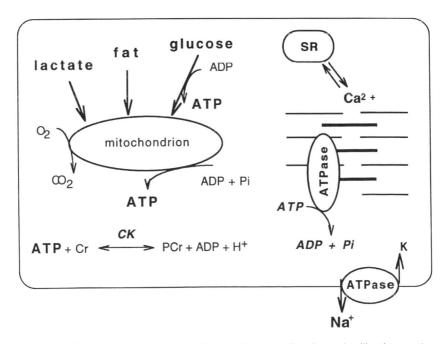

Figure 2. Diagram of adenosine triphosphate synthesis and utilization pathways. Drawn by Rong Tian, NMR Laboratory for Physiological Chemistry. Brigham and Women's Hospital, Boston, MA.

Thermodynamics

Another important principle essential for our understanding of bioenergetics is that the chemical reactions that use ATP are "driven" by high ratios of [ATP] to adenosine diphosphate concentration ([ADP]), while ATP synthesis reactions are "inhibited" by high [ATP]-to-[ADP] ratios. There are several ways that the energy state of the cell describing the balance between demand and synthesis can be quantitated. One expression that defines the energy state is the adenylate energy charge. It is defined as ([ATP]+1/2[ADP])/([ATP]+[ADP]+[AMP]), and it distinguishes between useable ATP (the numerator) and the total adenine nucleotide pool (the denominator). In well perfused tissue, the cytosolic [ATP], [ADP], and adenosine monophosphate concentration ([AMP]) are approximately 10 mmol/L, 30 μmol/L, and 0.1 μmol/L, respectively, and the energy charge is close to 1. Even when [ADP] and [AMP] increase (as in ischemia) to near mmol/L levels, the energy charge does not change very much.

A variation of the energy charge that is more relevant to biological conditions is the phosphorylation potential, defined as [ATP]/([ADP] × [Pi]). This term takes into account the ability of the end products of ATP hydrolysis, namely inorganic phosphate (Pi) and ADP, to inhibit ATPase activities on the one hand, and, on the other, to stimulate ATP synthesis pathways. The phosphorylation potential in well perfused myocardium is greater than 300 mmol/L^{-1} (ATP, ADP, and Pi concentrations of ~10 mmol/L, 30 μmol/L, and 1 mmol/L, respectively). Even a modest increase in ADP and Pi (say, a doubling of each at essentially constant [ATP]), lowers the phosphorylation potential to ~80 mmol/L^{-1}. Thus, the phosphorylation potential is a sensitive marker of the energy state of the cell. It is the critical component of the thermodynamic quantity representing the free energy of ATP hydrolysis, ΔG.

The free energy of ATP hydrolysis defines the driving force for all ATP-utilizing reactions in the cell for that set of conditions. It is calculated from the constant value for ATP hydrolysis under standard conditions of temperature and pressure for molar concentrations of reactants, ΔG°, corrected for the actual concentrations of ATP, ADP, and Pi in the cytosol. The expression is:

$$\Delta G = \Delta G^{\circ} - RT \, ln \, \frac{[ATP]}{[ADP] \, [Pi]} \qquad (2)$$

where ΔG° is the standard free energy change of ATP hydrolysis (−30.5 kJ/mol under standard conditions of molarity, temperature, pH, and Mg^{2+}), R is the gas constant (8.3 J/mol · K), and T is the absolute temperature in kelvin. The argument of the *ln* term is the phosphorylation potential. The value of ΔG for pyruvate-perfused rodent heart with a typical rate-pressure product of 28,000 mm Hg min^{-1} is -68 ± 2 kJ/mol; for a glucose-perfused heart, which has higher ADP and Pi concentrations, ΔG becomes less negative, -57.7 ± 0.6 kJ/mol. The less negative value means that the glucose-only perfused heart has a lower driving force for ATP-utilizing reactions (the value is closer to zero). Notice that the values of the two terms in the equation (ΔG° and the *ln* term) are about the same; thus, to change ΔG, there must be a large change in the *ln* term. Because it is often confusing to describe changes for a negative number, it is convenient to describe changes in ΔG in terms of its absolute value, $|\Delta G|$.

In order to know whether there is a high enough driving force for the ATP-utilizing reactions, we compare the values of ΔG obtained for the whole heart with the literature values for ΔG for the actomyosin ATPase and the sodium and calcium pumps. Values of $|\Delta G|$ for the AT-Pases calculated under well controlled conditions are ~52, 48, and 46 kJ/mol for the calcium, sodium, and the myofibrillar ATPases, respectively. Thus, even a heart perfused with only glucose as its carbon source for ATP synthesis has a $|\Delta G|$ (~58 kJ/mol) sufficient to drive these ATPase reactions.

The concept is analogous to the way a battery works. As long as the voltage is high enough to run the motor or to turn on the flashlight, the motor will function and the flashlight will turn on. With time, as the voltage runs down and becomes close to threshold, there is a brown-out. When the voltage falls below the threshold necessary to turn on the motor (or light), it will not turn on. Thus the sign (+, 0, or −) determines the direction of the reaction or, in the case of the motor and of the ATPases, whether they function. One other point is instructive. New batteries have more voltage than batteries nearing the threshold value for turning on the motor. The motor turns on for both conditions, but the new batteries have more *energy reserve*. For our biological studies, we refer to the difference between the ΔG for ATP hydrolysis measured for the tissue and the literature values for the ΔG needed to run the AT-Pase as the driving force for the reaction or the energy reserve. As shown below, an evaluation of the energy reserve of the heart can be useful for an understanding of metabolic and ionic events in the cell.

Enzyme Kinetics: The Developing Heart as a Model System Illustrating the Importance of Changing Enzyme Capacity

Enzymes are catalysts. They do not determine whether a reaction takes place. Instead, they determine how fast it takes place. Biochemists have developed quantitative expressions that allow calculation of the speed of the reaction; these expressions are called rate equations. One common feature of rate equations is that the velocity of the reaction is linearly dependent on the amount of enzyme present. This is usually determined as the capacity of the reaction (V_{max}), ie, the activity measured under conditions when none of the substrates for the reaction are limiting. Velocity of the reaction also depends (but not always linearly or even monotonically) on the amount of substrate available to drive the reaction. Thus, a useful estimate for the velocity of a reaction is the product of V_{max} and the concentration of its reactants.

The developing heart is the quintessential example of large changes in the velocity of reactions that are important for ATP synthesis. One developmentally regulated enzyme that has been studied in detail is CK. CK activity is highest in cells with high ATP turnover rates, namely nondividing differentiated skeletal and cardiac muscle cells and brain, and rapidly dividing cells. CK catalyzes the transfer of a phosphoryl group between PCr and ATP:

$$PCr + ADP + H \rightleftharpoons creatine + ATP \qquad (3)$$

The velocity of the CK reaction can be directly measured in the intact functioning heart by use of a nuclear magnetic resonance (NMR) technique called ^{31}P magnetization transfer. The opportunity to measure the velocity of a specific chemical reaction in the intact beating heart is unique. Velocity can also be calculated but this requires not only knowledge of the concentrations of all substrates and products of the reaction but also the binding constants for each entity, weighted for the amount of each of the five distinct CK isoenzymes present in the heart. We have found the estimation of the velocity as the product of V_{max}—the activity under saturating conditions—and the creatine (or PCr) concentrations to be a useful estimation of the directional change in measured reaction velocity. Below are three examples of developmental changes in energetics based on our work with mouse and rabbit hearts.

Example 1: Changes in Enzyme Capacity (mouse heart)[1]

Figure 3 shows values for the tissue activity of CK for fetal (filled circles), neonatal (open circles), and adult mouse hearts as a function of heart weight and age. Figure 4 shows values for the creatine pool (the sum of free creatine and PCr). During the last trimester of development, the fetal heart rapidly accumulates CK (here measured as activity) and creatine (remember that ATP stays constant). The rates of accumulation of both enzyme and substrate slow during neonatal development, but nonetheless both V_{max} and creatine pool continue to increase. Between 16 days' gestation and adulthood, V_{max} increases ~30-fold, the creatine pool increases ~50-fold, and the product of

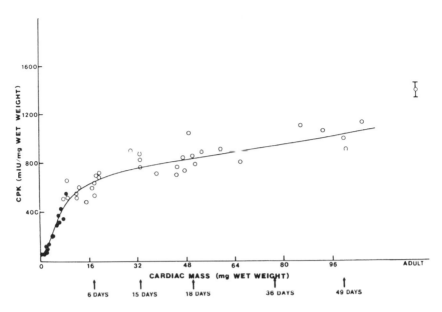

Figure 3. The relationship between tissue concentration of creatine kinase expressed as milli-international units (mIU) per milligram wet weight and cardiac mass. Values from 14- to 21-day-old fetuses are shown as filled circles; values for hearts from newborn to 49 days postpartum are shown in open circles. Average value for adult hearts (mean ± SEM for eight hearts) is also shown. Arrows indicate age of heart at various sizes. Reprinted from Reference 1.

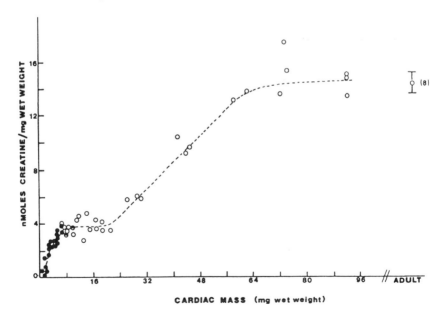

Figure 4. The relationship between tissue creatine concentration (nanomoles per milligram wet weight) in fetal (filled circles), neonatal (open circles), and adult mouse hearts and cardiac mass. Creatine concentration is measured in total creatine, ie, free creatine plus creatine phosphate. Reprinted from Reference 1.

V_{max} and creatine increases approximately ~1500-fold. This means that the capacity of this enzyme system increases 1500-fold during this period of maturation and that, if needed to replete the ATP pool, the rate of repletion would be 1500 times faster in the adult heart than in the fetal heart.

Example 2: Changes in Isoenzyme Diversity (rabbit heart)

CK is one of the classic examples of an isoenzyme family. The CK isoenzyme family displays remarkable diversity in terms of developmental regulation, tissue specificity, species distribution, self-assembly, and intracellular localization. CK exists as a family of five proteins, BB, MB, MM, and two mitochondrial isoenzymes, the ubiquitous uMtCK and sarcomere-specific sMtCK isoenzymes. The isoenzymes are named based on their source, B for brain, M for muscle, and the mitochondrial forms because they are located in mitochondria. CK isoenzyme distribution in the heart is developmentally regulated. Fetal myocardium contains primarily the BB isoenzyme. Genes encoding M and sMtCK are activated by unknown mechanism(s) at different times during terminal differentiation. MCK accumulates during fetal development at the same time that myofibrillar proteins rapidly accumulate; sMtCK accumulates when the inner mitochondrial membrane undergoes final maturation. Isoenzyme diversity is species-dependent. Adult hearts of large mammals with relatively slow metabolic rates contain 90% MMCK, 10% (or less) sMtCK, and only small amounts of B-containing isoenzymes while small animal hearts contain greater isoenzyme diversity, typically less than 1% BB, 6% to 14% MB, 25% to 35% sMtCK, and the balance as MM.

Using a combination of tissue biochemistry and whole organ enzymology, we performed a set of experiments testing whether the presence of sMtCK on the outer membrane of the mitochondria—the primary source of ATP in the heart—made a difference in the kinetics of the CK reaction in the intact heart.[2] For these experiments, we studied isolated hearts from 3- and 18-day-old neonatal rabbits (18-day-old hearts were subdivided into two groups). These times provided hearts that had 0%, 3.7%, or 9.3% of the total CK in the form of the sMtCK. Total CK activity was unchanged during this short period of development. The creatine pool increased approximately threefold, from 6 to 22.5 mmol/L, approximately 40% to 50% of which was phosphorylated. We found that the presence of sMtCK on the mitochondria *did* make a difference on the CK reaction velocity. As shown in Figure 5, for a given rate of ATP synthesis calculated

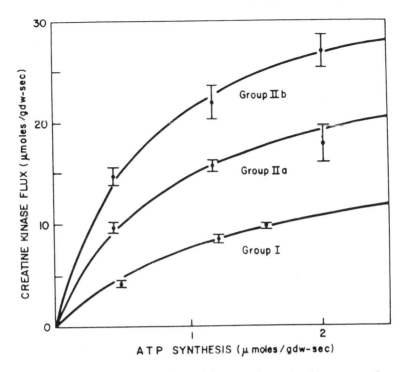

Figure 5. Relationship between the unidirectional creatine kinase reaction velocity (flux) (μmol [grams dry weight]$^{-1}$s^{-1}) measured by magnetization transfer and rate of adenosine triphosphate synthesis (μmol [grams dry weight]$^{-1}$s^{-1}) calculated from oxygen consumption measurements assuming a P:O ratio of 3. The curves are the result of fitting all of the data points (not the mean values, which are shown) for each group to the Michaelis-Menten equation. The three points shown for each group or curve represent means for each group at the three levels of cardiac performance. Error bars represent standard error. Group I = 3-day-old rabbit hearts; Group IIa = subgroup a of 18-day-old rabbit hearts; Group IIb = subgroup b of rabbit hearts. Reprinted from Reference 2.

from (independently made) oxygen consumption measurements, the velocity of the CK reaction (or unidirectional flux) measured using ^{31}P magnetization transfer increased with increasing concentrations of sMtCK in the heart (the change in creatine pool was taken into account). This was true at all levels of ATP synthesis rate. These data suggest that as the amount of this one isoenzyme increases in the heart, 1) the rate of ATP synthesis at which the reaction is half maximal decreases, and 2) the maximal reaction velocity of CK increases. This is an example of how localization of a specific enzyme in the cell can alter whole organ enzyme kinetics without a change in total enzyme activity.

Example 3: Changes in $|\Delta G|$ (rabbit heart)

These same experiments also provide results that illustrate an important principle about $|\Delta G|$ for ATP hydrolysis. In this experiment, the total amount of creatine increased threefold and the amount of PCr increased proportionately; the ATP and Pi concentrations stayed the same. Because the *ratio* of [PCr] to creatine concentration stayed about the same, there was no significant difference in the $|\Delta G|$ for ATP hydrolysis for these hearts: 59, 59, and 60 kJ/mol for 3-day-old, 18-day-old, and adult hearts, respectively.

Energetics and VF: An Example of Large Changes in the Free Energy of ATP Hydrolysis

The sodium gradient across the sarcolemma is $\sim$15: Na^+ concentration ($[Na^+]$) outside is 145 mmol/L and $[Na^+]$ inside is 5–15 mmol/L, depending on the species. The calcium gradient is much larger: Ca^{2+} concentration ($[Ca^{2+}]$) outside is $\sim$1 μmol/L and $[Ca^{2+}]$ inside varies during a beat from $\sim$80 nmol/L to 1 μmol/L. Maintaining these ion gradients across the sarcolemma requires energy: ATP is consumed by the Na^+, K^+, and Ca^{2+} ATPases. As indicated in the diagram showing the major pumps, channels, and exchangers in the sarcolemma (Figure 6), all of the ion gradients across the cell wall are maintained either directly or indirectly by these ATPases.[4] Thus, a cellular overload of either Na^+ or Ca^{2+} would drive these pumps, and would consume a large amount of energy to restore (if possible) normal cation homeostasis. Conversely, derangements in energetics could be severe enough to cause failure of these ion pumps, which, in turn, would lead to an inability to maintain normal ion gradients. There is little information about the energetics of ion movements in the fetal and neonatal heart. Below is a review of some of our work[3] using the adult rodent heart that demonstrates that VF increases energy expenditure of the heart and that derangements in energetics and ion homeostasis can lead to altered ion gradients, which can lead to VF.

In this experiment, isolated rat hearts were perfused isovolumically in the Langendorff mode and subjected to 30 minutes of hypoxia (pO_2 $\sim$20 torr). Approximately half of the hearts developed spontaneous VF at $\sim$19 minutes. This allowed us to determine retrospectively which (if any) parameters of isovolumic contractile performance, energetics assessed by ^{31}P NMR spectroscopy, and sodium ion homeostasis assessed by ^{23}Na NMR spectroscopy were made worse by VF, and which held predictive value. Figures 7 through 9 show

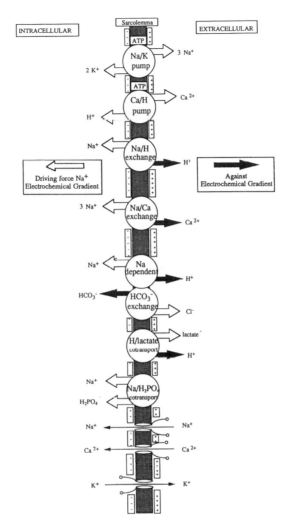

Figure 6. Diagram of sarcolemmal ion pumps and exchanger. Reprinted from Reference 4.

time-dependent indices of isovolumic contractile performance (namely, left ventricular developed pressure, heart rate, end-diastolic pressure), indices of cardiac energetics (namely, ATP, PCr, and Pi concentrations), and intracellular Na+ during 30 minutes of hypoxia for the two groups. In all cases, values for the VF hearts are shown as filled circles; values for the non-VF hearts are open circles. All data were fit to appropriate exponential functions to simplify analysis of the time-dependent data.

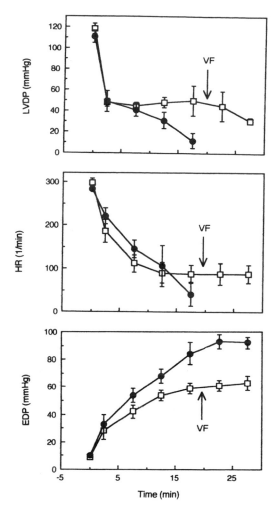

Figure 7. Plots of changes of left ventricular developed pressure (LVDP; mm Hg; top panel), heart rate (HR; min⁻¹; middle panel), and end-diastolic pressure (EDP; mm Hg; bottom panel) during control and hypoxia in nonventricular fibrillation (VF) (□) and VF (●) hearts. At time "0," hypoxia is initiated. Arrow indicates onset of VF. In the top and middle panels, there are no data points for VF hearts after the occurrence of VF. Reprinted from Reference 3.

Consequences of VF

VF exacerbated diastolic dysfunction in the hypoxic heart and accelerated the rate of depletion of ATP and PCr and, consequently, the rate of increase of Pi. VF also exacerbated the rise of intracellular Na^+

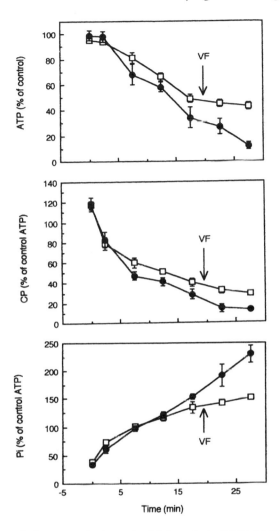

Figure 8. Plots of changes of adenosine triphosphate (ATP; percent of control; top panel), creatine phosphate (CP; percent of control ATP; middle panel), and inorganic phosphate (Pi; percent of control ATP; bottom panel) during control of hypoxia in nonventricular fibrillation (VF) (□) and VF (●) hearts. At time "0," hypoxia is initiated. Arrow indicates onset of VF. Reprinted from Reference 3.

in the hypoxic heart. It seems likely that the large fall in the sodium gradient observed in this experimental setting—in this case from ~10 to less than 2—at the time of onset of VF would be accompanied by a rise in intracellular calcium through reverse Na/Ca exchange, but this was not directly tested.

We also calculated the |ΔG| for ATP hydrolysis for the VF and non-

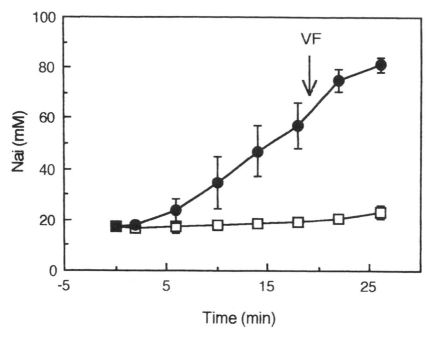

Figure 9. Plots of changes of intracellular Na$^+$ (Na$_i$; nmol/L) during control and hypoxia in nonventricular fibrillation (□) and ventricular fibrillation (●) (VF) hearts. Na$_i$ at control was set to 17.1 mmol/L. At time "0," hypoxia is initiated. Arrow indicates onset of VF. Reprinted from Reference 3.

VF hearts just before VF occurred and after 30 minutes of hypoxia, as well as for prehypoxic control hearts. During control perfusion just prior to imposing hypoxia, |ΔG| was 57 kJ/mol, well above the threshold |ΔG|s for any of the ATPases. Just prior to VF during the period of hypoxia, the hearts that would go on to fibrillate had a |ΔG| of 48.7 kJ/mol while the hearts that did not undergo VF had a higher energy reserve: |ΔG| ~50.3 kJ/mol. The energetic cost of VF was severe. In hearts that had been fibrillating for ~11 minutes, |ΔG| fell to 42.6 kJ/mol, while in those that did not, |ΔG| fell to only 48.7 kJ/mol. This author knows of no other example where it is possible to demonstrate such large changes in |ΔG| of ATP hydrolysis. The changes are not only severe, they are associated with large changes in cardiac performance (massive diastolic dysfunction) and in ion homeostasis (sodium accumulation). Even if the literature estimates for the ATPase reactions are inaccurate or even if the |ΔG| of the pumps could be "reset" to different levels depending on the energetic state of the cell, these changes in |ΔG| are so large that it is difficult to imagine how any of the ATPases in the cell could function normally.

Predictability

We also tested the predictability for VF of the functional and bio-chemical parameters measured. We found that end-diastolic pressure, rate-pressure product (which depends in part on end-diastolic pressure), and PCr content were predictors. The strongest predictor was intracellular sodium accumulation. These results suggest that changes in end-diastolic pressure, in energy reserve, and in the sodium gradient may contribute causally to VF.

Future Directions for Research on the Energetics of the Developing Heart

- establish guidelines for relevant models for the study of the developing heart, or at least define the advantages and limitations of existing models;
- exploit transgenic mouse models by developing ways to study myocytes from the developing heart and to study intact fetal and neonatal hearts;
- define steady state and dynamic aspects of the energetics of the immature heart (a daunting task without developing tools to study whole hearts);
- define consequences of the energy-poor state on cardiac function and its impact on disease;
- define predictors of an imbalance between energy supply and demand, especially in disease.

References

1. Jacobus WE, Ingwall JS (eds): *Heart Creatine Kinase. The Integration of Isozymes for Energy Distribution.* Baltimore: Williams & Wilkins; 1980.
2. Perry SB, McAuliffe J, Balschi JA, et al. Velocity of the creatine kinase reaction in the neonatal rabbit heart: Role of mitochondrial creatine kinase. *Biochemistry* 1988;27:2165–2172.
3. Neubauer S, Newell JB, Ingwall JS. Metabolic consequences and predictability of ventricular fibrillation in hypoxia. A 31 P- and 23 Na-nuclear magnetic resonance study of the isolated rat heart. *Circulation* 1992;86:302–310.
4. Ingwall JS, Clarke K, Stewart LC, Bernard M. Cation movements across the cell walls of intact tissues using MRS. In Grant D, Harris R (eds): *Encyclopedia of Nuclear Magnetic Resonance.* Norwell, Massachusetts: Kluwer Academic Publishers; 1996:1189–1197.

Chapter 2

Developmental Changes in Innervation and Autonomic Responses

Richard B. Robinson, PhD

Introduction

Newborn and adult hearts respond differently to autonomic agonists, whether endogenous neurotransmitters or synthetic analogs. These differences in response arise primarily from two sources. First, the signaling cascade activated by the agonist may differ developmentally. This includes differences at the level of the receptor with which the agonist directly interacts, as well as more distal elements that in turn interact with the activated receptor. Second, the substrate that is the ultimate target of the signaling cascade may differ between newborn and adult, or in fact may not even be present at one age. For example, many potential substrates, including contractile proteins, exhibit age-dependent isoform switches.[1,2] Ion channel expression and function also change significantly with age,[3] and these changes are likely to contribute to developmental differences in the effect of autonomic agonists on cardiac rhythm.

These developmental differences are significant because the sympathetic nervous system is known to modulate both normal cardiac rhythm and repolarization, as well as families of genetic,[4] exercise-induced, and catecholamine-induced arrhythmias,[5] all of which predominate in relatively young, otherwise healthy hearts. This chapter therefore focuses on developmental differences in ventricular responsiveness to autonomic agonists. It covers both the nature of the differ-

These studies were supported by USPHS-NHLBI grant HL-28958.

ences and, where data are available, the cause or developmental stimulus. As is shown, in many cases the onset of innervation itself plays a role in determining the response of the myocyte to neurotransmitters.

Receptor Targets for Neurotransmitters

The two neurotransmitters of interest are catecholamines (ie, norepinephrine and epinephrine) released by the sympathetic neurons in the heart, and acetylcholine released by the parasympathetic neurons. Catecholamines act at two broad classes of receptors, designated the α-and β-adrenergic receptors. Each group is now known to represent a family of receptor molecules. There are α_1- and α_2-adrenergic receptors, and each family is further divided into multiple subtypes. Here we only are concerned with the α_1 family, which includes the α_{1A}-, α_{1B}-, and α_{1D}-receptors. The β-adrenergic receptor represents a family that includes the β_1-, β_2-, and β_3-receptors. Of note, norepinephrine, which is the primary catecholamine released at sympathetic terminals, has relatively little β_2 activity compared to epinephrine, the primary catecholamine released into the circulation by the adrenal medulla. Acetylcholine also acts at two broad classes of receptors, the muscarinic and nicotinic receptors, but in the case of the heart we only need to be concerned with the muscarinic family. There have been five muscarinic receptor genes cloned to date, designated M_1 through M_5,[6] although subtype selective ligands are only available to readily distinguish among the M_1, M_2, and M_3.

The traditional view was that the heart responded to catecholamines via activation of cardiac β_1-adrenergic receptors, and to acetylcholine via activation of cardiac M_2 receptors. The β-adrenergic effect was considered purely excitatory and the muscarinic effect inhibitory. α-Adrenergic receptors, as well as the other subtypes of β-adrenergic and muscarinic cholinergic receptors, were considered not to be present on myocardial cells. We now know this to be an oversimplification, and we further know that it is these other subtypes and their signaling cascades that show some of the most marked developmental differences in responsiveness.

All of these receptors are membrane-bound proteins which, upon binding of an agonist, undergo a conformational change that facilitates interaction with another protein, called a guanine nucleotide regulatory protein or G protein. This G protein in turn interacts with a third element, referred to as the effector, usually to activate it but in some cases to reduce its activity. In many cases, this effector is an enzyme such as adenylyl cyclase or phospholipase C, although it also may be an ion channel. When the effector is an enzyme, the product of the subsequent reaction is a cytosolic molecule, referred to as a second messenger, which in turn interacts with other substrates within the myocyte. Both β_1- and β_2-adrenergic receptors couple to adenylyl cyclase via the stimulatory G protein G_s, leading to the formation of cyclic adenosine monophosphate (cAMP), the activation of protein kinase A (PKA), and the phosphorylation of numerous PKA-dependent substrates. $\alpha_{1A/D}$-Adrenergic receptors often couple to phospholipase C (PLC) via another G protein, typically G_q, resulting in the generation of two second messengers, inositol triphosphate (IP_3) and diacyl glycerol (DAG). IP_3 is associated with the release of calcium from intracellular stores in many cell types,[7] although the evidence in the heart is not compelling; DAG results in activation of protein kinase C (PKC) and the phosphorylation of PKC-dependent substrates. Finally, muscarinic M_2 cholinergic receptors have two well characterized actions in the heart. First, via the G protein $G_{i/o}$, they inhibit adenylyl cyclase, particularly after its activation by β-adrenergic agonists. Second, via the direct membrane-delimited interaction of the G protein with a potassium channel denoted $I_{K,Ach}$,[8] they increase potassium conductance and resting potential. This latter effect is much more pronounced in the atrium than it is in the ventricle.

The remainder of this chapter reviews each of these three signaling cascades in turn, focusing on developmental differences and the extent to which the ontogeny of sympathetic innervation contributes to these differences.

The α-Adrenergic Response

This discussion of the cardiac α-adrenergic response is based on studies in rat ventricular myocytes and tissue, but it should be noted that the conclusions apply equally well to canine Purkinje fibers, another preparation that has been extensively employed in studies of α-adrenergic signaling during development.[9–11] In the normal, mature heart, the response to activation of myocardial α-adrenergic receptor stimulation by catecholamines is modest, although it has been suggested that they contribute to arrhythmias during ischemia and reperfusion.[12] Of particular interest, there is a notably different α-adrenergic response in the immature heart compared to the adult heart. Figure 1 illustrates the response of ventricular tissue from neonatal (panel A) and adult (panel B) rat hearts to the α-adrenergic agonist phenylephrine, and demonstrates that at both ages the response is blocked with the α-adrenergic selective antagonist, prazosin. In this case, a ventricular septal preparation, which beats spontaneously, was used. What is apparent is that with age there is not simply a change in the magnitude of the response, but actually in its direction. That is, α-adrenergic agonists cause

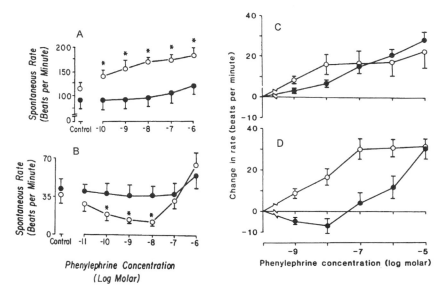

Figure 1. Chronotropic response to the α-adrenergic receptor agonist phenylephrine in neonatal and adult ventricular tissue and in cell culture. A and B. Spontaneously beating ventricular septal preparations from neonatal (A) and adult (B) rat ventricle were exposed to increasing concentrations of phenylephrine alone (open circles) and in the presence of 1×10^{-6} mol/L of the α_1-selective antagonist prazosin (filled circles). The neonatal response to phenylephrine is exclusively positive, while the adult is negative at lower concentrations; at both ages, prazosin blocks the response. Reprinted from Reference 13, with permission. C and D. Spontaneously beating cell culture of neonatal ventricular cells (C) and sympathetically innervated ventricular cells (D) exposed to increasing concentrations of phenylephrine. Filled circles represent control cultures in each case, while open circles are those pretreated for 16 to 24 hours with pertussis toxin. The innervated culture exhibits a negative chronotropic response (similar to the adult ventricular tissue), and this negative response is prevented by pretreatment with pertussis toxin. The positive response in the noninnervated culture is not sensitive to pertussis toxin. Reprinted with permission from Steinberg SF, Drugge ED, Bilezikian JP, Robinson RB. Innervated cardiac myocytes acquire a pertussis toxin-specific regulatory protein functionally linked to the alpha$_1$-receptor. Reprinted from Reference 14, with permission.

an increase in automaticity in the neonate but a decrease in the adult.[13] This observation leads to several questions: first, what is the developmental stimulus that results in expression of the inhibitory α-adrenergic response in the adult? Second, which elements of the signaling cascade differ in the adult versus the newborn? The ionic current that is the final target for any change in rate obviously must differ, but what of more proximal elements, including the receptor, G protein, and effector?

Addressing the question of the developmental stimulus first, Figure

1 (panels C and D) demonstrates that sympathetic innervation is that stimulus.[14] Neonatal ventricular myocytes were maintained in culture in the absence or presence of sympathetic neurons. When present, the neurons functionally innervated the myocytes in vitro. The noninnervated neonatal myocytes in culture respond to phenylephrine similarly to the intact neonatal tissue; that is, with an increase in spontaneous rate. In contrast, the innervated myocytes respond with a decrease in rate, just as the adult intact tissue. This experiment also demonstrates that the excitatory and inhibitory cascades involve distinct signaling cascades, since only the inhibitory response is sensitive to pertussis toxin pretreatment, which ADP-ribosylates and inactivates a subset of G proteins. Additional experiments have used an in vivo paradigm to confirm a role for innervation in evolution of the inhibitory α-adrenergic response.[15]

The mechanism by which innervation exerts this effect is via neurally released neuropeptide Y (NPY).[16] NPY is a peptide present in sympathetic terminals and released along with catecholamines upon nerve stimulation. Evidence for a neurotransmitter-like function of NPY and other neuropeptides has been inconsistent, but it has been suggested that these peptides may serve as long-term modulators of target tissue.[17] In the case of NPY and the cardiac α-adrenergic response, this appears to be the case. Figure 2 illustrates that myocytes maintained in culture in the sustained presence of NPY express an inhibitory α-adrenergic response typical of innervated cultures; short-term NPY exposure has no effect. In addition, the effect of innervation on α-adrenergic responsiveness is prevented if innervated cultures are maintained in the presence of an NPY antagonist. Recent experiments have found that this trophic or developmental action of NPY involves interaction with a particular NPY receptor subtype, most likely the NPY Y_2 receptor.[18]

Finally, a series of experiments has shown that the immature excitatory α-adrenergic response and the mature inhibitory response involve distinct signaling cascades, incorporating different receptor subtypes and different G proteins and effectors.[19] In the neonatal or immature ventricle, α-adrenergic agonists act at an α_1-adrenergic receptor subtype that is sensitive to blockade by WB4101. This receptor couples via a pertussis toxin-insensitive G protein (presumably G_q) to PLC, resulting in the generation of two second messengers, IP_3 and diacylglycerol. IP_3 is associated with release of Ca^{2+} from intracellular stores in some cell types, although the evidence in the heart is minimal. Diacylglycerol activates (isoforms of) PKC, resulting in phosphorylation of target proteins. This pathway persists in the adult heart, where an additional cascade is present. This second cascade, which appears with in vivo development or in vitro innervation or NPY exposure, involves a distinct receptor subtype (α_{1B}, sensitive to chloroethylclonidine) and G protein ($G_{i/o}$, sensitive to pertussis toxin). Activation of this

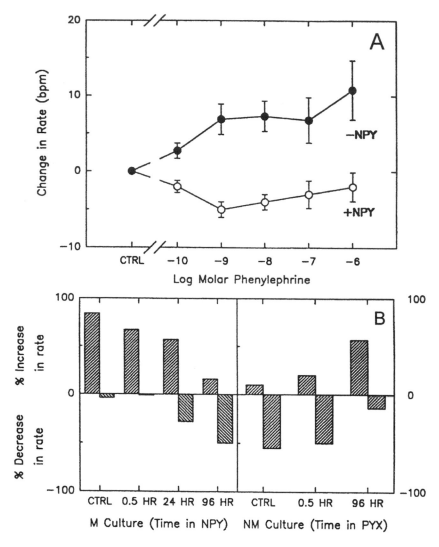

Figure 2. Effect of neuropeptide Y (NPY) and the NPY antagonist PYX-2 on response of neonatal ventricular cells in culture to phenylephrine. A. Chronotropic response of control culture (filled circles) and culture grown in the sustained presence of 10^{-7} mol/L NPY (open circles). Note the similarity of the response in the NPY culture to that of an innervated culture (Fig. 1, panel D). B. Percentage of cultures exhibiting a positive or negative chronotropic response to phenylephrine. The left panel illustrates that the ability of NPY to lead to expression of a negative chronotropic α-adrenergic response requires 24 to 96 hours of NPY exposure; 30 minutes of exposure was ineffective. The right panel similarly demonstrates that the ability of PYX-2 to interfere with the developmental effect of innervation requires sustained exposure; 30 minutes of exposure to PYX-2 was ineffective in preventing the action of innervation, while 96 hours of exposure prevented appearance of the typical negative chronotropic response in the innervated culture. Reprinted from Reference 40, with permission.

cascade is associated with stimulation of the Na/K pump and inhibition of automaticity, presumably via the hyperpolarization of the cell membrane expected from stimulation of the electrogenic pump.[19]

The β-Adrenergic Response

As stated earlier, the predominant β-adrenergic cascade in the normal adult heart is the β_1-adrenergic cascade, which results in elevation of cAMP levels and positive inotropy. However, the β_2-adrenergic cascade appears to take on increased importance in the failing or aged heart,[20,21] and recent evidence suggests the presence of a β_3-adrenergic response in the human heart as well.[22] An increased contribution of β_2-adrenergic receptors has been found in the neonate.[23] Further, although activation of both β_1- and β_2-adrenergic receptors results in elevation of cAMP levels in the neonatal heart, there appear to be important differences. Specifically, only the β_1-adrenergic response is susceptible to antagonism by acetylcholine (Figure 3), a response known as accentu-

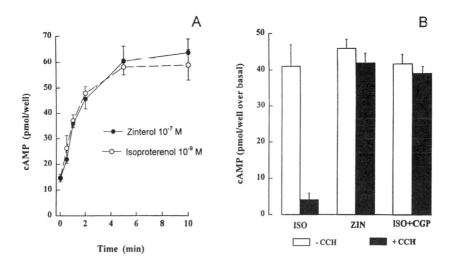

Figure 3. Effect of carbachol on β_2-receptor-dependent cyclic adenosine monophosphate (cAMP) accumulation. A. Kinetics of cAMP accumulation in response to the mixed agonist isoproterenol (ISO, 10^{-9} mol/L, open circles) and the β_2-selective agonist zinterol (ZIN, 10^{-7} mol/l, filled circles). At the concentrations used, the magnitude and kinetics of the cAMP accumulation in response to the two agonists was equivalent. B. Myocytes were exposed for 5 minutes to either ISO (10^{-9} mol/L), ZIN (10^{-7} mol/L), or ISO (2×10^{-8} mol/L) combined with the β_1-selective antagonist CGP-20712A (CGP, 10^{-7} mol/L). cAMP accumulation was determined in the absence (open bars) or presence (filled bars) of carbachol (10^{-6} mol/L). Carbachol significantly reduced only the ISO-dependent (ie, β_1) cAMP accumulation. Reprinted from Reference 24, with permission.

ated antagonism; the β_2-adrenergic response is resistant to antagonism by acetylcholine.[24] The β_2-adrenergic response is more modest in the adult, and exhibits other differences as well. The adult positive inotropic response appears to be independent of cAMP, and is not associated with enhanced relaxation (Figure 4).[23] This response has been

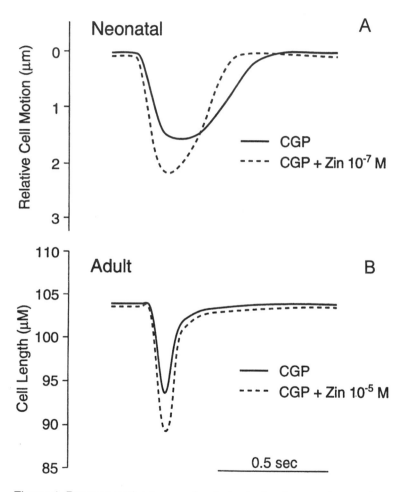

Figure 4. Representative traces of cell shortening in paced myocytes and the response to selective β_2-adrenergic stimulation. A. Example from a neonatal myocyte in culture first exposed to the β_1-selective antagonist CGP-20712A (CGP, 10^{-7} mol/L) and then exposed to the β_2-selective agonist zinterol (10^{-7} mol/L) in the continued presence of CGP. Zinterol caused both increased shortening and enhanced relaxation. B. Example from an adult myocyte first exposed to CGP and then to zinterol (10^{-5} mol/L) in the continued presence of CGP. Zinterol increased shortening without affecting relaxation. Reprinted from Reference 23, with permission.

shown to be secondary to cellular alkylinization via an HCO_3-dependent mechanism,[25] which most likely results in enhanced myofibrillar sensitivity to calcium and therefore a positive inotropic response. It also should be noted that interactions with the inhibitory G protein G_i may contribute to the effects in the adult,[26] while developmental changes in G_i may be a factor in age-dependent differences in β-adrenergic responsiveness.[27]

Besides developmental differences in the relative contribution of the different β-adrenergic receptor subtypes, there are differences in the substrates that are the likely targets of the β-adrenergic cascade. This includes isoform switches in contractile protein, and also differences in the density and characteristics of several ionic currents. The L-type calcium current is a well known target for cAMP-dependent enhancement, and this current itself changes developmentally. The delayed rectifier I_K is also enhanced by β-adrenergic agonists.[28] Interestingly, I_K is unresponsive to such stimulation in the neonatal canine ventricle, even though the L-type Ca^{2+} current is sensitive in the same preparation.[29] Another target of cAMP in the heart is the pacemaker current, I_f. cAMP shifts the voltage activation of I_f positive, and this appears to involve a direct interaction between cAMP and the channel,[30] although in some tissues PKA-dependent phosphorylation also plays a role.[31] A positive shift of I_f would be expected to enhance automaticity and excitability. Until recently, it was thought that I_f was only present in the normally automatic regions of the heart, specifically the sinoatrial node and the Purkinje system. It is now known that the current exists in most, if not all, regions of the heart. However, in the normal adult ventricle, the activation voltage is shifted extremely negative, outside the physiological range,[32] so that the current would not be activated. Interestingly, I_f is active at physiological voltages in the ventricles of hypertensive animals[33] and in the failing human myocardium.[34] Furthermore, I_f has been shown to be active at physiological voltages in the neonatal ventricle.[35] In the newborn, the activation threshold is -70 mV, comparable to the resting potential in these myocytes. In the adult it is shifted approximately 40 mV negative, to a mean value of -113 mV, well outside the physiological range.

The Muscarinic Cholinergic Response

The dominant cholinergic actions in the mature heart are supraventricular and relate to the two effects described earlier, namely inhibition of adenylyl cyclase and direct activation of $I_{K,Ach}$. Both of these effects follow from activation of M_2 muscarinic receptors and both are inhibitory in nature, decreasing automaticity via membrane hyperpolarization, a negative shift of I_f, and possible inhibition of L-type calcium current. There is, however, evidence of excitatory effects of acetylcholine in the neonatal canine and rat hearts.[36,37] In the rat, Sun et al[37,38] report an excitatory neonatal response in intact ventricular tissue[37] and in cell culture.[38] The response in culture was found to involve a non-M_2 muscarinic receptor, most probably M_1 or M_3 (based on its sensitivity to pirenzepine), and was lost upon in vitro innervation with sympathetic neurons. The excitatory muscarinic response in the neonatal canine heart also involves a pirenzepine-sensitive receptor.[39] Other than the fact that a non-M_2 receptor subtype is involved, little is known concerning the nature of this excitatory signaling cascade.

Conclusion

It is apparent from the preceding review that autonomic signaling cascades in the neonate tend to favor excitation over inhibition. The α-adrenergic response is entirely excitatory in the neonate, but it is mixed (ie, both excitatory and inhibitory) in the adult. The β-adrenergic response is excitatory at all ages, but has an additional β_2 contribution in the newborn (and in the failing and aged heart).[20,21] Given that neurally released norepinephrine is largely ineffective at β_2-adrenergic receptors, while circulating epinephrine is equally effective at both β_1- and β_2-adrenergic receptors, this would result in a greater dependence of the newborn on circulating sources of catecholamines. Finally, the muscarinic response is entirely inhibitory in the adult, via M_2 muscarinic receptors, but in the neonate there is an additional non-M_2 muscarinic excitatory response.

The parasympathetic nervous system innervates the heart earlier than the sympathetic system, with the sympathetic nervous system not being fully developed until well after birth.[40] In addition, sympathetic-parasympathetic interactions that act to inhibit vagal activity mature postnatally.[41] Thus, early in development there is at least the potential for excess parasympathetic tone. The age-dependent differences in the autonomic signaling cascades and responses described here would tend to mitigate any deleterious aspects of such an imbalance. That is, the greater excitatory tendency of each of these cascades would protect against excess influence from a parasympathetically activated inhibitory M_2 cascade. On the other hand, failure of the mature, less excitatory responses to appear at the appropriate developmental time points, or failure of the immature excitatory responses to disappear on schedule, could well lead to a situation of excess susceptibility to excitability. In this regard, it is worth noting that in a German shepherd model of sudden death there appears to be reduced ventricular sympathetic innervation in the region associated with electrophysiological anomalies and lethal arrhythmias.[42,43] It is therefore important to fully elucidate the factors that regulate and control the expression of these signaling cascades during normal development, and to understand the types of problems that may result from any deviation from normal autonomic development.

References

1. Chizzonite RA, Zak R. Regulation of myosin isoenzyme composition in fetal and neonatal rat ventricle by endogenous thyroid hormones. *J Biol Chem* 1984;259:12628–12632.
2. Anderson PAW, Malouf NN, Oakeley AE, et al. Troponin T isoform expression in humans: A comparison among normal and failing adult heart, fetal heart, and adult and fast skeletal muscle. *Circ Res* 1991;69:1226–1233.
3. Wetzel GT, Klitzner TS. Developmental cardiac electrophysiology: Recent advances in cellular physiology. *Cardiovasc Res* 1996;31:E52–E60.
4. Roden DM, Lazzara R, Rosen MR, et al. Multiple mechanisms in the long-QT syndrome (for the SADS foundation Task Force on LQTS). *Circulation* 1996;94:1996–2012.
5. Breithardt G, Camm AJ, Campbell RWF, et al. *Antiarrhythmic Therapy: A Pathophysiologic Approach.* Armonk, NY: Futura Publishing Co., Inc.; 1994:129–148.
6. Hulme EC, Birdsall NJM, Buckley NJ. Muscarinic receptor subtypes. *Ann Rev Pharmacol Toxicol* 1990;30:633–673.
7. Berridge MJ, Irvine RF. Inositol triphosphate, a novel second messenger in cellular signal transduction. *Nature* 1984;312:315–321.
8. Nair LA, Inglese J, Stoffel R, et al. Cardiac muscarinic potassium channel activity is attenuated by inhibitors of G beta gamma. *Circ Res* 1995;76: 832–838.
9. Rosen MR, Hordof AJ, Ilvento JP, Danilo P Jr. Effects of adrenergic amines on electrophysiological properties and automaticity of neonatal and adult canine Purkinje fibers: Evidence for alpha- and beta-adrenergic actions. *Circ Res* 1977;40:390–400.
10. Reder RF, Danilo P Jr, Rosen MR. Developmental changes in alpha adrenergic effects on canine Purkinje fiber automaticity. *Dev Pharmacol Ther* 1984;7:94–108.
11. Rosen MR, Steinberg SF, Chow Y-K, et al. The role of a pertussis-toxin sensitive protein in the modulation of canine Purkinje fiber automaticity. *Circ Res* 1988;62:315–323.
12. Sheridan DJ, Penkoski PA, Sobel BE, Corr PB. Alpha adrenergic contributions to dysrhythmia during myocardial ischemia and reperfusion in cats. *J Clin Invest* 1980;65:161–171.
13. Drugge ED, Rosen MR, Robinson RB. Neuronal regulation of the development of the cardiac alpha adrenergic chronotropic response. *Circ Res* 1985;57:415–423.
14. Steinberg SF, Drugge ED, Bilezikian JP, Robinson RB. Innervated cardiac myocytes acquire a pertussis toxin-specific regulatory protein functionally linked to the alpha$_1$-receptor. *Science* 1985;230:186–188.
15. Malfatto G, Rosen TS, Steinberg SF, et al. Sympathetic neuronal modula-

tion of cardiac impulse initiation and repolarization in the newborn rat. *Circ Res* 1990;66:427–437.

16. Sun LS, Ursell PC, Robinson RB. Chronic exposure to neuropeptide Y determines cardiac alpha$_1$ adrenergic responsiveness. *Am J Physiol* 1991;261:H969-H973.

17. Hokfelt T. Neuropeptides in perspective: The last ten years. *Neuron* 1991;7:867–879.

18. Sun LS, Rybin VO, Steinberg SF, Robinson RB. Characterization of the α_1-adrenergic chronotropic response in neuropeptide Y treated cardiomyocytes. *Eur J Pharmacol* 1998;349:377–381.

19. Rosen MR, Robinson RB, Cohen IS, et al. Alpha-adrenergic modulation of cardiac rhythm in the developing heart. In Sperelakis N (ed): *Physiology and Pathophysiology of the Heart*. Hingham: Kluwer Academic Publishers; 1995:457–465.

20. Bristow MR, Ginsburg R, Umans V, et al. β_1- and β_2-Adrenergic receptor subpopulations in nonfailing and failing human ventricular myocardium: Coupling of both receptor subtypes to muscle contraction and selective β_1-receptor down-regulation in heart failure. *Circ Res* 1986;59:297–309.

21. White M, Roden R, Minobe W, et al. Age-related changes in b-adrenergic neuroeffector systems in the human heart. *Circulation* 1994;90:1225–1238.

22. Gauthier C, Tavernier G, Charpentier F, et al. Functional β_3-adrenoceptor in human heart. *J Clin Invest* 1996;98:556–562.

23. Kuznetsov V, Pak E, Robinson RB, Steinberg SF. β_2-Adrenergic receptor actions in neonatal and adult rat ventricular myocytes. *Circ Res* 1995;76:40–52.

24. Aprigliano O, Rybin VO, Pak E, et al. β_1- and β_2-Adrenergic receptors exhibit differing susceptibility to muscarinic accentuated antagonism. *Am J Physiol* 1997;272:H2726–H2735.

25. Jiang T, Steinberg SF. β_2-Adrenergic receptors enhance contractility by stimulating HCO_3-dependent intracellular alkalinization. *Am J Physiol* 1997;273:H1044–H1047.

26. Xiao R-P, Ji X, Lakatta EG. Functional coupling of the β_2-adrenoceptor to a pertussis toxin-sensitive G protein in cardiac myocytes. *Mol Pharmacol* 1995;47:322–329.

27. Osaka T, Joyner RW. Developmental changes in the beta-adrenergic modulation of calcium currents in rabbit ventricular cells. *Circ Res* 1992;70:104–115.

28. Walsh KB, Kass RS. Distinct voltage-dependent regulation of a heart-delayed I_K by protein kinases A and C. *Am J Physiol* 1991;261:C1081–C1090.

29. Charpentier F, Liu Q-Y, Rosen MR, Robinson RB. Age-related differences in β-adrenergic regulation of repolarization in canine epicardial myocytes. *Am J Physiol* 1996;271:H1174–H1181.

30. DiFrancesco D, Tortora P. Direct activation of cardiac pacemaker channels by intracellular cyclic AMP. *Nature* 1991;351:145–147.

31. Chang F, Cohen IS, DiFrancesco D, et al. Effects of protein kinase inhibitors on canine Purkinje fibre pacemaker depolarization and the pacemaker current i_f. *J Physiol (Lond)* 1991;440:367–384.

32. Yu H, Chang F, Cohen IS. Pacemaker current exists in ventricular myocytes. *Circ Res* 1993;72:232–236.

33. Cerbai E, Barbieri M, Mugelli A. Characterization of the hyperpolarization-activated current, I_f, in ventricular myocytes isolated from hypertensive rats. *J Physiol (Lond)* 1994;481:585–591.

34. Cerbai E, Pino R, Porciatti F et al. Characterization of the hyperpolarization-activated current, I_f, in ventricular myocytes from human failing heart. *Circulation* 1997;95:568–571.
35. Robinson RB, Yu H, Chang F, Cohen IS. Developmental change in the voltage-dependence of the pacemaker current, i_f, in rat ventricle cells. *Pflugers Arch* 1997;433:533–535.
36. Danilo P Jr, Rosen MR, Hordof AJ. Effects of acetylcholine on the ventricular specialized conducting system of neonatal and adult dogs. *Circ Res* 1978;43:777–784.
37. Sun LS, Roberts LA, Rosen MR, Robinson RB. The positive chronotropic effect of acetylcholine has muscarinic and nicotinic components in the neonatal rat heart. *J Pharmacol Exp Ther* 1988;247:585–589.
38. Sun LS, Vulliemoz Y, Huber F, et al. An excitatory muscarinic response in neonatal rat ventricular myocytes and its modulation by sympathetic innervation. *J Mol Cell Cardiol* 1994;26:779–787.
39. Rosen MR, Steinberg SF, Danilo P Jr. Developmental changes in the muscarinic stimulation of canine Purkinje fibers. *J Pharmacol Exp Ther* 1990;254:356–361.
40. Robinson RB. Autonomic receptor-effector coupling during post-natal development. *Cardiovasc Res* 1996;31:E68–E76.
41. Pickoff AS, Stolfi A. Postnatal maturation of autonomic modulation of heart rate. *J Electrocardiol* 1996;29:215–222.
42. Dae MW, Lee RJ, Ursell PC, et al. Heterogeneous sympathetic innervation in German shepard dogs with inherited ventricular arrhythmia and sudden cardiac death. *Circulation* 1997;96:1337–1342.
43. Moise NS, Meyers-Wallen V, Flahive WJ, et al. Inherited ventricular arrhythmias and sudden death in German shepherd dogs. *J Am Coll Cardiol* 1994;24:233–243.

Chapter 3

Pediatric Animal Models of Ventricular Fibrillation

Robert A. Berg, MD

Investigators have used many animal models to study various aspects of ventricular fibrillation (VF) and cardiopulmonary resuscitation (CPR). This chapter describes the most common animal models of VF and addresses some of the advantages and disadvantages of these models.

As a reference point, the ideal animal model for the study of pediatric VF should simulate the clinical circumstances of pediatric VF cardiac arrests. Such a model should also be reproducible and practical, and should use animals that have thoracic and cardiovascular anatomy and physiology similar to that of a child.

Generally, VF is induced in animals by rapid right ventricular pacing or by direct current countershock. The animals are young and healthy. They do not have coronary artery disease or obstruction or other comorbidities. These features allow for less variability than clinical VF in adult patients (eg, variability of coronary obstruction, variability of vessels involved, presence or absence of myocardial infarction, size of infarction, etc.), and thereby allow greater uniformity and reproducibility. Investigators can therefore delineate various aspects of the pathophysiology of VF and its treatment that are difficult to study in humans. Ironically, many of the features in these models are more consistent with VF in pediatric patients than that in adult patients.

The early studies by Redding and Pearson[1,2] regarding the efficacy of various medications for modern CPR with chest compressions and positive pressure ventilation used canine asphyxial models. The au-

Research for this paper has been funded by the American Heart Association Southwest Affiliate and Arizona Disease Control Research Commission.

From: Quan L, Franklin WH (eds). Ventricular Fibrillation: A Pediatric Problem. Armonk, NY: Futura Publishing Company, Inc.; ©2000.

thors were anesthesiologists, and their experience suggested that most cardiac arrests were secondary to asphyxial episodes. They induced cardiac arrest by asphyxia alone (endotracheal tube clamping) in one set of animals and asphyxia followed by induction of VF via alternating current electroshock in another set. These landmark studies established the value of epinephrine and phenylephrine during CPR in both models. Animals treated with these two medications had superior initial resuscitation rates compared with animals provided with CPR without medications or with animals treated with calcium chloride or isoproterenol. Successful initial resuscitation was defined as return of spontaneous circulation within 20 minutes of resuscitative efforts. Similarly, the original studies by Otto and colleagues[3,4] that established that the efficacy of epinephrine during CPR was due to α-agonist effects used canine asphyxial models. These models, asphyxial cardiac arrests, and VF after an asphyxial episode are especially pertinent models for pediatric cardiac arrests. When epidemiological studies demonstrated that most sudden cardiac arrests in adults were due to sudden VF, CPR investigators modified their animal models to acute VF without a pre-VF asphyxial episode.

The species most commonly used in animal CPR studies have been dogs and pigs. Early VF studies generally used dogs due to their easy availability, the general similarity of their size and shape to that of humans, low cost, and familiarity with the species in medical laboratories. However, it is now well established that the thoracic and coronary anatomy of swine are more similar than the canine thoracic and coronary anatomy to that of humans.[5–8] The physiology of CPR in dogs with keel-shaped chest walls is markedly different from that in humans and in swine. Chest compressions in these animals are usually directed from the lateral aspect of the thorax rather than in an anterior-to-posterior direction.[9–12] In addition, the extensive collateral coronary circulation in dogs differs from that of humans and swine. Not surprisingly, in comparison to dogs, swine regional blood flow during CPR and cardiac electrophysiology are more similar to humans.[5–7] Some laboratories continue to use dogs because of their familiarity with the species and the ability to compare the results with their previous studies (without the problem of interspecies variability).[10–12] Over the last decade, investigators have focused increasingly on swine models.[8,13–19]

Many other species have been used in VF studies. Rats are becoming increasingly popular for VF models, primarily due to cost advantages.[20–22] However, the cardiorespiratory biomechanics of rats are quite different from those of humans. CPR at chest compression rates of 200 per minute and rescue breathing rates of 100 per minute obviously differ from human rates. The thorax of a rat differs dramatically from that of a human, thereby affecting differently relative transmission of external compressions. Importantly, the rat heart can spontaneously defibrillate. Such issues may confound experimental results in unexpected ways. Although primates would be the ideal species for a VF model, ethical considerations and prohibitive costs have generally precluded their use.

Perinatal asphyxial arrest models have used rabbits and sheep.[23–27] Although rabbit models have been useful for perinatal asphyxia studies, the issues noted above regarding rat VF models are similarly problematic with rabbits. Ovine models are advantageous for perinatal studies because of the well established elegant techniques of intrauterine and postpartum hemodynamic monitoring of fetal and newborn sheep.[27]

Due to practical considerations of cost and personnel availability, most CPR laboratory investigations have evaluated the effects of various interventions on physiological, or process, variables rather than clinically important outcome variables. Such physiological variables include coronary perfusion pressures, cerebral perfusion pressures, coronary and cerebral blood flows, cardiac outputs, myocardial and cerebral oxygen delivery and consumption, blood gases, myocardial and cerebral bioenergetics, and initial defibrillation efficacy. These variables are important in terms of understanding and establishing pathophysiological mechanisms and the response to various treatment regimens. In addition, it is easier to demonstrate differences in the continuous variables than discrete outcome variables because of the large β-error involved in comparing discrete outcomes with the small numbers of animals usually studied. However, the clinical relevance of differences in physiological variables may be questionable (see discussion on high dose/standard dose below).

Long-term neurologically intact survival is the gold standard of CPR research. Other endpoints, such as return of spontaneous circulation, 1-hour survival, and 24-hour survival, have been used as practical outcome measures. Animal investigations that include 24-hour or 48-hour survival and evaluation of neurologic and cardiac sequelae have demonstrated that initial successful resuscitation does not guarantee long-term survival or good neurologic outcome.[13,14,28,29] Moreover, continued observation of animals after initial successful resuscitation has allowed delineation of postarrest cardiomyopathy,[30–32] a common phenomenon after prolonged cardiac arrest, and a postarrest hyperadrenergic state after high-dose epinephrine.[13–15] Postarrest cardiac and neurologic dysfunctions are important clinical phenomena that are ignored in short-term physiological studies (eg, whether a drug improves myocardial perfusion pressure), and often impact the gold standard of long-term neurologically intact survival. These observations in animal studies are consistent with clinical experience.

Although survival and neurologically normal survival are important outcomes, most animal investigations are underpowered to demonstrate moderate differences in these clinically important outcome differences between experimental groups. For example, assuming 20 animals in two groups and 30% survival in one of the groups, an experiment would have a statistical power of 0.85 to detect an increase in survival in the other group to 80% or a power of 0.62 to detect an increase in survival to 60%, with an α-error of 5%. However, the power to detect an increase in survival to 40% (ie, a 33% increase in survival) would only be 0.07. Conversely, more than 200 animals would be needed in each group to increase the power to 0.80 of determining an increase in survival from 30% to 40%.[33] Not surprisingly, investigators prefer to evaluate continuous variables with narrow confidence intervals (eg, physiological endpoints) to increase the power of their studies.

Critics have suggested that animal studies have led us astray in the field of clinical cardiac arrest and CPR. For example, they claim that animal studies suggested that higher doses of epinephrine were superior to the standard dose, yet clinical trials did not demonstrate any benefit. In fact, animal studies clearly established that higher epinephrine dosage resulted in greater myocardial perfusion pressure and greater myocardial blood flow during CPR (Figure 1).[8,15,17,34–36] However, cardiac output during CPR decreased with higher epinephrine dosage, presumably due to excessive peripheral vasoconstriction increasing afterload (Figure 1).[36] Human studies confirmed the improvement in myocardial perfusion pressure with higher epinephrine dosage.[37] Unfortunately, these physiological benefits were overinterpreted as strong evidence that higher dosages of epinephrine were indicated during CPR. Of note, the clinically important outcome measure, survival, was not used.

Clinicians with high expectations for high-dose epinephrine based on these initial physiological studies were disappointed when several large, randomized, controlled clinical trials were unable to demonstrate improved outcome with higher epinephrine doses.[38–42] Consistent with these human data, our two swine randomized, controlled studies[13,14] also showed no differences in 24-hour survival or neurologic outcome with higher epinephrine doses, one with a VF model[14] and one with an asphyxial model (Tables 1 and 2).[13] In both studies, the high-dose epinephrine groups experienced a severe hyperadrenergic state with tachycardia, hypertension, and recurrent VF within 10 minutes of the initial return of spontaneous circulation. Several other laboratories have now demonstrated that high-dose epinephrine during CPR can have deleterious effects, including a postarrest hyperadrenergic state,[15] myocardial necrosis,[20] and worsening of postarrest cardiomyopathy.[43]

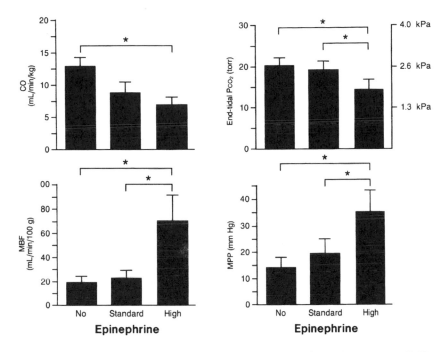

Figure 1. *Top left:* Graded doses of epinephrine and cardiac output (CO). Changes in cardiac output in mL/min/kg of body weight after infusion of standard and high-dose epinephrine. The 5-minute period after resuscitative efforts were initiated and before standard-dose epinephrine infusion served as the control period. Only high-dose epinephrine infusion resulted in a significant decrease in cardiac output. *Top right:* Graded doses of epinephrine and end-tidal PCO_2. End-tidal PCO_2 levels were unchanged after infusion of standard-dose epinephrine. The infusion of high-dose epinephrine resulted in significantly lower end-tidal PCO_2 when compared with either no or standard-dose epinephrine. Bottom right: Graded doses of epinephrine and myocardial perfusion pressure (*MPP*). MPP pressure was greatly enhanced after infusion of high-dose epinephrine when compared with either the control period or infusion of standard dose epinephrine. Bottom left: Graded doses of epinephrine and myocardial blood flow (*MBF*). MBF was significantly improved after infusion of high-dose epinephrine. The infusion of standard-dose epinephrine did not significantly increase MBF, a finding that is similar to the results of MPP. Significant change at $P<0.05$. Reprinted with permission.

What lessons are to be learned from the high-dose/standard-dose epinephrine saga? Animal studies did not lead us astray. Physiological studies in animals and humans were consistent and encouraging with respect to myocardial hemodynamics. The decreased cardiac output during animal studies was concerning. When animal studies focused on the important outcome variables of 24-hour survival and postresuscitation neurologic and cardiac function, high-dose epinephrine was

Table 1

HDE versus SDE: 15-Minute VF

Epi dose	ROSC	2-hour ICU mortality	24-hour survival
0.02 mg/kg (N = 15)	14	0*	6
0.20 mg/kg (N = 15)	14	4*	4

*P<0.05. Epi = epinephrine; HDE = high-dose epinephrine; ICU = intensive care unit; ROSC = restoration of spontaneous circulation; SDE = standard-dose epinephrine; VF = ventricular fibrillation. From Reference 14.

not beneficial. Animal outcome studies would have predicted the disappointing clinical trials; however, they were not completed and published until after the clinical trials. One important message is that well controlled animal outcome studies should be performed prior to embarking on large-scale expensive human clinical trials. Perhaps more poignantly, as in all scientific endeavors, the investigator must ask the right question to get the right answer.

Although it is axiomatic that animal models should attempt to replicate the clinical situation, most animal VF models replicate pediatric VF better than adult VF (young, healthy animals without coronary obstruction or other comorbidities). Clinically relevant animal models of adult VF and VF in special circumstances do exist. Models for VF with coronary obstruction have been established.[29,44–46] Asphyxial models to investigate asphyxial cardiac arrests, the more common etiology of cardiac arrest in children, have established that VF often occurs during the asphyxial event or during CPR for the asphyxial cardiac arrest.[1–4,13,47–51] Such a model may be particularly pertinent for many pediatric VF cardiac arrests.

Ventricular ectopy, including VF and ventricular tachycardia, with

Table 2

HDE versus SDE: 10-Minute Asphyxial Cardiac Arrest

Epi dose	ROSC	2-hour ICU mortality	24-hour survival
0.02 mg/kg (N = 15)	13	0*	3
0.20 mg/kg (N = 15)	10	4*	3

*P<0.05. Epi = epinephrine; HDE = high-dose epinephrine; ICU = intensive care unit; ROSC = restoration of spontaneous circulation; SDE = standard-dose epinephrine; VF = ventricular fibrillation. From Reference 13.

tricyclic poisoning, behaves quite differently from ventricular ectopy in other circumstances, and has been investigated in appropriate animal models.[52,53] VF in the setting of hypothermia is also quite distinct in terms of pathophysiology and outcome, and has been studied in a clinically relevant model.[54] Similarly, VF due to a lightning strike has unique characteristics, and has been investigated with a clinically relevant model.[55]

A final example of the importance of asking the right question is the issue of optimal initial treatment for VF. Most adult cardiac arrests occur in the prehospital setting and countershock therapy is not immediately available. It is well known that immediate countershock shortly after the occurrence of VF is very effective and is clearly the medical intervention of choice. It is less clear whether immediate countershock is the medical treatment of choice after prolonged VF. Following a 7.5-minute interval of untreated VF, Niemann and colleagues[10] randomly treated dogs with immediate countershocks per the American Heart Association recommendations, versus manual CPR and epinephrine prior to countershock. Return of spontaneous circulation occurred in 3 of 14 animals treated with immediate countershocks, versus 9 of 14 treated with CPR and epinephrine first ($P=0.014$). Is immediate countershock the correct treatment for prolonged untreated VF in adults or children? This issue deserves further investigation.

In conclusion, animal VF models provide a preclinical arena for VF research. Most of these models appear to have more relevance to pediatric VF than to adult VF. It is important to study physiological variables in order to better understand mechanisms. However, improving physiology does not necessarily improve outcome. Examples are cited to emphasize that careful modeling of the specific clinical question is paramount in order to yield clinically meaningful answers.

References

1. Redding JS, Pearson JW. Evaluation of drugs for cardiac resuscitation. *Anesthesia* 1963;24:203–207.
2. Pearson JW, Redding JS. Peripheral vascular tone in cardiac resuscitation. *Anesth Analg* 1965;44:746–752.
3. Otto CW, Yakaitis RW, Blitt CD. Mechanism of action of epinephrine resuscitation from asphyxial arrest. *Crit Care Med* 1981;9:321–324.
4. Yakaitis RW, Otto CW, Blitt CD. Relative importance of α and β adrenergic receptors during resuscitation. *Crit Care Med* 1979;7:293–296.
5. Howe BB, Fehn PA, Pensinger RR. Comparative anatomical studies of the coronary arteries of canine and porcine hearts. *Acta Anat* 1968;71:13–21.
6. Schaper W, Jageneau A, Xhonneux R. The development of collateral circulation in the pig and dog heart. *Cardiologia* 1967;51:321–335.
7. Bowman TA, Hughes HC. Swine as an in vivo model for electrophysiologic evaluation of cardiac pacing parameters. *PACE* 1984;7:187–194.

8. Brown CG, Werman HA, Davis EA, et al. The effects of graded doses of epinephrine on regional myocardial blood flow during cardiopulmonary resuscitation in swine. *Circulation* 1987;75:491–497.
9. Yakaitis RW, Ewy GA, Otto CW, et al. Influence of time and therapy on ventricular defibrillation in dogs. *Crit Care Med* 1980;8:157–163.
10. Niemann JT, Cairns CB, Sharma J, et al. Treatment of prolonged ventricular fibrillation: Immediate countershock versus high-dose epinephrine and CPR preceding countershock. *Circulation* 1992;85:281–287.
11. Ditchey RV, Slinker BK. Phenylephrine plus propranolol improves the balance between myocardial oxygen supply and demand during experimental cardiopulmonary resuscitation. *Am Heart J* 1994;127:324–330.
12. Vukmir RB, Bircher NG, Radovsky A, et al. Sodium bicarbonate may improve outcome in dogs with brief or prolonged cardiac arrest. *Crit Care Med* 1995;23:515–522.
13. Berg RA, Otto CW, Kern KB, et al. A randomized, blinded trial of high-dose epinephrine versus standard-dose epinephrine in a swine model of pediatric asphyxial cardiac arrest. *Crit Care Med* 1996;24:1695–1700.
14. Berg RA, Otto CW, Kern KB, et al. High-dose epinephrine results in greater early mortality after resuscitation from prolonged cardiac arrest in pigs: A prospective, randomized study. *Crit Care Med* 1994;22:282–290.
15. Hornchen U, Lussi C, Schuttler J. Potential risks of high-dose epinephrine for resuscitation from ventricular fibrillation in a porcine model. *J Cardiothorac Vasc Anesth* 1993;7:184–187.
16. Berkowitz ID, Gervais H, Schleien CL, et al. Epinephrine dosage effects on cerebral and myocardial blood flow in an infant swine model of cardiopulmonary resuscitation. *Anesthesiology* 1991;75:1041–1050.
17. Koehler RC, Michael JR, Guerci AD, et al. Beneficial effect of epinephrine infusion on cerebral and myocardial blood flows during CPR. *Ann Emerg Med* 1985;14:744–749.
18. Lindner KH, Strohmenger HU, Prengel AW, et al. Hemodynamic and metabolic effects of epinephrine during cardiopulmonary resuscitation in a pig model. *Crit Care Med* 1992;20:1020–1026.
19. Idris AH, Becker LB, Fuerst RS, et al. Effect of ventilation on resuscitation in an animal model of cardiac arrest. *Circulation* 1994;90:3063–3069.
20. Neumar R, Bircher N, Radovsky M, et al. Myocardial necrosis after high-dose epinephrine during CPR. *Ann Emerg Med* 1993;22:892–893.
21. Tang W, Weil MH, Sun S, et al. Cardiopulmonary resuscitation by precordial compression but without mechanical ventilation. *Am J Respir Crit Care Med* 1994;150:1709–1713.
22. Duggal C, Weil MH, Tang W, et al. Effect of arrest time on the hemodynamic efficacy of precordial compression. *Crit Care Med* 1995;23:1233–1236.
23. Dawes GS, Jacobson HN, Mott JC, et al. The treatment of asphyxiated, mature foetal lambs and rhesus monkeys with intravenous glucose and sodium carbonate. *J Physiol* 1963;169:167–184.
24. Dawes GS, Mott JC, Shelley HJ, et al. The prolongation of survival time in asphyxiated immature foetal lambs. *J Physiol* 1963;168:43–64.
25. Campbell AGM, Cross KW, Dawes GS, et al. A comparison of air and O_2 in a hyperbaric chamber or by positive pressure ventilation, in the resuscitation of newborn rabbits. *J Pediatr* 1966;68:153–163.
26. Cross KW, Dawes GS, Hyman A, et al. Hyperbaric oxygen and intermittent positive-pressure ventilation in resuscitation of asphyxiated newborn rabbits. *Lancet* 1964;2:560–562.

27. Burchfield DJ, Preziosi MP, Lucas VW, et al. Hemodynamic effects of graded doses of epinephrine in asphyxiated newborn lambs. *Resuscitation* 1993;25:235–244.
28. Berg RA, Kern KB, Hilwig RW, et al. Assisted ventilation does not improve outcome in a porcine model of single-rescuer bystander cardiopulmonary resuscitation. *Circulation* 1997;95:1635–1641.
29. Berg RA, Kern KB, Hilwig RW, et al. Assisted ventilation during 'bystander' CPR in a swine acute myocardial infarction model does not improve outcome. *Circulation* 1997;96:4364–4371.
30. Tang W, Weil MH, Sun S, et al. Progressive myocardial dysfunction after cardiac resuscitation. *Crit Care Med* 1993;21:1046–1050.
31. Kern KB, Hilwig RW, Rhee KH, et al. Myocardial dysfunction after resuscitation from cardiac arrest: An example of global myocardial stunning. *J Am Coll Cardiol* 1996;28:232–240.
32. Kern KB, Hilwig RW, Berg RA, et al. Postresuscitation left ventricular systolic and diastolic dysfunction: Treatment with dobutamine. *Circulation* 1997;95:2610–2613.
33. Dupont WD, Plummer JR. Power and sample size calculations: A review and computer program. *Control Clin Trials* 1990;11:116–128.
34. Lindner KH, Ahnefeld FW, Bowdler IM. Comparison of different doses of epinephrine on myocardial perfusion and resuscitation success during cardiopulmonary resuscitation in a pig model. *Am J Emerg Med* 1991;9:27–31.
35. Brown CG, Werman HA, Davis EA, et al. Comparative effect of graded doses of epinephrine on regional brain blood flow during CPR in a swine model. *Ann Emerg Med* 1986;15:1138–1144.
36. Chase PB, Kern KB, Sanders AB, et al. The effects of graded doses of epinephrine on both noninvasive and invasive measures of myocardial perfusion and blood flow during cardiopulmonary resuscitation. *Crit Care Med* 1993;21:413–419.
37. Gonzalez ER, Omato JP, Garnett AR, et al. Dose-dependent vasopressor response to epinephrine during CPR in human beings. *Ann Emerg Med* 1989;18:920–926.
38. Stiell IG, Hebert PC, Weitzman BN, et al. High-dose epinephrine in adult cardiac arrest. *N Engl J Med* 1992;327:1045–1050.
39. Brown CG, Martin DR, Pepe PE, et al. A comparison of standard-dose and high-dose epinephrine in cardiac arrest outside the hospital. *N Engl J Med* 1992;327:1051–1055.
40. Callaham M, Madsen CD, Barton CW, et al. A randomized clinical trial of high-dose epinephrine and norepinephrine vs standard-dose epinephrine in prehospital cardiac arrest. *JAMA* 1992;268:2667–2672.
41. Lindner KH, Ahnefeld KFW, Prengel AW. Comparison of standard and high-dose adrenaline in the resuscitation of asystole and electromechanical dissociation. *Acta Anaesthesiol Scand* 1991;35:253–256.
42. Lipman J, Wilson W, Kobilski S, et al. High-dose adrenaline in adult in-hospital asystolic cardiopulmonary resuscitation: A double-blind randomised trial. *Anaesth Intensive Care* 1993;21:192–196.
43. Tang W, Weil MH, Sun S, et al. Epinephrine increases the severity of postresuscitation myocardial dysfunction. *Circulation* 1995;92:3089–3093.
44. Kern KB, Ewy GA. Minimal coronary stenoses and left ventricular blood flow during CPR. *Ann Emerg Med* 1992;21:1066–1072.
45. Kern KB, Lancaster L, Goldman S, et al. The effect of coronary artery lesions on the relationship between coronary perfusion pressure and my-

ocardial blood flow during cardiopulmonary resuscitation in pigs. *Am Heart J* 1990;120:324–333.

46. Kern BK, Lancaster LD, Olajos M, et al. A closed-chest porcine model of chronic left ventricular systolic and diastolic dysfunction after myocardial infarction. *Coron Artery Dis* 1991;2:685–689.

47. Berg RA, Kern KB, Otto CW, et al. Ventricular fibrillation in a swine model of acute pediatric asphyxial cardiac arrest. *Resuscitation* 1996;33:147–153.

48. Caputo G, Delgado-Paredes C, Swedlow D, et al. Anoxic cardiopulmonary arrest in a pediatric animal model: Clinical and laboratory correlates of duration. *Pediatr Emerg Care* 1985;1:57–60.

49. DeBehnke DJ. Effects of vagal tone on resuscitation from experimental electromechanical dissociation. *Ann Emerg Med* 1993;22:1789–1794.

50. Hickey RW, Karasic RB, Bircher NG. ATP-MgCl$_2$ pre-treatment in an animal model of asphyxial arrest. *Resuscitation* 1993;25:109–118.

51. Nadkarni V, Tice L, Hofmann B, Jasani M. Etiology of experimental pediatric porcine arrest influence epinephrine and blood gas values and gradients. *Crit Care Med* 1998;26:A96. Abstract.

52. Nattel S, Mittleman M. Treatment of ventricular tachyarrhythmias resulting from amitriptyline toxicity in dogs. *J Pharmacol Exp Ther* 1984;231:430–435.

53. Sasyniuk BI, Jhamandas V, Valois M. Experimental amitriptyline intoxication: Treatment of cardiac toxicity with sodium bicarbonate. *Ann Emerg Med* 1986;15:1052–1059.

54. Murphy K, Nowak RM, Tomlanovich MC. Use of bretylium tosylate as prophylaxis and treatment in hypothermic ventricular fibrillation in the canine model. *Ann Emerg Med* 1968;15:1160–1166.

55. Ishikawa T, Miyazawa T, Ohashi M, et al. Experimental studies on the effect of artificial respiration after lightning accidents. *Res Exp Med* 1981;179:59–68.

Chapter 4

Ventricular Fibrillation in the Asphyxiated Piglet Model

Vinay Nadkarni, MD

Introduction

Pediatric cardiac arrest most frequently results from initial respiratory compromise that leads to pulmonary failure, hypoxemia, hypercarbia, and subsequent bradyasystolic arrest. A small but significant subset of children with underlying congenital heart disease or predisposing condition (toxin, drug overdose, electrolyte abnormality, hypothermia) may arrest with ventricular fibrillation (VF), but the neurologic/functional outcome in these children is generally better than the poor neurologic and functional outcome associated with a bradyasystolic arrest. Walsh and Krongrad[1] studied the terminal electrical activity in 100 pediatric patients and found bradyasystole in 88% of newborns, 67% of infants, and 64% of children. VF or ventricular tachycardia (VT) was seen in up to 22% of patients at some point during their monitored course. Prevalence of VF was related to heart mass and the presence of concomitant congenital heart disease. Meny et al[2,3] studied cardiorespiratory recordings from infants on apnea and bradycardia monitors who died unexpectedly at home while on the monitors (n=6), as well as 161 infants monitored at home for dysrhythmias. There were no reported cases of VF or VT. Additionally, Losek et al[4] report an initial rhythm of VF in 6% of 117 pulseless, nonbreathing children resuscitated out-of-hospital. In contrast, Milner et al[5] observed ambulatory continuous electrocardiogram recordings at the time of fatal cardiac arrest, with terminal rhythms of VT in 12 of 13, and VF in 1 of 13, adult victims.

From: Quan L, Franklin WH (eds). *Ventricular Fibrillation: A Pediatric Problem.* Armonk, NY: Futura Publishing Company, Inc.; ©2000.

The incidence and prevalence of VF during pediatric asphyxial injury is unknown. Most porcine cardiac arrest research explores therapeutic interventions and outcomes in electrically induced VF, without antecedent periods of hypoxia and hypercarbia relevant to infants and children. Why study VF in a piglet asphyxial arrest model? As mentioned in Chapter 3 of this volume, piglets provide an important anatomic and physiological similarity to humans, particularly in relation to cardiopulmonary resuscitation (CPR) mechanics and circulation. Airway obstruction, hypercarbia, and hypoxemia are easy to induce with appropriate attention to anesthesia and analgesia, and are well tolerated in swine with healthy, young hearts.

The important features of VF in the asphyxial arrest model are discussed with the following objectives:

1. Review existing porcine asphyxial arrest models and the factors affecting prevalence of VF with emphasis on relevance to infants and children.
2. Identify common limitations of existing asphyxial animal models for the study of VF.
3. Identify critical experimental factors, outcome measures, and timing of outcome reporting that contrast asphyxial versus VF models.

Background of Pediatric Porcine Asphyxial Cardiac Arrest Models

Holliman and Bates[6] reviewed all animal models of CPR presented in the EM literature from 1982 to 1992 and found that only 3 of 96 models used asphyxia to induce cardiac arrest. Many current models are based on earlier observations that canine models of asphyxia-induced cardiac arrest require artificial ventilation, closed-chest cardiac massage, and vasopressors for return of spontaneous circulation (ROSC).[7] Yakaitis, Otto, and Blitt[8,9] implicated the relative importance of the α- and β-adrenergic agonists in resuscitation from asphyxial arrest, and identified key mechanisms of action of epinephrine in canine resuscitation. Similar studies in puppies by Caputo et al[10] suggest that cardiopulmonary arrest outcome measures are closely linked with duration of anoxia preceding cardiac arrest. A typical pattern emerges of catecholamine release and initial rise in blood pressure with narrowed pulse pressure, followed by diastolic hypotension, widened pulse pressure, and finally significant systolic and diastolic hypotension. A typical blood pressure tracing from an anesthetized piglet during paralysis without ventilation is demonstrated in Figure 1. Endogenous catecholamines are

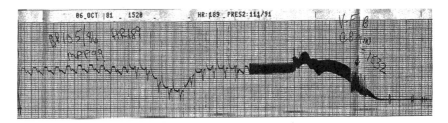

Figure 1. Sample blood pressure tracing during anesthesia and paralysis without ventilation. Note initial systolic and diastolic hypertension during hypoxia with a catecholamine surge (α-adrenergic predominant), followed by hypercarbia-induced vasodilatation and exhaustion of catechol stores resulting in widening of pulse pressure and systemic hypotension. This piglet exhibited ventricular fibrillation 8 minutes after respiratory arrest induction.

prominent during this period of asphyxia, hypoxia, and hypercarbia. Measured venous plasma catecholamine levels rise 30 to 100 times baseline levels, which may lead to cardiac irritability and risk for dysrhythmia.[11] Pediatric porcine asphyxial arrest models allow investigation to try to determine whether there is a window of opportunity during asphyxial-induced arrest to intervene with dysrhythmia interventions, whether outcome from VF is superior to other presenting rhythms with equivalent prearrest hypoxia/hypercarbia, and whether the philosophy of "call first" for adults versus "call fast" (after 1 minute of CPR) for children is appropriate for identified asphyxial versus dysrhythmic arrests.

How Frequently Does VF Occur During Asphyxia-Induced Cardiac Arrest in Piglet Models?

Berg et al[12] observed the development of VF after anesthesia with isoflurane and clamping of the endotracheal tube without paralysis in 36 piglets. None of the 36 developed VF during approximately 8 to 12 minutes of arrest induction (until loss of aortic pulsation), but 14 showed VF during a 10-minute nonintervention interval, and 4 progressed on from VF to asystole without intervention. This suggests that there may be opportunity for VF intervention early after asphyxial cardiac arrest if one can assess and intervene before degeneration into asystole. A similar model of pediatric porcine asphyxial arrest in Yucatan minipiglets with cardiac arrest induction by anesthesia, paralysis, and cessation of ventilation without endotracheal tube clamping demonstrated an overall VF incidence of 8 of 24 (33%). The anesthetic agent used, ketamine more than pentobarbital or isoflurane, correlated with VF risk.[13]

Key Aspects of Asphyxia versus VF Induction of Cardiac Arrest in Piglet Models

A major difference between circulatory arrest induced by sudden onset of electrically induced VF and gradual asphyxial arrest induction is the period of hypoxia, hypercarbia, and sluggish blood flow that precedes cardiac arrest. Both hypoxia and hypercarbia have been demonstrated to have independent negative effects on ROSC and survival outcome in experimentally induced models of VF.[14] When comparing asphyxia for 7 minutes followed by 10 minutes of VF versus induction of VF arrest for 10 minutes alone in dogs, Vaagenes et al[15] demonstrated differential patterns of brain damage and neuroprotective medication response. Most animal/piglet models of VF resemble the pediatric paradigm of a young, healthy heart not associated with coronary artery disease. Various factors can be identified that should be taken into account when evaluating the relevance of a particular porcine asphyxial or VF arrest model: age-related factors, prearrest interventions (including anesthesia), method of asphyxial arrest induction, definition of arrest, duration of nonintervention interval, sites of invasive and noninvasive monitoring, time sequence for reporting outcomes, appropriateness of interventions, and clinical applicability.

Age-Related Factors

Maturation of autonomic control may play a major role in baseline heart rate and response to stress or vagal stimulation.[16] Metabolic needs and metabolic response to stress are quite variable, particularly in piglets of 1 day to 3 months of age. Obvious attention must be paid to relevance of size and physiology for clinical application.

Prearrest Intervention Impact

Lindner and Ahnefeld[17] demonstrated that the risk for postresuscitation VF was significantly higher in piglets subjected to 3 minutes of asphyxial cardiac arrest after treatment with epinephrine than in those resuscitated without prior asphyxial insult. Control of such factors as body temperature, hypoxia, hyperoxia, exposure to myocardial depressants, and steroid use may influence both early and late resuscitation outcomes. One particularly dramatic example is the effect of an anesthetic regimen on pediatric porcine asphyxial arrest. Dramatic and significant influences of anesthetic agents on time from onset of asphyxia to onset of cardiac arrest, incidence of VF during arrest induction and nonintervention interval, metabolic stress, plasma epinephrine levels, and arterial-venous epinephrine gradients can be demonstrated.[13]

Method of Asphyxial Arrest Induction

Most protocols employ anesthesia combined with endotracheal tube clamping[8,9,12] or paralysis with central apnea.[11,13] Endotracheal tube clamping may result in retention of functional residual capacity and gasping typical of airway obstruction, with a potential effect on intrathoracic pressure and hemodynamics. Apnea induced with paralysis precludes gasping ventilation during arrest induction and nonintervention but may predispose to atelectasis and mimics central apneic etiologies of hypoxia and hypercarbia. Hart et al[18] report that catecholamine stress responses in 31 animal species were dramatic with decapitation, hypoxia, hemorrhage, and hypothermia stresses, even in very primitive species. These findings suggest that the method of asphyxial arrest induction may exert a great influence in determining the hemodynamic and catecholamine background upon which resuscitation intervention outcomes are measured.

Definition of Arrest and Nonintervention

Prospective definition of "cardiac arrest" is important.[19] During asphyxial arrest in porcine models, loss of aortic pulsations, as measured by invasive arterial blood pressure monitoring, is generally accepted as the cardiac arrest endpoint. However, cardiac dysfunction is a continuum, with a usual progression from tachycardia and hypertension to bradycardia, hypotension, and eventually asystole. There may be prolonged periods of relative bradycardia (heart rate 40 to 60 bpm) with variable pulsatile blood pressure over 8 to 12 minutes of asphyxia prior to loss of arterial pulsation. Time of onset of electrically induced VF cardiac arrest is generally abrupt and easily defined, while asphyxial cardiac arrest is usually gradually progressive. The duration of nonintervention following defined cardiac arrest is dictated by the question and intervention being studied. Early interventions for basic life support versus late interventions including advanced life support (ALS) should be applied at appropriate intervals to mimic clinical settings. The duration of nonintervention may clearly influence resuscitation outcome.

Monitoring and Reporting

Sites of invasive and noninvasive monitoring and time sequence for reporting outcomes are critically important in pediatric asphyxial and VF arrest models. Berg et al[20] demonstrated that end-tidal carbon dioxide levels ($ETCO_2$ = 92) were markedly elevated in the first five breaths after CPR in pigs subjected to asphyxia-induced arrest and 10 minutes of nonintervention compared with levels of 34 in pigs with electrically induced VF arrest and 15 minutes of nonintervention. Similarly, Bhende et al[21] demonstrated an equivalent rise in $ETCO_2$ during asphyxial arrest induction in puppies, followed by a fall in levels after arrest until just prior to ROSC. This emphasizes the critical importance of prospectively selecting time sequence and location of monitoring and reporting. Direct comparison of blood gas values, plasma epinephrine levels, and venous/arterial epinephrine gradients demonstrate that asphyxial versus VF etiology of arrest may exert great influence on experimental resuscitation outcomes.[22] A study of 31 anesthetized and paralyzed immature piglets evaluated 8-minute periods of pure respiratory arrest (apnea) with intact circulation (respiratory arrest; n=12) versus 8 minutes of cardiac arrest following this period of apnea (respiratory arrest + cardiac arrest; n=12) versus VF cardiac arrest induced by electrical stimulation of the right ventricle without preceding respiratory arrest (VF + cardiac arrest; n=19). These 8-minute nonintervention intervals were then followed by mechanical CPR (50% duty cycle, 5:1 compression:ventilation ratio, depth of compression 1.5 inches), ventilation pressure 30 cm H_2O, with 100% FiO_2. Figure 2 (respiratory arrest followed by cardiac arrest) and Figure 3

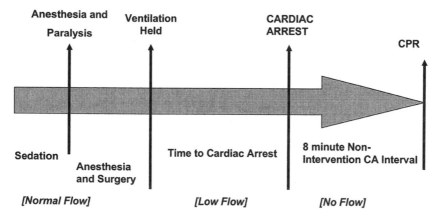

Figure 2. Time line for asphyxial porcine arrest induction model (Nadkarni 1998). Note variable interval of "Low Flow" (hypoxia and hypercarbia) during cardiac arrest induction following anesthesia and surgery, paralysis, and apnea. This is followed by an 8-minute period of cardiac arrest ("No Flow") without intervention.

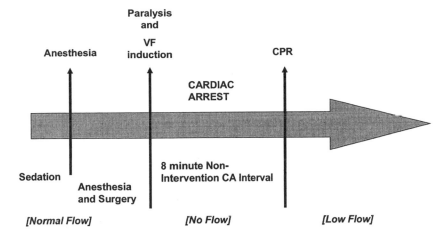

Figure 3. Time line for ventricular fibrillation porcine arrest induction model (Nadkarni 1998). Note abrupt onset of "No Flow" from "Normal Flow" following electrical stimulation of the right ventricle, without preceding hypoxic/hypercarbic and low circulatory flow.

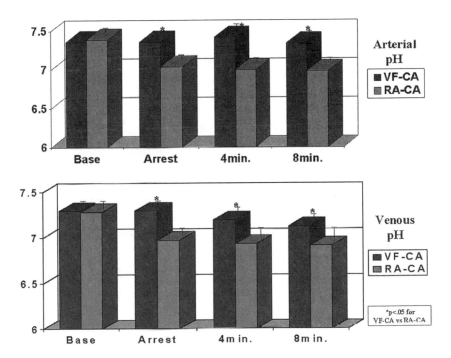

Figure 4. Comparison of arterial and venous pH in respiratory arrest followed by cardiac arrest (RA-CA) versus ventricular fibrillation-induced cardiac arrest (VF-CA) piglets during arrest and nonintervention intervals. RA-CA piglets exhibit markedly lower pH in both arterial and venous circuits during cardiac arrest without intervention.

(cardiac arrest) present the time lines for these experimental interventions. Figure 4 (pH), Figure 5 (pCO_2), Figure 6 (pO_2), and Figure 7 (venous/arterial epinephrine ratio) suggest that during 8 minutes of cardiac arrest without intervention, VF-induced cardiac arrest induction resulted in only modest decreases in pH and pO_2 and a mild increase in pCO_2, but rapid venous pooling of epinephrine. In contrast, respiratory arrest followed by cardiac arrest induction resulted in significant elevation of pCO_2 with a decrease in pH and in pO_2. Ratios of venous/arterial epinephrine were markedly different: respiratory arrest (1:1) versus respiratory arrest followed by cardiac arrest (5:1) versus VF-induced cardiac arrest (160:1). This suggests that even with carefully controlled anesthetic technique and definition of cardiac arrest, the etiology of experimental cardiac arrest induction exerts great influence on arterial and venous blood gas values, epinephrine levels, and venous/arterial epinephrine gradients. These factors may have a great impact on experimental cardiac arrest outcome and should be considered in research design.

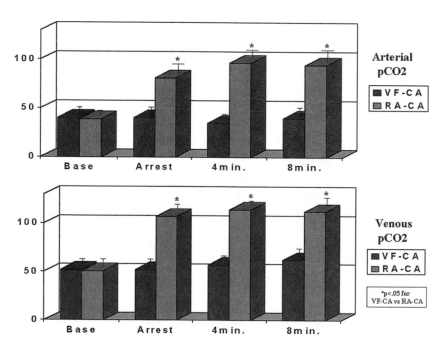

Figure 5. Comparison of arterial and venous pCO_2 in respiratory arrest followed by cardiac arrest (RA-CA) versus ventricular fibrillation-induced cardiac arrest (VF-CA) piglets during arrest and nonintervention intervals. RA-CA piglets exhibit markedly higher pCO_2 in both arterial and venous circuits during cardiac arrest without intervention.

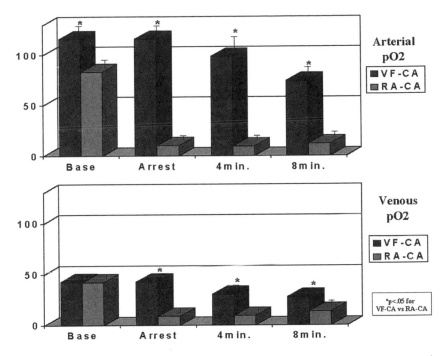

Figure 6. Comparison of arterial and venous pO_2 in respiratory arrest followed by cardiac arrest (RA-CA) versus ventricular fibrillation-induced cardiac arrest (VF-CA) piglets during arrest and nonintervention intervals. RA-CA piglets exhibit markedly lower pO_2 in both arterial and venous circuits during arrest without intervention.

Interventions and Timing of Outcome Measures

In addition to the primary outcome measures of ROSC and immediate survival, secondary outcome measures of postresuscitation myocardial depression, long-term survival, neurologic outcome, and prevalence of VF following resuscitation outcomes may be affected by asphyxia versus VF cardiac arrest induction. For example, in a randomized and blinded trial of high-dose versus standard-dose epinephrine in porcine asphyxial arrest (n=30) with a 10-minute nonintervention cardiac arrest interval, equivalent numbers of piglets developed initial ROSC.[23] However, 4 of 13 high-dose versus zero of 10 standard-dose epinephrine-treated pigs developed VF within 10 minutes of resuscitation, and all deaths in the high-dose group were attributable to VF. Similarly, Lindner and Ahnefeld[17] compared response to epinephrine versus norepinephrine in pigs subjected to short nonintervention intervals after asphyxial arrest (n=7; 3 minutes) versus VF arrest (n=7; 4 minutes). Equivalent time to ROSC was seen with both drugs after asphyxial arrest, but

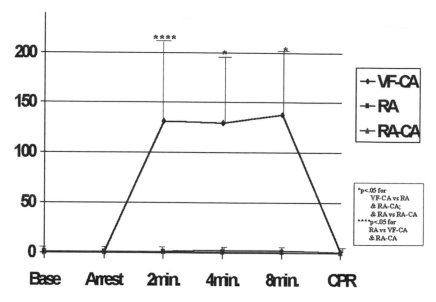

Figure 7. Comparison of venous/arterial epinephrine gradients during respiratory arrest induction with low flow (RA) versus respiratory arrest followed by cardiac arrest (RA-CA) versus ventricular fibrillation-induced cardiac arrest (VF-CA) piglets during arrest and nonintervention intervals. Venous/arterial epinephrine ratio was 1:1 for RA versus 5:1 for RA-CA versus 160:1 for VF-CA during arrest induction and nonintervention. All ratios reverted to approximately 1:1 within 2 minutes of cardiopulmonary resuscitation intervention.

significantly shorter times to ROSC were seen with norepinephrine than with epinephrine in the VF pigs. In the same model, interposed abdominal compression demonstrated similar advantage over standard CPR technique in both asphyxia- and VF-induced arrested pigs with regard to CPR hemodynamics, early ROSC, and time to ROSC.[24] These examples emphasize the importance of prospective selection of critical outcome measures related to resuscitation intervention and specific attention to etiology of arrest impact on resuscitation outcome.

Model Selection

Asphyxial porcine cardiac arrest models are relevant to many pediatric resuscitation scenarios. As discussed above, the challenge is to select a model that is physiologically sound and measurable but still relevant to clinical application. Models that mimic hypoxic and hypercarbic intervals prior to cardiac arrest followed by 4- to 10-minute nonintervention interval prior to basic life support or ALS arrival, and a short interval of CPR prior to ALS intervention, are most relevant to the most commonly encountered pediatric scenario. Models of sudden on-set of VF with short intervals prior to ALS and defibrillation are most relevant to infants in hospital settings with underlying cardiac disease and short ALS intervention intervals. Outcome measures and applicability of conclusions from asphyxial animal models to the "real world" depend on an understanding of the critical differences between asphyxial and VF cardiac arrest induction techniques discussed above.

Summary

Pediatric cardiac arrest most frequently results from initial respiratory compromise leading to pulmonary failure, hypoxemia, hypercarbia, and subsequent bradyasystolic arrest, with resultant poor neurologic and functional outcome. A review of current pediatric porcine cardiac arrest and resuscitation models suggests that asphyxial versus electrical VF induction of cardiac arrest may have major impact on arrest, early and late resuscitation outcome measures. In addition, VF may present during asphyxial-induced arrest induction or nonintervention interval, and after interventions such as high-dose epinephrine. Asphyxial models suggest that there may be a window of opportunity to apply VF interventions in some children during asphyxial arrest, with the potential for alternative therapy and improved outcome. Experimental factors such as age, health status, prearrest management, anesthetic regimen, definition of arrest, duration of nonintervention, site and timing of monitoring, type of intervention, and specific outcome measure monitored play a large role in assessment of VF prevalence and treatment outcome. These critical factors and limitations must be acknowledged before relevance to infants and children can be inferred. Outcome measures and applicability of conclusions from asphyxial animal models to the "real world" depend on an understanding of the critical differences between asphyxial and VF cardiac arrest induction models.

References

1. Walsh CK, Krongrad E. Terminal electrical activity in pediatric patients. *Am J Cardiol* 1983;31:557–561.
2. Meny RG, Carroll JL, Carbone MT, Kelly DH. Cardiorespiratory recording findings from infants dying suddenly and unexpectedly at home. *Pediatrics* 1994;93:44–49.
3. Meny RG, Currey K, Scheel JN, et al. Asystoles during infancy recorded by home monitors. *Arch Pediatr Adolesc Med* 1996;150:901–905.
4. Losek JD, Hennes H, Glaeser PW, et al. Prehospital countershock treatment of pediatric asystole. *Am J Emerg Med* 1989;7:571–575.

5. Milner PG, Platia EV, Reid PR, Griffith LS. Ambulatory electrocardiographic recordings at the time of fatal cardiac arrest. *Am J Cardiol* 1985;56: 588–592.
6. Holliman CJ, Bates MA. Review of all studies of cardiopulmonary resuscitation in animal models reported in the emergency medicine literature for the past 10 years. *Am J Emerg Med* 1992;10:347–353.
7. Redding JS, Pearson JW. Resuscitation from asphyxia. *JAMA* 1962;182: 283.
8. Yakaitis RW, Otto CW, Blitt CD. Relative importance of alpha and beta receptors during resuscitation. *Crit Care Med* 1979;7:293–296.
9. Otto CW, Yakaitis RW, Blitt CD. Mechanism of action of epinephrine in resuscitation from asphyxial arrest. *Crit Care Med* 1981;9:364–365.
10. Caputo G, Delgado-Paredes C, Swedlow D, Fleisher G. Anoxic cardiopulmonary arrest in a pediatric animal model: Clinical and laboratory correlates of duration. *Pediatr Emerg Care* 1985;1:57–60.
11. Jasani MS, Nadkarni VM, Finkelstein MS, et al. Effects of different techniques of endotracheal epinephrine administration in pediatric porcine hypoxic-hypercarbic cardiopulmonary arrest. *Crit Care Med* 1994;22:1174–1180.
12. Berg RA, Kern KB, Otto CW, et al. Ventricular fibrillation in a swine model of acute pediatric asphyxial cardiac arrest. *Resuscitation* 1996;33:147–153.
13. Jasani MS, Salzman SK, Tice LL, et al. Anesthetic regimen effects on a pediatric porcine model of asphyxial arrest. *Resuscitation* 1997;35:69–75.
14. Idris AH, Wenzel V, Becker LB, et al. Does hypoxia or hypercarbia independently affect resuscitation from cardiac arrest? *Chest* 1995;108:522–528.
15. Vaagenes P, Safar P, Moossy J, et al. Asphyxiation versus ventricular fibrillation cardiac arrest in dogs. Differences in cerebral resuscitation effects—a preliminary study. *Resuscitation* 1997;35:41–52.
16. Buckley NM, Gootman PM, Yellin EL, Brazeau P. Age-related cardiovascular effects of catecholamines in anesthetized piglets. *Circ Res* 1979; 45(2):282–292.
17. Lindner KH, Ahnefeld FW. Comparison of epinephrine and norepinephrine in the treatment of asphyxial or fibrillatory cardiac arrest in a porcine model. *Crit Care Med* 1989;17:437–441.
18. Hart BB, Stanford GG, Ziegler MG, et al. Catecholamines: Study of interspecies variation. *Crit Care Med* 1989;17:1203–1222.
19. Idris AH, Becker LB, Ornato JP, et al. Utstein-style guidelines for uniform reporting of laboratory CPR research. *Resuscitation* 1996;33:69–84.
20. Berg RA, Henry C, Otto CW, et al. Initial end-tidal CO_2 is markedly elevated during cardiopulmonary resuscitation after asphyxial cardiac arrest. *Pediatr Emerg Care* 1996;12:245–248.
21. Bhende MS, Karasic DG, Karasic RB. End-tidal carbon dioxide changes during cardiopulmonary resuscitation after experimental asphyxial cardiac arrest. *Am J Emerg Med* 1996;14:349–350.
22. Nadkarni VM, Tice L, Hofmann W, Jasani M. Etiology of experimental pediatric porcine arrest influence epinephrine and blood gas values and gradients. *Crit Care Med* 1998;26:A96.
23. Berg RA, Otto CW, Kern KB, et al. A randomized, blinded trial of high-dose epinephrine versus standard-dose epinephrine in a swine model of pediatric asphyxial cardiac arrest. *Crit Care Med* 1996;24:1695–1700.
24. Lindner KH, Ahnefeld FW, Bowdler IM. Cardiopulmonary resuscitation with interposed abdominal compression after asphyxial or fibrillatory cardiac arrest in pigs. *Anesthesiology* 1990;72:675–681.

Sudden Death in the Pediatric Patient with an Ostensibly Normal Heart:

Developmental Expression of Lethal Arrhythmias in Children

Chapter 5

Ventricular Fibrillation in Pediatric Out-of-Hospital Cardiac Arrest

Linda Quan, MD

When the initial rhythms in cardiac arrest were first described in a pediatric in-hospital population, bradycardia and asystole were the most frequent dysrhythmias.[1] In this study, ventricular fibrillation (VF) was far less common, although it heralded cardiac arrest in all pediatric age groups. The fact that the prevalence was lowest in neonates supported the belief that VF requires a larger cardiac mass. That VF occurred only in those pediatric patients with congenital heart disease supported the belief that VF does not occur in normal pediatric hearts. Subsequently, VF has been virtually ignored in most pediatric cardiac arrest studies. Some studies do not even describe the prevalence of VF, and fewer still describe outcome of VF. This chapter seeks to describe the unique epidemiology of VF in the pediatric victim in out-of-hospital cardiac arrest (OHCA), to compare this and outcome data with the adult experience, and to make recommendations on directions for future research of this pediatric problem.

In marked contrast to pediatric cardiac arrest studies, adult cardiac arrest studies have focused on the diagnosis and treatment of VF in both in-patient cardiac arrest and OHCA. This adult focus on VF developed because of reports from emergency medical service (EMS) systems on their experience treating adult cardiac arrest. These studies showed that VF was the most common initial dysrhythmia in adults with sudden death; in some reports, the prevalence of VF was 60% to 85%. It must be noted, however, that the patient population of most adult out-of-hospital reports included only patients with nontraumatic cardiac arrests; this patient population reflected the interest and focus of the internists who directed early EMS systems. This medical group

From: Quan L, Franklin WH (eds). *Ventricular Fibrillation: A Pediatric Problem.* Armonk, NY: Futura Publishing Company, Inc.; ©2000.

of patients had atherosclerotic heart disease as the major cause of death. These studies specifically excluded traumatic causes of cardiac arrest.

Increasingly, studies of EMS system experiences with OHCA in Belfast, Ireland, and King County and Seattle, Washington, USA, showed that adults with VF had significantly better outcomes than patients with asystole. An initial rhythm of VF in the adult was associated with significantly greater survival rates, as high as 63%.[2] Survival rates from out-of-hospital VF became the basis upon which EMS systems defined themselves and were rated.

The exciting prospect of good outcomes following cardiac arrest spurred evaluation of the experiences of multiple EMS systems; in 1990, Eisenberg et al[3] were able to identify 74 individual papers from EMS systems, each reporting on more than 100 patients. Further studies, primarily of and by EMS systems, defined outcome predictors for adult OHCA. Good outcome in adults was associated with witnessed or monitored arrests that reflected early recognition of the collapse, victims less than 60 years old (this reflected patients with ischemic heart disease and without terminal or other severe illnesses), early bystander cardiopulmonary resuscitation (CPR), rapid arrival of emergency personnel trained in defibrillation, early defibrillation (treatment within 5 minutes of collapse), and advanced life support interventions including endotracheal intubation and intravenous pharmacology. In 1986, Weaver et al[4] showed that the best outcome predictors for successful resuscitation were in witnessed VF in younger adults; the best system variables were short time intervals from collapse to CPR and from collapse to defibrillation. Using logistic regression, Valenzuela et al[5] recently elegantly confirmed that these parameters remain the key determinants of outcome. Time is the key to outcome in adults.

By the 1970s, it was already obvious to the EMS community that CPR provided to the OHCA victim by EMS was too late. Cobb's audacious Seattle EMS Medic II program showed communities how to achieve high levels of penetration of CPR capabilities in the citizenry; an estimated 40% of Seattleites have had CPR training. CPR courses and public education were made widely available and inexpensive in order to increase the public's recognition of and response to cardiac collapse and pre-cardiac-arrest states such as chest pain.[6] With CPR-trained citizenry, EMS systems were able to demonstrate the key role of CPR in VF. Studies from multiple countries showed that patients in VF who received bystander CPR prior to the arrival of EMS did better than those who did not.[7] Data have led to a consensus that CPR sustains VF, preventing its deterioration to asystole.[7,8] Significant efforts to increase early intervention of OHCA with citizen CPR have been made based on these findings. While public education efforts to increase the training in CPR of high-risk adult populations have met with minimal success, efforts to increase training in middle school and high school have just begun; Emergency Medical Services for Children, a federal agency under Maternal Child Health Bureau and National Highway and Transportation Agency, has set a 5-year goal for states to require CPR training for high school graduation.[9]

Early studies from multiple centers showed that delay in EMS response led to decreased survival from cardiac arrest. EMS systems sought ways to achieve shorter response times to provide defibrillator therapy and advanced life support by improving strategic placement of EMS responders, adding second responders/paramedics, and using 911 technology to better locate and reach victims. Further research showed that the key variable actually was the time interval to defibrillation provided by the EMS responder; for every minute of delay to defibrillation of VF, survival rates dropped 10%. Late defibrillation, defined as greater than 10 minutes from collapse to defibrillation, was associated with decreased survival. Increasing knowledge of these predictors of good outcome from OHCA drove EMS systems, the American Heart Association (AHA), local communities, and technology to make additional changes to improve outcome from VF causes of cardiac arrest. By 1992, the AHA guidelines set forth by the Emergency Cardiac Care Committee recommended a "call first" approach to the adult. The "adult" approach applies to unresponsive patients over age 8. This approach has the single rescuer first assess whether the victim is truly unconscious, apneic, and pulseless, and then call EMS before initiating CPR. This approach therefore has the rescuer, at the earliest possible moment, activate a system that would provide defibrillation. It is predicated on the reasonable likelihood of VF in the pulseless adult victim.

Recognizing the enormous cost of adding EMS ambulances and paramedics, the EMS community sought alternative, more efficient approaches to provide earlier defibrillation. In the 1980s, the EMS community started equipping first responders, who were lesser trained than paramedics, with defibrillators because first responders were more ubiquitous personnel in EMS systems and therefore had shorter response times than paramedics. In rural communities, EMS systems may not include paramedics; first responders may be the only prehospital personnel. This new cadre of EMS personnel, first responders trained in defibrillation, proved that they saved lives when VF was present.[10]

In the 1990s, with the advent of the automated external defibrillator (AED), recognition of VF in adults, treatment with defibrillation, and training in defibrillation became astoundingly sensitive, simple, and safe. The AED facilitated rhythm recognition more quickly than systems that require lead placement and rhythm strips. It was more sensitive in diagnosing VF than were physicians, and it proved highly accurate and specific.[11] These features allowed large groups of trained personnel outside the EMS system, including police officers, airline personnel, and families, to use automated defibrillators and save lives.[12] Major systems changes placed the defibrillators near the patients at risk, be it in the setting of an international exposition, an airplane, or a casino.[5] Thus, the collapsed patient no longer has to get to the hospital to be treated, nor does he or she have to wait for someone to call EMS and for EMS to respond. Increasingly in our communities, treatment is potentially steps away for the VF victim. Efforts to ensure this level of care for most Americans culminated in the Cardiac Arrest Bill, which awaits Congressional support; the state of Washington and others have passed similar laws allowing training of nonmedical personnel in AED use and encouraging widespread placement and use of AEDs in public places.

The lessons learned from the adult experience with VF can be best summarized in the "chain of survival" concept. Successful resuscitation of adult OHCA requires that every sequence of the process occur within tight time limits. The sequences are early recognition of impending cardiac arrest, early bystander basic CPR, early defibrillation, and provision of intubation and intravascular medication. Short time differences, on the order of 1 minute, are important determinants of survival, and bystander CPR and response interval from call to arrival of the prehospital ambulance are independent factors in survival.[13,14] Any weakness in any link decreases survival and thus explains the varying success rates for out-of-hospital adult VF reported by varying EMS systems.[15]

In pediatric OHCA studies that note the initial rhythm, the prevalence of VF, which varies from 6% to 22%, is lower than that in most adult reports.[16–21] Diverse prevalences have even come from data sets that included the same large EMS system.[17,19,20] The different findings demonstrate several of the vagaries in the epidemiology of pediatric VF.

In contrast to adult OHCA, pediatric OHCAs are not well characterized. A lack of uniform case definitions has thwarted the ability to draw conclusions from multiple studies to an even greater extent than the adult studies.[22] Difficulties with studying VF in the pediatric patient occur at every level: case ascertainment, the population studied versus the populations excluded, and outcome, since treatment is problematic. Furthermore, few pediatric cardiac arrest studies have evaluated time intervals, the key factor identified by studies of adult series. Instead, pediatric studies continue to report on presentation or outcome in the emergency department or intensive care unit with patients whose cardiac arrest was out-of-hospital. Not surprisingly, these studies show that VF is rare and with poor outcome.[23,24]

Importantly, the small size of published case series has precluded in-depth analyses that would elucidate factors associated with VF and good outcome from VF. For example, analyzing the largest published series to date of 158 cases, Mogayzel et al[19] were unable to show significant differences in VF prevalence by age; in a larger series involving 940 cases from the same region, Paris et al[21] were able to demonstrate significant differences. Thus, variations in the numerator as well as the denominator make prevalence of VF a varying number.

Denominator Issues

Pediatric OHCA series, in contrast to adult studies, have tended to be inclusive rather than exclusive. Variations in the populations studied in existing case series have included two important groups of patients not included in most adult OHCA studies: victims of trauma and those of sudden infant death syndrome (SIDS). SIDS is a major cause of pediatric arrests, accounting for the great majority of OHCAs in infants less than 1 year of age. It is always unwitnessed with unknown and often long down times (time from arrest to call). Despite recent evidence suggesting that VF due to prolonged QT syndromes may be the cause of death for a subset of SIDS victims, most victims are found in asystole and, by definition, all die.[25] Thus, inclusion of SIDS victims in a pediatric OHCA series lowers the VF prevalence, and exclusion increases it.[26] For instance, when SIDS was excluded from the study by Mogayzel and colleagues,[19] the prevalence of VF was 19%; when SIDS was included, the prevalence decreased to 13%. However, survival was so strongly associated with VF compared with asystole or pulseless electrical activity in that series when SIDS was excluded (RR 4.5; 95% confidence interval 2, 8.1) that outcome from VF remained significantly better, even when the SIDS group was included (RR 2.0; 95% confidence interval 1.2, 34).

Traumatic cardiac arrest is also a major cause of pediatric OHCA. In general, a traumatic etiology is associated with a dismal outcome; however, survival, especially in victims with VF, has been noted.[19,27] Thus, inclusion of patients with SIDS and trauma, two large etiologic population subsets in the denominator, lowers the prevalence of VF and good outcome from VF. However, if adult OHCA studies included traumatic cardiac arrest, successful outcomes would be so low as to approach survival rates in pediatric OHCA series that include trauma.

To further complicate the denominator, there is no consensus as to the definition of a pediatric patient. Therefore, the age groups included vary among studies. Many studies often exclude older adolescents, the second largest pediatric age group at risk for cardiac arrest and the group at highest risk for VF.[21] The increased prevalence of VF in adolescents may be due to their use of substances of abuse, especially cocaine or amphetamines, and inhalants, as well as medications used in suicide, such as tricyclic antidepressants. In addition, the expression of several of the conditions that predispose to conduction defects and hypertrophic cardiomyopathy become manifest at this age. Thus, there may be a lower prevalence of VF in studies of younger pediatric populations or in rural populations or regions with less drug use.

The definition of cardiac arrest has also varied, with some studies unclear as to whether patients are pulseless.[28] Moreover, variability has been noted among EMS systems' approaches to the pediatric patient in cardiac arrest. Possibly because of the young age of the victims or the parental reaction and expectation to finding their well baby dead, in one system EMS personnel attempted CPR or even provided advanced life support to victims with rigor or livido reticularis, and included these in their resuscitation studies.[29] In another system, EMS personnel seemed more willing to forego an attempted resuscitation in a child who was obviously dead.

The question of who is being resuscitated has also been a problem for adult OHCA studies. Valenzuela and colleagues[30] addressed the effect of changing the denominator on outcomes of adult OHCA studies; the change in denominators may be even more pronounced in pediatric studies, in which small numbers are easily overwhelmed.

Numerator Issues

Causes of VF in the pediatric OHCA population can be categorized into injury, pharmacologic injury, or "sudden cardiac death." In the pediatric patient, the most common injury is from hypoxia. Respiratory causes remain the major cause of OHCA in all pediatric studies. In one pediatric OHCA community in the western United States, drowning was the most common respiratory cause.[19,31] Asphyxia, from strangulation, croup, epiglottitis, and, increasingly, asthma are other respiratory conditions that cause hypoxia-induced VF. Less commonly, ischemia may cause VF; this is more likely to be global ischemia in the pediatric patient than in the adult, in whom it is usually from local myocardial vessel occlusion. Thus, hypovolemia and acidosis causing shock can precipitate VF even in young pediatric patients. Other physical injuries include electrocution or a direct blow to the sternum during the T wave rise or resulting in myocardial contusion.[32] Hypothermia remains a feared cause of VF. Pharmacologic agents—either substances of abuse, such as cocaine, or the ingestion of medications or other agents such as tricyclic antidepressants or inhalants—may cause VF.

The pediatric "sudden cardiac death" population, that in which death is not due to injury or drugs, continues to be elucidated. Unfortunately, most series represent cohorts of pediatric cardiology patients rather than community-based populations. Most studies exclude infants of less than 1 year, thereby avoiding the SIDS group.[33] The study by Driscoll and Edwards[34] remains a landmark as a community-based descriptive study. In that 1985 series, the largest (33%) subgroup population was patients with structural cardiac lesions, especially anomalous coronary postoperative repair. In an EMS systems-/community-based series, when initial rhythm at cardiac arrest was identified, causes of VF were equally distributed among cardiac and noncardiac causes.[19] Patients with inherited and postoperatively acquired conduction defects comprise another subgroup of sudden cardiac death victims. With advances in pediatric cardiac surgery, increasing numbers of patients with repaired cardiac defects have reentered their communities. Specific groups of patients, such as those post repair of tetralogy of Fallot, have demonstrated increased risk for sudden death in their communities. In addition, patients known to have prolonged QT syndrome, autosomal dominant syndromes, Romano-Ward, and Jervell and Lange-Nielsen syndromes are always present in these series. Patients with acquired heart disease such as hypertrophic cardiomyopathy, myocarditis, and, more rarely, arrhythmogenic right ventricular dysplasia comprise the majority of sudden cardiac death victims when evaluated in other series. More current population-based studies are needed to determine if the prevalence of cardiac disorders causing OHCA have increased and if the types of cardiac disorders associated with OHCA and VF have changed with improved outcome for many cardiac conditions.

It must be noted that the true prevalence of nonstructural cardiac disorders continues to be underestimated by any study. Unexplained VF in a child or young adult who may have been swimming or engaged in some other activity is often attributed to that activity, such as drowning or falling. Family history of sudden death and syncope, and genetic evaluation, are not routine; viral studies and PCR evaluation for myocarditis are not regularly obtained. Greater recognition of the causes of VF are needed. This would require increased vigilance among medical examiners and pediatric fatality review teams. Thus, VF prevalence may be determined but remains poorly understood.

The most pressing unresolved issue in VF prevalence studies is the timing of rhythm identification. Until the advent of the AED and its use by first responders, rhythm identification was accomplished by the second responder in most EMS systems—in other words, paramedics using a cardiac monitor, placing leads, and reading a rhythm strip. With the AED, however, identification of VF could be accomplished by the first responding EMS unit, which typically arrives several to many minutes earlier than the second responder, the paramedic. The result of this was not only earlier recognition but also identification of more cases of VF, since VF is known to degenerate over time to asystole.

Early recognition and ensuing earlier treatment are not, however, in the purview of the pediatric patient. The use of AEDs was limited to those patients older than 12 years in the 1986, and then to those older than 8 years in the 1992 AHA Adult Advanced Life Support guidelines. This means that pediatric OHCA has been managed in the field with lesser technology than has adult OHCA, and that patients with pediatric OHCA are less likely to be diagnosed with VF. In rural or volunteer EMS systems without paramedic capabilities or with long response time intervals, the diagnosis of VF, though rare, would never be made in a child younger than 12 years old, given the decay rate of VF.

In 1992, the AHA AED guidelines changed, lowering the age limit and recommending its use in children older than 8 years. Unfortunately, very large multicenter series would be needed to prove any effect on the prevalence, given the low frequency of pediatric VF, especially in this age group. Eisenberg and Becker[35] calculated that a suburban EMS system with rapid response times and an active AED program would only see one to two cases per year; even if it was assumed that the prevalence rate would double with earlier detection, the number of cases per year would still be very small.

Does Prevalence Matter?

The importance of early VF recognition lies in the better outcome of this rhythm in pediatric arrest. Several studies have shown that the pediatric patient in VF, like the adult in VF, has a significantly better outcome than the pediatric patient in pulseless electrical activity (PEA) or asystole.[18,19,36] Paris et al,[21] reporting the largest series—940 patients in the Seattle/King County EMS systems—make clear the abysmal survival rate from asystole/PEA (2%) versus survival from VF (19%). While most pediatric studies have reported dismal overall survival rates of 5% to 10% in OHCA, they have generally failed to analyze the factors associated with survival. Reporting a very low prevalence of VF (4%) and a 1.7% survival rate from pediatric OHCA, the recent in-depth analysis of Dallas' EMS system by Sirbaugh and colleagues[37] identified a low prevalence of bystander CPR and pediatric advanced life support interventions. Interestingly, the highest frequency and survival rates from pediatric VF have been reported in the Seattle/King County EMS systems, which report the highest consistent adult survival rates (30%) from VF. It is not surprising that relatively high VF prevalence and save rates in the pediatric population would occur in an EMS system where patients are most likely to receive bystander CPR, short EMS response intervals, and pediatric advanced life support, with documented greater than 90% intubation and vascular access rates.[19]

Out-of-hospital adult resuscitation studies make clear that a short time interval from arrest to call and from call to defibrillation are the key determinants of survival of VF.[5] These issues have enormous implications for the pediatric patient younger than 8 years old. First, the AHA pediatric basic life support guidelines recommend that CPR be provided for 1 minute before the rescuer calls EMS. This prolongs the arrest-to-call interval. It is unknown if a parent really provides only 1 minute of CPR. Second, rhythm identification and treatment are delayed until the arrival of the paramedic, usually the second responder, who will interpret the rhythm. This delays the call-to-defibrillation interval. With a 4% decrease in successful defibrillation for every minute of delay in defibrillation, outcome in the pediatric patient with VF would understandably be less favorable than that of an adult in VF cared for by the same EMS system. Thus, the true prevalence of VF and, more importantly, the best outcome from VF, regardless of the denominator used, remain undefined in the child younger than 8 years old.[19]

For out-of-hospital pediatric cardiac arrests, the major challenge is early recognition of VF in the victim. Groups at high risk for VF include adolescents, patients with known heart disease (structural and nonstructural), and those with chest trauma. The second and more difficult challenge to pediatric OHCA is early defibrillation of the pediatric patient. The needed data driving the research agenda are:

1. Determination of the prevalence of VF early in OHCA. Large multicenter pediatric OHCA studies are needed, given the infrequency of the condition. Longitudinal and community-based studies are needed to determine the risk for sudden death among different cardiac patient populations too.

2. Better understanding of the etiologies of VF, to include why VF occurs in various types of injury as well as to recognize the etiologies of VF in sudden cardiac death. Better evaluations of victims of VF are needed. This would require coordination between EMS and medical examiners' offices and pediatric cardiologists, and would include thorough evaluation for viral myocarditis and genetic structural and nonstructural cardiac conditions, including detailed family histories. Pediatric fatality review

committees are needed to coordinate and review findings and to identify families at risk.

3. Open minded, fresh approaches to the identification and treatment of pediatric VF are needed to identify ways to assess and approach the pediatric patient in arrest that will result in higher save rates. Consideration must be given to earlier identification of cardiac versus respiratory arrest in the pediatric patient and rapid progression to rhythm assessment versus CPR.

4. Research on treatment must focus on identification of effective, safe defibrillation doses for OHCA that are technologically easy to deliver; the most important question remains that of how the AED can be modified to be accurate and safe for the younger, smaller patient.

References

1. Walsh CK, Krongrad E. Terminal cardiac electrical activity in pediatric patients. *Am J Cardiol* 1983;51:557–561.
2. Mayer J. Paramedic response time and survival from cardiac arrest. *Soc Sci Med* 1979;13:267–271.
3. Eisenberg M, Cummins R, Damon S, et al. Survival rates from OOH cardiac arrest: Recommendations for uniform definitions and data to report. *Ann Emerg Med* 1990;19:1249–1259.
4. Weaver W, Cobb L, Hallstrom A, et al. Considerations for improving survival from out-of-hospital CA. *Ann Emerg Med* 1986;15:1181–1186.
5. Valenzuela TD, Roe DJ, Cretin S, et al. Estimating effectiveness of cardiac arrest interventions: A logistic regression survival model. *Circulation* 1997;96:3308–3313.
6. Cobb L, Hallstrom A. Community based cardiopulmonary resuscitation: What have we learned? *Ann N Y Acad Sci* 1982;382:330–342.
7. Cummins RO, Eisenberg MS, Hallstrom AP, Litwin PE. Survival of out-of-hospital cardiac arrest with early initiation of cardiopulmonary resuscitation. *Am J Emerg Med* 1985;3:114–119.
8. Weaver WD, Cobb LA, Dennis D, et al. Amplitude of ventricular fibrillation waveform and outcome after cardiac arrest. *Ann Intern Med* 1985;102:53–55.
9. U.S. Department of Health and Human Services, Health Resources and Services Administration, Maternal and Child Health Bureau. *5 Year Plan: Emergency Medical Services for Children, 1995–2000.* Washington DC: Emergency Medical Services for Children National Resource Center; 1995.
10. Auble T, Menegazzi J, Paris P. Effect of out-of-hospital defibrillation by basic life support providers on cardiac arrest mortality: A metaanalysis. *Ann Emerg Med* 1995;25:642–648.
11. Cummins RO. From concept to standard-of-care? Review of the clinical experience with automated external defibrillators. *Ann Emerg Med* 1989;18:1269–1275.
12. Mosesso VN Jr, Davis EA, Auble TE, et al. Use of automated external de-

fibrillators by police officers for treatment of out-of-hospital cardiac arrest. *Ann Emerg Med* 1998;32:200–207.

13. Stiell IG, Wells GA, DeMaio VJ, et al. Modifiable factors associated with improved cardiac arrest survival in a multicenter basic life support/defibrillation system: OPALS Study Phase I results. Ontario Prehospital Advanced Life Support. *Ann Emerg Med* 1999;33:44–50.

14. White RD, Hankins DG, Bugliosi TF. Seven years' experience with early defibrillation by police and paramedics in an emergency medical services system. *Resuscitation* 1998;39:145–151.

15. Cummins R, Ornato J, Thies W, et al. The "chain of survival" concept. *Circulation* 1991;83:1832–1847.

16. Hickey R, Cohen D, Strausbaugh S, Dietrich A. Pediatric patients requiring CPR in the prehospital setting. *Ann Emerg Med* 1994;25:495–501.

17. Appleton GO, Cummins RO, Larson MP. CPR and the single rescuer: At what age should you "call first" rather than "call fast"? *Ann Emerg Med* 1995;25:492–494.

18. Losek JD, Hennes H, Glaeser P, et al. Prehospital care of the pulseless, nonbreathing pediatric patient. *Am J Emerg Med* 1987;5:370–374.

19. Mogayzel C, Quan L, Graves J, et al. Out-of-hospital ventricular fibrillation in children and adolescents: Causes and outcomes. *Ann Emerg Med* 1995;25:484–491.

20. Safranek D, Eisenberg M, Larsen MP. The epidemiology of cardiac arrest in young adults. *Ann Emerg Med* 1992;21:1102–1105.

21. Paris C, Quan L, Fahrenbruch C, Copass M. Predictors of survival after pediatric cardiac arrest. *39th Annual Meeting of the Ambulatory Pediatric Association Program and Abstracts.* 1999.

22. Cummins R, Chamberlain D, Hazinski M, et al. Recommended guidelines for reviewing, reporting, and conducting research on in-hospital resuscitation: The in-hospital "Utstein style." A statement for healthcare professionals from the American Heart Association, the European Resuscitation Council, the Heart and Stroke Foundation of Canada, the Australian Resuscitation Council, and the Resuscitation Councils of Southern Africa. *Circulation* 1997;95:2213–2239.

23. Schindler MB, Bohn D, Cox PN, et al. Outcome of out-of-hospital cardiac or respiratory arrest in children. *N Engl J Med* 1996;335:1473–1479.

24. Schoenfeld P, Baker D. Management of cardiopulmonary and trauma resuscitation in the pediatric emergency department. *Pediatrics* 1993;91:726–729.

25. Schwartz P, Stramba-Badiale M, Segantini A, et al. Prolongation of the QT interval and the sudden infant death syndrome. *N Engl J Med* 1998;338:1709–1761.

26. Hazinski M. Is pediatric resuscitation unique? Relative merits of early CPR and ventilation versus early defibrillation for young victims of cardiac arrest. *Ann Emerg Med* 1995;25:540–543.

27. Suominen P, Rasanen J, Kivioja A. Efficacy of cardiopulmonary resuscitation in pulseless paediatric trauma patients. *Resuscitation* 1998;36:9–13.

28. Young KD, Seidel JS. Pediatric cardiopulmonary resuscitation: A collective review. *Ann Emerg Med* 1999;33:195–205.

29. Quan L. Editorial reply: Ventricular fibrillation in pediatric cardiac arrest. *Ann Emerg Med* 1995;26:658–659.

30. Valenzuela TD, Spaite DW, Meislin HW, et al. Case and survival definitions in out-of-hospital cardiac arrest. Effect on survival rate calculation [see comments]. *JAMA* 1992;267:272–274.

31. Eisenberg M, Bergner L, Hallstrom A. Epidemiology of cardiac arrest and resuscitation in children. *Ann Emerg Med* 1983;12:672–674.
32. Maron BJ, Poliac LC, Kaplan JA, Mueller FO. Blunt impact to the chest leading to sudden death from cardiac arrest during sports activities. *N Engl J Med* 1995;333:337–341.
33. Steinberger J, Lucas R, Edwards J, Titus JL. Causes of sudden unexpected cardiac death in the first two decades of life. *Am J Cardiol* 1996;77:992–995.
34. Driscoll DJ, Edwards WD. Sudden unexpected death in children and adolescents. *J Am Coll Cardiol* 1985;5:118B-121B.
35. Eisenberg M, Becker L. Abstract, Presented at American Heart Association symposium, Dallas, TX: 1998.
36. Ronco R, King W, Donley D, Tilden S. Outcome and cost at a children's hospital following resuscitation for out-of-hospital cardiopulmonary arrest. *Arch Pediatr Adolesc Med* 1995;149:210–214.
37. Sirbaugh PE, Pepe PE, Shook JE, et al. A prospective, population-based study of the demographics, epidemiology, management, and outcome of out-of-hospital pediatric cardiopulmonary arrest [see comments]. *Ann Emerg Med* 1999;33:174–184.

Chapter 6

Ventricular Fibrillation from Hypothermia

Howard M. Corneli, MD

Introduction

Severe hypothermia commonly causes ventricular fibrillation (VF) in otherwise healthy adults and children. This dysrhythmia is a common fatal endpoint in accidental hypothermia.[1,2] VF is probably more common than asystole is in severe hypothermia[3,4]; in a recently published series of patients with severe hypothermia,[5] VF was twice as common as asystole. Although hypothermic children are said to be more prone to asystole than are adults,[4] VF is commonly reported in children with hypothermia.[6–10]

The presence of hypothermia offers unique insights into the etiology and treatment of VF. At the same time, the development of VF may be a fatal event for many hypothermic patients. VF can be triggered by both avoidable and unavoidable interventions in the rescue[11] and resuscitation[12] of victims of hypothermia. The treatment of VF in the hypothermic patient is difficult and varies in several regards from standard treatment in normothermia.

Definitions

Hypothermia is defined as a core body temperature below 35°C (95°F). Mild hypothermia is typically considered a core temperature between approximately 31°C and 35°C. In this range, the physiological changes of hypothermia are mostly those of compensation, such as

From: Quan L, Franklin WH (eds). *Ventricular Fibrillation: A Pediatric Problem.* Armonk, NY: Futura Publishing Company, Inc.; ©2000.

vasoconstriction and shivering, and VF is not a typical consequence. Moderate hypothermia is typically defined as a core temperature between 29°C and 31°C. In this narrow range, many compensation mechanisms begin to fail. Severe hypothermia is defined as core temperature below 29°C. It is in this range that VF most commonly develops. Profound hypothermia occurs at core temperatures below 25°C. In the controlled setting of induced hypothermia for cardiac surgery, asystole may be associated with colder temperatures, on average, than VF.[13]

The Electrocardiogram in Severe Hypothermia

VF is just one of several cardiac rhythms described in severe hypothermia. As mentioned, asystole is also seen. Sinus bradycardia is common as the core temperature decreases below 32°C. Severely hypothermic patients may manifest profound bradycardia with heart rates below 15 bpm.[14] Dysrhythmias seen in hypothermia are many: atrial fibrillation is perhaps most common, but does not usually require treatment beyond rewarming.[15] Atrioventricular block has also been reported.[16]

A specific electrocardiographic (ECG) change seen in 10% to 80% of hypothermic patients is the J or Osborn wave.[17,18] Other ECG changes may include T wave inversion, PR, QRS, and QT interval prolongation, and nodal and junctional rhythms.[19,20]

Pulseless electrical activity (PEA) is commonly noted in severe hypothermia, but this term may be misleading. A host of factors may render the pulse difficult to detect in severe hypothermia. These include profound hypovolemia, increased blood viscosity, paradoxical vasodilatation, decreased cardiac ejection velocity, and muscular rigidity. Because of markedly reduced metabolic needs, patients with no detectable pulse have survived long periods of severe hypothermia.[21]

Clinical Aspects

A complete exploration of hypothermia is beyond the scope of this chapter. The reader is referred to reviews of this problem in adults[22] and children.[23] The relative preponderance of VF over asystole in hypothermia deserves some comment. First, untreated VF in hypothermia will terminate in asystole. VF could be reported more commonly if its presence was more likely than asystole to trigger recognition that a patient was not in fact irredeemably dead. Then too, fine muscular tremor artifact is common in hypothermic patients who are not overtly shivering.[15,16] This might be misinterpreted as VF in some cases.

VF may develop in two distinct ways during hypothermia. Both may shed some light on the etiology of VF in hypothermia. In the first, VF develops from some more functional cardiac rhythm, often sinus bradycardia.[24,25] Besides cooling, other clinical precipitating factors are discussed below. The second form of onset is, however, more striking. In many cases of severe hypothermia, VF develops out of asystole during rewarming.[6–8,76] This may be associated in some cases with the administration of epinephrine.[27] VF has alternated with asystole below 20°C.[9,28] Rapid rewarming using extracorporeal circulation has been associated with spontaneous transition from asystole to fine VF, to coarse VF, and then to normal sinus rhythm in a span of less than 30 minutes.[10] Such spontaneous defibrillation with rewarming has been reported in a number of other cases.[9,11,28]

VF frequently develops in hypothermia during rescue and resuscitation.[11,12,28] This nonperfusing rhythm impairs rewarming[29] and may prove refractory to treatment.[30] Several causes may be involved.[31]

The name given to the almost universal phenomenon by which core temperature continues to decrease after removal from a cold environment is "afterdrop." In part, this drop is due to simple conduction of heat from the core to the periphery.[32] Nevertheless, the return of blood from chilled surface areas and extremities to the core circulation would clearly potentiate the severity of the afterdrop.[33] Afterdrop could trigger VF. Afterdrop would be increased by factors such as exertion on the part of the patient and by measures, such as peripheral rewarming, which increase the return of cold blood to the core. Both are discouraged during rescue and rewarming of severe hypothermia victims.

Another important precipitant of VF during resuscitation may be so-called rewarming shock. Vascular volume is severely depleted in hypothermia, due to several mechanisms. In addition, bradycardia and the reduced cardiac output associated with a cold myocardium are aggravated by paradoxical vasodilatation and loss of circulatory autoregulation. The result is that an increase in metabolic demand during rewarming produces a profound inadequacy of the circulation. Factors associated with rewarming shock (such as increased acidosis) might potentiate VF.

The "dumping" of stagnant blood from the muscle and skin beds during patient exertion or external rewarming could also worsen acidosis, hyperkalemia, and other potential precipitants of VF. Room-temperature intravenous fluid (at approximately 21°C) is colder than all but the coldest hypothermia patients and has been blamed for the onset of VF.

More controversial is the role of rough handling. Although much of the evidence is circumstantial or based on cases in which several variables interacted, most experts feel that both exertion and unnecessary vigor in moving and jostling the patient may be associated with the onset of VF. This is presumed to be due to mechanical stimulation of the myocardium[30] as well as an increase in afterdrop, rewarming shock, and dumping. Mechanical irritation of the myocardium is also blamed for development of VF during insertion of intracardiac wires and transcardiac catheters.[4] Ventricular pacing for hypothermic brady-cardia has been associated with the onset of VF.[1]

A particular form of mechanical myocardial insult is that associated with chest compressions. CPR performed for bradycardia or PEA has been anecdotally linked to the onset of VF. Many patients with severe hypothermia have been rewarmed from bradycardia or PEA with no se-quelae. Given the difficulties described above in measuring a pulse or blood pressure, and given the extreme reduction in cellular metabolism, severe hypotension, bradycardia, or even pulselessness may be toler-ated for some time. The development of VF is associated with a worse prognosis and more difficulty in rewarming. For this reason, many ex-perts recommend withholding CPR in the presence of bradycardia (or even pulselessness with a documented narrow ECG complex) when it is known that a patient has a core temperature below 28°C.[34-36]

A long-standing controversy of similar nature involved the role of endotracheal intubation. Individual case reports seemed to associate this procedure with the onset of VF.[12] More recently, however, both an-imal experiments[37] and experience with a large series of human pa-tients[38] suggest that the risk of VF during intubation is low.

Pathophysiology

VF appears to be an almost inevitable consequence of severe cool-ing in homeothermic animals. True hibernators, whose core tempera-tures may drop to temperatures just above freezing, have evolved spe-cial adaptations to prevent VF.[39] Despite several decades of investigation, the exact mechanism or mechanisms by which VF devel-ops during hypothermia remain unclear.

Most authors cite decreased cardiac conduction and increased my-ocardial irritability as primary factors in the development of VF.[19] As discussed by Bjørnstad et al,[40] much of the original work on this subject dates to the 1950s and early 1960s. They note that a decreased rate of membrane depolarization slows myocardial conduction. This is re-flected in QRS widening on the ECG. Further, the duration of the ven-tricular action potential lengthens. This is reflected in a prolonged QT interval (and refractory period). It is also accepted that hypothermia de-creases the VF threshold[40,41] as measured by determination of the min-imum current required to produce VF during the vulnerable period.

Hypoxia has been blamed for the onset of VF in hypothermia.[42] In addition, acid-base balance appears to play a role. The complex topic of the pH and blood gases in hypothermia is reviewed elsewhere.[43,44] Both acidosis and alkalosis may occur. Sudden shifts in pH, especially sudden decreases, are held to provoke VF. As noted by Swain and coworkers,[41] acidosis lowers the VF threshold. These investigators found that the reduction in VF threshold seen in hypothermia could be avoided if the pH were allowed to remain relatively alkalotic.

Both hypokalemia and hyperkalemia are seen in hypothermia, the former being more common. As discussed by Wong,[3] hypokalemia and the loss of intracellular potassium have been implicated in the development of VF.

An increase in circulating catecholamines has been documented in hypothermia.[45] This could increase the risk of VF.[46] Evidence suggests, however, that the increased catecholamine levels occur during the compensatory phase of mild hypothermia, and normalize before severe hypothermia is reached.[47] Recent work tends to confirm that catecholamine levels may be depressed rather than elevated in severe hypothermia.[40] Furthermore, animal studies have found that catecholamine infusion is effective in reversing the cardiodepressant effects of hypothermia and is not associated with the development of dysrhythmias.[48,49]

Other mechanisms for VF have been proposed, including differential conduction within the myocardium[50] as well as differential cooling or warming of the myocardium with resultant discrepancies in action potential duration and, thus, a setting for reentry.[51]

Other physiological factors continue to be explored. Recent work suggests that the mean frequency of fibrillation in hypothermia is reduced, and that this reduction in frequency is associated with refractoriness to countershock.[52] Further insight may be gained from work on the VF of postcardioplegia reperfusion,[53] on spectral analysis of VF in normothermia and hypothermia,[54] and on the mechanisms by which drugs can reverse hypothermic VF.[51]

Treatment

It is commonly accepted that VF may prove refractory to therapy during severe hypothermia, and rewarming is recommended to achieve cardioversion.[55] Case reports document this contention,[8,27,56] and some patients have been warmed to 35°C before being successfully cardioverted.[26] Other case reports, however, document successful cardioversion at core temperatures of 18°C (in a child),[9] 20°C,[28] and 24°C.[7]

The electrical current and energy required to achieve cardioversion in hypothermia have been studied. It does not appear that transchest or transcardiac impedance is increased by hypothermia, or that increased energy is required or helpful for defibrillation during hypothermia.[57,58]

As noted, epinephrine administration has been associated with some cases of spontaneous defibrillation[27] as well as some cases of successful cardioversion.[6] Evidence suggests that sympathomimetic agents may be both desirable and efficacious in hypothermic conditions.[47–49]

Many other drugs are less effective in the hypothermic patient, and such may be the case with lidocaine. Case reports of its apparent failure to aid in conversion of VF are quite common; those of its efficacy are rare. This does not prove that it is of no value; however, it is not considered especially effective.[59]

Bretylium tosylate appears to be a different case. Theory,[60] animal work,[25,40,45,61 62] and experience with human case reports[56,63] support its efficacy. These studies suggest that it may be effective not only for treatment of VF (so-called "chemical defibrillation"), but also for prophylaxis against VF during hypothermia. Bretylium appears to increase the VF threshold during hypothermia. This action appears to be due the drug's antiarrhythmic properties and not its potential suppression of catecholamine levels.[40,45]

Two cautionary notes, however, are in order regarding bretylium. In a study that found bretylium effective in preventing VF during hypothermic manipulations of dogs, it was noted that 3 of 11 dogs receiving bretylium fibrillated "within minutes of its administration."[25] At least one other study was unable to demonstrate a beneficial effect of bretylium in promoting the success of countershock during hypothermic VF: 7 of 10 dogs were successfully converted from VF in both bretylium- and placebo-treated groups.[64]

To summarize the current state of knowledge regarding treatment of VF in hypothermia, it seems worthwhile to make one or two attempts at cardioversion using standard current, perhaps after administration of epinephrine.[19] If this is unsuccessful, bretylium tosylate in standard dosage could be administered. At the same time, aggressive rewarming (discussed below) should be undertaken. Countershock could then be attempted at intervals during rewarming, recalling that successful defibrillation has occurred at temperatures from 18°C to 35°C. The potential for spontaneous defibrillation during rewarming is not remote. Finally, it must be noted that failure to achieve a perfusing rhythm after more than approximately 30 minutes at a core temperature greater than 32°C is synonymous with death. Hypothermic protection of vital organs is absent at this temperature.

Prevention of Hypothermic VF

The primary prevention of hypothermic VF implies prevention of accidental hypothermia, which in children especially stems from immersion mishaps. This is clearly a priority in pediatric injury prevention.

The secondary prevention of VF once a victim is hypothermic requires several measures. First, all possible steps should be taken to reduce the afterdrop and prevent rewarming shock. Administration of copious warmed intravenous fluid is specifically indicated. Most fluid warming equipment is ineffectual; special large countercurrent fluid warmers and plumbed tubing systems are required.

Rescuers should avoid unnecessary patient exertion, rough handling, and procedures. It is important to determine the core temperature as early as possible, since not only the risk of VF but also the specific treatment measures required and the prognosis depend heavily on the degree of hypothermia.

External warming methods should be avoided in severe hypothermia. Use of core rewarming techniques is doubly helpful in this setting. First, these measures prevent dumping of cold, acidotic blood from the periphery, and rewarm the core (including the myocardium) before increasing peripheral circulatory demands. Second, specific circulatory warming methods (extracorporeal circulation with rewarming) unload the myocardium, dilute, circulate, and oxygenate the blood, and provide extremely rapid rewarming. The provision of circulation makes these methods especially effective when VF or asystole are present.

Research Agenda Issues

The topic of VF in hypothermia seems ripe for further exploration. More work is required to elucidate the electrophysiology of hypothermic VF. It is striking that many of the current reviews on this topic must refer to work conducted 40 years ago. Large advances in our ability to study electrophysiological events and cardiocellular physiology should allow further progress in this area. Insight into the spontaneous defibrillation seen during rewarming could conceivably shed light on the treatment of VF in normothermia.

The role of interventional procedures, especially CPR, in provoking hypothermic VF begs further study. The research done on the role of endotracheal intubation in animals and in review of human series forms an excellent model for this work.

An especially fertile area for investigation seems to be the role of pH regulation in preventing hypothermic VF. If Swain and coworkers[41] are correct, this relatively simple intervention could prevent the lowering of the VF threshold typically seen in hypothermia. Further work is required to confirm this result and to apply it in the clinical arena.

The concept of chemical prophylaxis against VF in hypothermia, for instance with bretylium, also seems promising and requires further investigation. An effective means of preventing deterioration of the cardiac rhythm to VF would be a boon to those treating hypothermia.

References

1. Towne WD, Geiss WP, Yanes HO, et al. Intractable ventricular fibrillation associated with profound accidental hypothermia—successful treatment with partial cardiopulmonary bypass. *N Engl J Med* 1972;287:1135–1136.
2. White JD. Hypothermia: The Bellevue experience. *Ann Emerg Med* 1982; 11:417–424.
3. Wong KC. Physiology and pharmacology of hypothermia. *West J Med* 1983;138:227–232.
4. Southwick FS, Dalglish PH Jr. Recovery after prolonged asystolic cardiac arrest in profound hypothermia. A case report and literature review. *JAMA* 1980;243:1250–1253.
5. Walpoth BH, Walpoth-Aslan BN, Mattle HP, et al. Outcome of survivors of accidental deep hypothermia and circulatory arrest treated with extracorporeal blood warming [see comments]. *N Engl J Med* 1997;337:1500–1505.
6. Dominguez de Villota E, Barat G, Peral P, et al. Recovery from profound hypothermia with cardiac arrest after immersion. *Br Med J* 1973;4:394–395.
7. Siebke H, Breivik H, Rød T, et al. Survival after 40 minutes' submersion without cerebral sequelae. *Lancet* 1975;1:1275–1277.
8. Bristow G, Smith R, Lee J, et al. Resuscitation from cardiopulmonary arrest during accidental hypothermia due to exhaustion and exposure. *Can Med Assoc J* 1977;117:247–249.
9. Kelly KJ, Glaeser P, Rice TB, et al. Profound accidental hypothermia and freeze injury of the extremities in a child. *Crit Care Med* 1990;18:679–680.
10. Bolte RG, Black PG, Bowers RS, et al. The use of extracorporeal rewarming in a child submerged for 66 minutes. *JAMA* 1988;260:377–379.
11. Cohen DJ, Cline JR, Lepinski SM, et al. Resuscitation of the hypothermic patient. *Am J Emerg Med* 1988;6:475–478.
12. Osborne L, Kamal E, Smith JE. Survival after prolonged cardiac arrest and accidental hypothermia. *Br Med J [Clin Res]* 1984;289:881–882.
13. Rittenhouse EA, Mori H, Dillard DH, et al. Deep hypothermia in cardiovascular surgery. *Ann Thorac Surg* 1974;17:63–98.
14. Solomon A, Barish RA, Browne B, et al. The electrocardiographic features of hypothermia. *J Emerg Med* 1989;7:169–173.
15. Okada M. The cardiac rhythm in accidental hypothermia. *J Electrocardiol* 1984;17:123–128.
16. Bashour TT, Gualberto A, Ryan C. Atrioventricular block in accidental hypothermia—a case report. *Angiology* 1989;40:63–66.
17. Gould L, Gopalaswamy C, Kim BS, et al. The Osborn wave in hypothermia. *Angiology* 1985;36:125–129.
18. Okada M, Nishimura F, Yoshino H, et al. The J wave in accidental hypothermia. *J Electrocardiol* 1983;16:23–28.
19. Reuler JB. Hypothermia: Pathophysiology, clinical settings, and management. *Ann Intern Med* 1978;89:519–527.

20. Fitzgerald FT, Jessop C. Accidental hypothermia: A report of 22 cases and review of the literature. *Adv Intern Med* 1982;27:127–150.
21. Althaus U, Aeberhard P, Schüpbach P, et al. Management of profound accidental hypothermia with cardiorespiratory arrest. *Ann Surg* 1982; 195:492–495.
22. Jolly BT, Ghezzi KT. Accidental hypothermia. *Emerg Med Clin North Am* 1992;10:311–327.
23. Corneli HM. Accidental hypothermia. *J Pediatr* 1992;120:671–679.
24. Coniam SW. Accidental hypothermia. *Anaesthesia* 1979;34:250–256.
25. Murphy K, Nowak RM, Tomlanovich MC. Use of bretylium tosylate as prophylaxis and treatment in hypothermic ventricular fibrillation in the canine model. *Ann Emerg Med* 1986;15:1160–1166.
26. Seuffert G. An Alaskan experience with cardiopulmonary bypass in resuscitating patients with profound hypothermia and cardiac arrest. *Alaska Med* 1984;26:31–33.
27. Nordrehaug JE. Sustained ventricular fibrillation in deep accidental hypothermia. *Br Med J [Clin Res]* 1982;284:867–868.
28. DaVee TS, Reineberg EJ. Extreme hypothermia and ventricular fibrillation. *Ann Emerg Med* 1980;9:100–102.
29. White JD. Cardiac arrest in hypothermia. *JAMA* 1980;244:2262. Letter.
30. Wickstrom P, Ruiz E, Lija GP, et al. Accidental hypothermia: Core rewarming with partial bypass. *Am J Surg* 1976;131:622–625.
31. Lloyd EL. The cause of death after rescue. *Int J Sports Med* 1992;13:S196–S199.
32. Webb P. Afterdrop of body temperature during rewarming: An alternative explanation. *J Appl Physiol* 1986;60:385–390.
33. Hayward JS, Eckerson JD, Kemna D. Thermal and cardiovascular changes during three methods of resuscitation from mild hypothermia. *Resuscitation* 1984;11:1–2.
34. Zell SC, Kurtz KJ. Severe exposure hypothermia: A resuscitation protocol. *Ann Emerg Med* 1985;14:339–345.
35. Steinman AM. Cardiopulmonary resuscitation and hypothermia. *Circulation* 1986;74:IV29–IV32. Review.
36. Ornato JP. Special resuscitation situations: Near drowning, traumatic injury, electric shock, and hypothermia. *Circulation* 1986;74:IV23–IV26. Review.
37. Gillen JP, Vogel MF, Holterman RK, et al. Ventricular fibrillation during orotracheal intubation of hypothermic dogs. *Ann Emerg Med* 1986;15:412–416.
38. Danzl DF, Pozos RS, Auerbach PS, et al. Multicenter hypothermia survey. *Ann Emerg Med* 1987;16:1042–1055.
39. Johansson BW. The hibernator heart—nature's model of resistance to ventricular fibrillation. *Cardiovasc Res* 1996;31:826–832.
40. Bjørnstad H, Mortensen E, Sager G, et al. Effect of bretylium tosylate on ventricular fibrillation threshold during hypothermia in dogs. *Am J Emerg Med* 1994;12:407–412.
41. Swain JA, White FN, Peters RM. The effect of pH on the hypothermic ventricular fibrillation threshold. *J Thorac Cardiovasc Surg* 1984;87:445–451.
42. Keatinge WR. Accidental immersion hypothermia and drowning. *Practitioner* 1977;219:183–187.
43. Swain JA. Hypothermia and blood pH. A review. *Arch Intern Med* 1988; 148:1643–1646. Review.

44. Delaney KA, Howland MA, Vassallo S, et al. Assessment of acid-base disturbances in hypothermia and their physiologic consequences. *Ann Emerg Med* 1989;18:72–82.
45. Orts A, Alcaraz C, Delaney KA, et al. Bretylium tosylate and electrically induced cardiac arrhythmias during hypothermia in dogs. *Am J Emerg Med* 1992;10:311–316.
46. Warner WA, Anton AH, Andersen TW, et al. Ventricular fibrillation and catecholamine responses during profound hypothermia in dogs. *Anesthesiology* 1970;33:43–51.
47. Chernow B, Lake CR, Zaritsky A, et al. Sympathetic nervous system "switch off" with severe hypothermia. *Crit Care Med* 1983;11:677–680.
48. Nicodemus HF, Chaney RD, Herold R. Hemodynamic effects of inotropes during hypothermia and rapid rewarming. *Crit Care Med* 1981;9:325–328.
49. Riishede L, Nielsen KF. Myocardial effects of adrenaline, isoprenaline and dobutamine at hypothermic conditions. *Pharmacol Toxicol* 1990;66:354–360.
50. Lloyd EL, Mitchell B. Factors affecting the onset of ventricular fibrillation in hypothermia. *Lancet* 1974;2:1294–1296.
51. Bjørnstad H, Tande PM, Refsum H. Cardiac electrophysiology during hypothermia. Implications for medical treatment. *Arctic Med Res* 1991;6: 71–75.
52. Strohmenger HU, Hemmer W, Lindner KH, et al. Median fibrillation frequency in cardiac surgery: Influence of temperature and guide to countershock therapy. *Chest* 1997;111:1560–1564.
53. Holman WL, Spruell RD, Vicente WV, et al. Electrophysiological mechanisms for postcardioplegia reperfusion ventricular fibrillation. *Circulation* 1994;90:II293-II298.
54. Marble AE, Landymore RW, Cameron C. Measurement and spectral analysis of fibrillation in the normothermic and hypothermic myocardium. *Med Biol Eng Comput* 1986;24:630–636.
55. Baumgartner FJ, Janusz MT, Jamieson WR, et al. Cardiopulmonary bypass for resuscitation of patients with accidental hypothermia and cardiac arrest. *Can J Surg* 1992;35:184–187.
56. Kochar G, Kahn SE, Kotler MN. Bretylium tosylate and ventricular fibrillation in hypothermia. *Ann Intern Med* 1986;105:624. Letter.
57. Arredondo MT, Armayor MR, Clavin OE, et al. Effect of body hypothermia on transventricular simple-capacitor-discharge defibrillation thresholds. *Am J Physiol* 1980;238:H675-H681.
58. Tacker WA Jr, Babbs CF, Abendschein DR, et al. Transchest defibrillation under conditions of hypothermia. *Crit Care Med* 1981;9:390–391.
59. MacLean D, Emslie-Smith D. *Accidental Hypothermia.* Philadelphia: J.B. Lippincott; 1977.
60. Dronen S, Nowak RM, Tomlanovich MC. Bretylium tosylate and hypothermic ventricular fibrillation. *Ann Emerg Med* 1980;9:335.
61. Nielsen KC, Owman C. Control of ventricular fibrillation during induced hypothermia in cats after blocking the adrenergic neurons with bretylium. *Life Sci* 1968;7:159–168.
62. Buckley JJ, Bosch OK, Bacaner MB. Prevention of ventricular fibrillation during hypothermia with bretylium tosylate. *Anesth Analg* 1971;50: 587–593.
63. Danzl DF, Sowers MB, Vicario SJ, et al. Chemical ventricular defibrillation in severe accidental hypothermia. *Ann Emerg Med* 1982;11:698–699. Letter.
64. Elenbaas RM, Mattson K, Cole H, et al. Bretylium in hypothermia-induced ventricular fibrillation in dogs. *Ann Emerg Med* 1984;13:994–999.

Section III

Sudden Death in the Pediatric Patient with an Ostensibly Normal Heart:

In-Hospital Ventricular Fibrillation

Chapter 7

Who Will Have an Arrest In-Hospital?

Arno L. Zaritsky, MD

Introduction

To answer the rhetorical question in the title of this chapter, the chapter reviews the available data on in-hospital resuscitation of children, the rhythms associated with arrest in the hospital, and the outcome following cardiac arrest. In addition, the research implications derived from this review and recommendations for reporting results on in-hospital resuscitation are emphasized.

Epidemiology of Pediatric In-Hospital Resuscitation

There are relatively few studies on in-hospital pediatric resuscitation, and differences in study design make comparisons between studies difficult, even when the studies are only descriptive. In addition, it is likely that the etiology and epidemiology of in-hospital cardiac arrest is changing over time in response to advances such as an effective vaccine against Hemophilus influenza and the wide availability of pediatric critical care units, which provide improved monitoring of critically ill and injured children. Since in-hospital care has changed substantially, studies more than a decade old are largely ignored in this chapter.

A 1-year retrospective review of all cardiac arrests occurring on the pediatric ward found only 42 cases among 22,531 admissions (0.186%) to the 600-bed Hospital for Sick Children in Toronto.[1] This group included 33 cardiac arrest (defined as absence of detectable blood pressure and

From: Quan L, Franklin WH (eds). *Ventricular Fibrillation: A Pediatric Problem*. Armonk, NY: Futura Publishing Company, Inc.; ©2000.

femoral pulse) patients and 11 respiratory arrest patients, but excluded neonates and children in the pediatric intensive care unit (PICU). Cardiac disease (in 14 children), neurologic conditions (in 7), neoplasm (in 6), and congenital malformations (in 3) were the most common causes of cardiac arrest. In the 33 children with cardiac arrest, the first recorded rhythm was asystole in 30 children and ventricular fibrillation (VF) in 3 (9.1%). All of the latter patients had an underlying cardiac condition.

One of the early attempts to collect prospective data on pediatric in-hospital resuscitation was conducted over a 1-year period at the Children's Hospital National Medical Center in Washington, DC, a 240-bed acute care hospital.[2] Cardiac arrest was defined by the absence of detectable cardiac activity leading to the need for chest compressions. Respiratory arrest was defined as the need for assisted ventilation in a child without respiratory effort, but who still had a detectable pulse. There were 53 cardiac arrests and 40 respiratory arrests. Most (33 arrests) occurred in the emergency department, the PICU (22), or the ward (19). The median patient age was 11 months.

Most of the children had an underlying condition on admission to the hospital: cardiac in 30.5%, respiratory in 17%, chromosomal in 10.5%, and prematurity in 10.5%. Overall, 87% of the cardiac arrest victims and 87.5% of the respiratory arrest victims had an underlying condition. The admission diagnoses were classified as cardiac in 39%, respiratory in 20%, sepsis in 13%, neurologic in 17%, and other in 11%. The initial arrest rhythm was not reported. Overall, 9.4% of the children with cardiac arrest and 67.5% of the children with respiratory arrest survived to hospital discharge.

In another prospective study,[3] 12 British hospitals collected in-hospital and out-of-hospital cardiac arrest data for at least 1 year in both children and adults. Of the 3765 patients included in this report, it is noteworthy that only 2% were in the 0- to 14-years age group. Analysis of the data in this study is limited, since voluntary reporting and follow-up was required. The authors note that some resuscitation attempts were probably missed and some false arrests were probably included. Their data show, however, the relative infrequency of pediatric arrests compared with arrests in adults.

In a study examining differences in outcome in children with in-hospital cardiac arrest and receiving standard-dose epinephrine versus high-dose epinephrine, Denver investigators identified 64 children who experienced a cardiac arrest over a 54-month period.[4] Of these, 13 (20%) were excluded from the report because the dose of epinephrine was not clearly recorded. These data are a bit difficult to summarize because demographics were reported based on the number of arrests (58) rather than on the 51 total patients analyzed. The median age was approximately 11.5 months. Most arrests (72.4%) occurred in the PICU; 13.8% occurred on the ward, and 6.9% occurred in the emergency department (children who arrived in the emergency department in cardiac arrest were excluded). The initial rhythm recorded was bradyasystolic in 55.1%, pulseless electrical activity in 29.3%, ventricular tachycardia (VT) in 5.1%, and VF in 3.4% of patients. No rhythm was recorded in 6.9% of the episodes.

Similar to other studies, the most frequently recorded diagnosis at the time of cardiac arrest was a cardiac disorder in 46.5% of patients; of these, two thirds had recently (defined as within 2 weeks) undergone surgical repair of a congenital heart lesion. Sepsis accounted for 13.8% of episodes, as did malignancy. Neurologic conditions accounted for 10.3% of episodes, respiratory for 5.2%, and miscellaneous conditions were recorded in 10.3%.

The PICU appears to be the most common place for in-hospital cardiac arrest to occur; but what do we know about arrest in that setting? The largest study by far evaluated data from 11,165 consecutive admissions to 32 PICUs.[5] A total of 205 children (1.8% of intensive care unit admissions) experienced a cardiac arrest, defined as greater than 2 minutes of chest compression. Initial rhythms were not reported, but underlying conditions were common, with cardiovascular conditions in 36.6%, neurologic conditions in 13.6%, respiratory conditions in 13.2%, and multiple organ system failure in 6.8% of patients. Heart disease (35.1%) was the most common etiologic group for cardiac arrest; infectious conditions (21.5%), trauma (12.2%), and miscellaneous conditions (15.1%) were other common etiologies.

In a single-center study of PICU cardiac arrest, 121 episodes of cardiopulmonary resuscitation (CPR) were provided to 81 children over a 30-month period in a 10-bed unit.[6] A much higher rate of cardiac arrest was observed in children admitted to the unit (6.0%) than in the multicenter study.[5] Based on the number of days of care, one cardiac arrest was observed for every 63 days of care during the 30-month study. Of note, however, is that cardiac arrest was defined in this study as the need for chest compressions and/or emergency drugs. This suggests that a number of the patients studied were not in cardiac arrest as defined by the pediatric Utstein guidelines,[7] and this conclusion is supported by the high survival to discharge rate (31%). As in other studies, cardiac disease was a common underlying condition, occurring in approximately 52% of the children.

What Have We Learned?

A review of the published data leads to a number of conclusions about in-hospital pediatric cardiac arrest. The most obvious is that it is difficult to compare studies because of differences in the populations evaluated, in the definitions of cardiac arrest, in the lack of critical data, and in the changing demographics within the hospital setting. In-hospital arrests occur most commonly in children younger than 1 year of age. It also is clear that most children who are at high risk for cardiac arrest have an underlying chronic condition; cardiac diseases are the most frequently associated condition.

There are few data on the initial rhythm in cardiac arrest. It appears that VF is most frequently observed in hospitalized children who have an underlying cardiac condition. This conclusion is consistent with the often-cited study reporting the terminal cardiac rhythms in children experiencing a cardiac arrest.[8] This was a prospective study of 100 hospitalized children at Babies Hospital in New York. Of these, 54 were newborn infants, 24 were of ages 28 days to 1 year, and 22 children were of ages 1 to 18 years. Overall, 46% of the children had congenital heart disease; 68% of the children 1 year of age or older had congenital heart disease. VT or VF was reported in 22% of the children; the remainder evolved from bradycardia to asystole. Ventricular arrhythmias were seen only in children with congenital heart disease.

A wide variety of conditions are associated with in-hospital cardiac arrest; a partial list is seen in Table 1. Clearly, the "type" of patients admitted to the hospital influences the likelihood of cardiac arrest and the type of rhythm seen during the arrest. For example, a center that operates on high-risk infants and children with complex congenital heart disease will experience a higher rate of cardiac arrest, especially in the PICU, as well as a relatively high rate of ventricular arrhythmias.

Most studies suggest that cardiac arrest occurs most commonly in the PICU. Fortunately, few arrests occur on the wards, and most of these are respiratory rather than cardiac arrests. The most common

---

Table 1

Possible Causes of Cardiac Arrest in Hospitalized Children

- Postsurgical, especially cardiac surgery
- Congenital conditions, especially cardiac and chromosomal
- Respiratory failure: numerous causes
- Metabolic: hperkalemia, hyper- and hypomagnesemia, hypoglycemia, inborn errors of metabolism
- Cardiac conditions: cardiomyopathy, myocarditis, congenital prolongation of the QT interval
- Sepsis
- Neurologic: seizures, stroke, shunt obstruction, tumor
- Drug toxicity: digoxin, tricyclic antidepressants, drug interactions, drug errors
- Munchausen by proxy

rhythms observed are a bradycardic rhythm or asystole. The overall occurrence of VF and VT appears to be approximately 10% of cases, but it is likely to be higher in centers with a higher proportion of children with cardiac conditions.

Research Implications

Based on a review of the available data, this author believes that there are three general research implications: 1) in-hospital cardiac arrest data must be collected in a consistent manner using a common set of definitions and reporting tools; 2) data collection should ideally be multicentered to adjust for differences in patient mix between centers and to account for the low prevalence of cardiac arrest; and 3) a mechanism of ongoing, prospective data collection is desirable, since new technologies, new vaccines, public health interventions, and changes in patient ethics are likely to influence CPR occurrence and outcome. Changes in the ethics regarding end-of-life decisions in children are likely to change the frequency of "do not attempt resuscitation" orders.

To improve data collection, the reader is referred to the pediatric Utstein guidelines[7] and to guidelines on reporting in-hospital resuscitation,[9] which were written for adults but can be easily adapted to children as well. The types of data to collect can be divided into patient variables, arrest variables, outcome variables, and hospital variables.[9] Patient variables include factors such as age, location of the arrest, and advanced life support interventions in place at the time of the event, such as mechanical ventilation and vasoactive drug infusions. Other patient variables include the child's pre-event functional capacity, the presence of comorbidities, and the severity of illness determined by an objective scoring system.

Event variables include the precipitating cause of the event, which is categorized as cardiac, respiratory, or cardiorespiratory. Ideally, more detailed information on the presence of underlying conditions should be included and may be obtained from the diseases coded at the time of hospital discharge, although hospital ICD-9 coding is often driven by reimbursement rather than by accurate coding of the presence of important comorbid conditions.[10,11] The initial rhythm and patient condition at the time of the event (eg, apneic, pulseless) should be recorded. Interventions administered during the resuscitation constitute additional event variables. These interventions include endotracheal intubation, administration of medications (including dose and time), defibrillation, and the application of advanced life support devices such as extracorporeal membrane oxygenation.

Outcome variables include the rate of return of spontaneous circulation and survival to 24 hours, to 7 days, and to hospital discharge. Information regarding mortality and functional outcome at 6 months to 1 year after discharge could provide helpful data on the ultimate effects of cardiac arrest on patient outcome. When death occurs, however, few studies have attempted to report its attributable cause; such data are needed to accurately determine the effectiveness of CPR. For example, a child with leukemia may suffer an arrest secondary to hyperkalemia during tumor lysis by chemotherapy. The child may respond appropriately to interventions to treat hyperkalemia and recover initially without sequelae but then die 3 months later from sepsis. Clearly, it would not be appropriate to conclude that the child's arrest directly contributed to the child's subsequent death, and that the CPR efforts were ineffective in changing the child's outcome.

When children survive, their subsequent quality of life should be reported using an objective scale such as the pediatric overall and cerebral performance categories.[12] The economic impact of CPR has been reported for out-of-hospital cardiac arrest in children,[13,14] but not specifically in the hospitalized population. In the latter setting, the cost-effectiveness can be quantified by calculating the cost per adjusted quality of life year, a measurement of anticipated outcome based on a patient's age and functional outcome.[15]

Hospital variables include providing data on the number of hospital and PICU beds for children, the number of admissions and days of care, the resuscitation response team composition, training and protocols used, and the overall experience of the team. The latter is quantified by the number of code responses.

Summary

There are few data on in-hospital resuscitation in children, and the available data are difficult to analyze secondary to differences in study design and the use of inconsistent definitions. Based on available data, cardiac arrest is an uncommon occurrence in hospitalized children. When arrest occurs, it often occurs in children with underlying chronic conditions; however, a large number of causes for cardiac arrest must be considered. There are insufficient data to conclude that VF or VT occur more frequently in the hospitalized child than reported in the out-of-hospital setting (around 10%), but their occurrence is likely to be higher in hospitals with a high proportion of children with cardiac conditions.

The outcome following resuscitation of cardiac arrest in hospitalized children is also difficult to determine, particularly since few studies report the attributable cause of subsequent mortality in children who experience a cardiac or respiratory arrest. Moreover, since most studies include relatively few patients in subgroup analysis, it is important to report the confidence intervals for the descriptive data to permit the reader to make an informed decision on how likely the patient would have the outcome reported. Finally, uniform guidelines for collecting and publishing data on arrest in children are available and should be more widely implemented.

References

1. Gillis J, Dickson D, Rieder M, et al. Results of inpatient pediatric resuscitation. *Crit Care* Med 1986;14:469–471.
2. Zaritsky A, Nadkarni V, Getson P, et al. CPR in children. *Ann Emerg Med* 1987;16:1107–1110.
3. Tunstall-Pedoe H, Bailey L, Chamberlain DA, et al. Survey of 3765 cardiopulmonary resuscitations in British hospitals (the BRESUS study): Methods and overall results. *Br Med J* 1992;304:1347–1351.
4. Carpenter TC, Stenmark KR. High-dose epinephrine is not superior to standard-dose epinephrine in pediatric in-hospital cardiopulmonary arrest. *Pediatrics* 1997;99:403–408.
5. Slonim AD, Patel KM, Ruttimann UE, et al. Cardiopulmonary resuscitation in pediatric intensive care units. *Crit Care Med* 1997;25:1951–1955.
6. Von Seggern K, Egar M, Fuhrman B. Cardiopulmonary resuscitation in a pediatric ICU. *Crit Care Med* 1986;14:275–277.
7. Zaritsky A, Nadkarni V, Hazinski MF, et al. Recommended guidelines for uniform reporting of pediatric advanced life support: The Pediatric Utstein Style. *Pediatrics* 1995;96:765–779.
8. Walsh CK, Krongrad E. Terminal cardiac electrical activity in pediatric patients. *Am J Cardiol* 1983;51:557–561.
9. Cummins RO, Sanders A, Mancini E, et al. In-hospital resuscitation: A statement for healthcare professionals from the American Heart Association Emergency Cardiac Care Committee and the Advanced Cardiac Life Support, Basic Life Support, Pediatric Resuscitation, and Program Administration Subcommittees. *Circulation* 1997;95:2211–2212.
10. Jollis JG, Ancukiewicz M, DeLong ER, et al. Discordance of databases designed for claims payment versus clinical information systems. Implications for outcomes research. *Ann Intern Med* 1993;119:844–850.
11. Iezzoni LI. Using administrative diagnostic data to assess the quality of hospital care: Pitfalls and potential of ICD-9-CM. *Int J Technol Assess Health Care* 1990;6:272–281.
12. Fiser DH. Assessing the outcome of pediatric intensive care. *J Pediatr* 1992;121:68–74.
13. Ronco R, King W, Konley DK, et al. Outcome and cost at a children's hospital following resuscitation for out-of-hospital cardiopulmonary arrest. *Arch Pediatr Adolesc Med* 1995;149:210–214.
14. Sheikh A, Brogan T. Outcome and cost of open- and closed-chest cardiopulmonary resuscitation in pediatric cardiac arrests. *Pediatrics* 1994;93:392–398.
15. Ebell MH, Kruse JA. A proposed model for the cost of cardiopulmonary resuscitation. *Med Care* 1994;32:640–649.

Section IV

At-Risk Pediatric Cardiac Populations

Chapter 8

Molecular Genetics of Structural Pediatric Cardiac Disease

Charles I. Berul, MD

Introduction

Cardiac arrhythmias and conduction disturbances are responsible for significant morbidity and mortality in children with structural heart disease. Nonuniform conduction delay due to chronic ventricular hypertrophy, myocardial surgical scars, areas of ischemia or infarction, and artificial patch materials may all promote reentry circuits and ventricular arrhythmias. Additionally, regionally inhomogeneous ventricular repolarization may also promote ventricular ectopy and arrhythmias, suggesting multiple potential mechanisms for the arrhythmias, conduction disturbances, and sudden death seen in these patients.

The molecular and genetic bases for electrophysiological disorders are increasingly being recognized. Molecular biological and genetic approaches to the evaluation of pediatric sudden cardiac death have led to new insights regarding mechanisms and therapies for arrhythmias associated with structural heart disease. These technological advances have led to the creation of genetically manipulated animal models for human electrophysiological disease processes.[1,2] This chapter provides a concise review of some inherited pediatric structural cardiac diseases associated with ventricular arrhythmias and sudden cardiac death, and the ability to characterize these disorders using murine genetic models.

The miniaturized in vivo mouse electrophysiology study methods have been described.[3] The cardiac rhythm is recorded and a 12-lead electrocardiogram (ECG) is obtained for measurement of axes and in-

From: Quan L, Franklin WH (eds). *Ventricular Fibrillation: A Pediatric Problem.* Armonk, NY: Futura Publishing Company, Inc.; ©2000.

This work was supported in part by NIH Clinical Investigator Development Award HL03607 and a grant from the Charles H. Hood Foundation.

tervals. Electrophysiological pacing protocols and pharmacologic manipulations are used to assess cardiac conduction parameters.[3] Long-term ambulatory ECG monitoring, exercise stress testing, and echocardiography add important diagnostic components to the complete murine heart station approach.

Inherited Structural Pediatric Heart Disease

Cardiomyopathies and Electrophysiological Abnormalities

Cardiomyopathies account for the most common cause of sudden death in the young. This multifactorial group of diseases has in common abnormal ventricular structure or function as well as a predisposition to conduction abnormalities, ventricular arrhythmias, and sudden death. Positional cloning has recently been used to identify specific gene products that cause some forms of familial cardiomyopathies and other inheritable heart developmental malformations associated with arrhythmia syndromes and pediatric sudden cardiac death.

Familial Hypertrophic Cardiomyopathy

Familial hypertrophic cardiomyopathy (FHC) is usually inherited in an autosomal dominant fashion with variable penetrance. Mutations in sarcomeric protein genes such as cardiac myosin, α-tropomyosin, and other genes responsible for regulation of the contractile apparatus lead to the characteristic cardiomyopathy phenotype.[4-6] Features of FHCs are manifold, but include ventricular hypertrophy, myocyte disarray and hypertrophy, interstitial fibrosis, atrial and ventricular arrhythmias, and sudden cardiac death. The clinical course of FHC can range from the asymptomatic carrier to premature sudden death in childhood. Risk factors for early sudden death in FHC patients include young age at presentation, syncope, inducible ventricular tachycardia during electrophysiological study, and a malignant family history.[7-9] Clinical electrophysiological testing demonstrates a high prevalence of sinus node dysfunction, electrogram fractionation, and inducible ventricular arrhythmias.[10-12] Particular FHC mutations appear to correlate with a higher risk of ventricular hypertrophy and left ventricular outflow tract obstruction,[13] ventricular arrhythmias and other electrophysiological abnormalities,[14,15] or sudden cardiac arrest.[16] However, echocardiography and cardiac catheterization are not accurate predictors of sudden death in FHC patients, and clinical electrophysiological testing has had variable predictive value, possibly because it has not been feasible to perform these studies in large human cohorts with similar genotypes.

Murine models of human diseases can be used to correlate the relationship between a specific genotype and its electrophysiological phenotype. The cardiac myosin heavy chain mutation Arg^{403}Gln has been engineered to create a murine model of FHC.[17] The homozygous defect (α-MHC$^{403/403}$) is fatal in neonatal life, while heterozygous α-MHC$^{403/+}$ mice develop the characteristic histologic and hemodynamic FHC phenotype.[17]

Using the mouse electrophysiological method, these animals have been shown to have distinct abnormalities in their ECGs (right axis deviation and prolonged repolarization times) and electrophysiology studies (prolonged sinus node recovery times, heterogeneous ventricular conduction properties, and inducible ventricular ectopy).[18,19] These specific electrophysiological abnormalities associated with the α-MHC$^{403/+}$ mutation raise the possibility that prospective evaluation of ECG and electrophysiological findings may be useful for risk stratification in FHC patients. There are multiple mutations in cardiac myosin heavy chain and other sarcomeric protein genes that cause FHC. Determination of specific electrophysiological abnormalities associated with FHC mutations may be assessed and potential therapies systematically evaluated.

Dilated Cardiomyopathy

Inherited dilated cardiomyopathies are associated with varying degrees of risk for sudden cardiac death secondary to ventricular arrhythmia and cardiac dysfunction. Familial dilated cardiomyopathy (FDC) encompasses a spectrum of distinct genetic disorders with overlapping phenotypes. FDC accounts for 20% to 30% of "idiopathic" dilated cardiomyopathy cases.[20,21] The clinical presentation typically includes cardiomegaly, congestive heart failure, and ventricular arrhythmias. Pathologic features include ventricular dilatation, myocyte hypertrophy, intracardiac thrombi, and fibrosis. There are abnormalities in immune regulatory antibodies in some forms of FDC, with autoantibodies against specific sarcomeric proteins identified in a subgroup of patients. Additionally, the β-adrenergic receptor pathways may be altered, with downregulation of β_1-receptor density in the heart as well as modulation of myocardial β_2-receptor response. The FDC syndromes have multiple genetic etiologies. One interesting form of FDC is inherited in an autosomal dominant fashion, and affected individuals have sinus node dysfunction, supraventricular tachycardias, cardiac conduction abnormalities, and dilated cardiomyopathy. Linkage analysis has identified the gene responsible in this pedigree to be in the region of chromosome 3p.[22] Additional mutations have been mapped to chromosomes 1q and 9q.[20,23] There are also X-linked recessive forms of FDC that present in males, often due to mitochondrial DNA defects[24,25] or deletions in the dystrophin gene.[26] More severe X-linked FDC phenotypes may present in infancy with congestive heart failure and unexplained sudden infant death; linkage analysis has allowed mapping to distinct locations on chromosome X.[27] These disorders have been modeled in mice that lack the gene encoding for the muscle LIM protein (MLP). These MLP-deficient mice develop disrupted cytoskeletal architecture leading to neonatal dilated cardiomyopathy.[28] As the genetic causes for these diseases are further elucidated, murine models can be engineered, and electrophysiological data may be systematically obtained.

Arrhythmogenic Right Ventricular Cardiomyopathy

This familial syndrome, also known as arrhythmogenic right ventricular dysplasia (ARVD), often presents with ventricular arrhythmias or sudden death in late childhood or young adulthood. It is primarily inherited in an autosomal dominant pattern, with variable penetrance, although a recessive form has also been reported. The pathology involves patchy fibro-fatty infiltration of the ventricular myocardium, typically affecting focal areas of the right ventricle. Recently, two distinct chromosomal loci have been identified in ARVD: one on chromosome 14 (ARVD1) and another milder form (ARVD2), which has been mapped to chromosome 1.[29,30] An additional mutation on chromosome 17 has been linked to ARVD with palmoplantar keratoderma and wooly hair, and is known as Naxos disease.[31]

Storage Diseases

There are numerous disorders of glycogen metabolism that lead to childhood cardiomyopathy, and are beyond the scope of this chapter. The most severe example is Pompe's Disease (glycogen storage disease type II), which has an autosomal recessive inheritance pattern and has been mapped to human chromosome 17. This defect in the lysosomal enzyme α-glucosidase results in massive tissue accumulation of glycogen in the heart, which causes severe cardiomyopathy.[32] In its most severe form, Pompe's disease leads to infantile sudden death, either from severe hypertrophic cardiomyopathy with left ventricular outflow obstruction or from malignant ventricular arrhythmias in the first year of life. Thus far, there are no genetic animal models of Pompe's disease or similar cardiac glycogen storage diseases and there is no effective therapy or prevention of sudden cardiac death.

Conotruncal Developmental Defects and Arrhythmia Vulnerability

Sudden death remains a major concern for patients with tetralogy of Fallot and other conotruncal abnormalities. The etiology is likely secondary to malignant ventricular arrhythmias of multifactorial origin, conceivably due to the development of a reentry circuit involving areas of ischemia, scar, or patch material. Right ventricular outflow tract patches, ventricular septal defect patches, infundibulotomy incisions, residual hemodynamic derangements (volume and/or pressure overloads), and Purkinje system distal conduction disturbances may contribute to nonuniform ventricular depolarization and heterogeneous repolarization times. Each of these abnormalities may lead to exposure of nonuniform anisotropy, providing multiple substrates for late-onset arrhythmia development. Moreover, regional differences in repolarization within the right ventricular free wall and outflow tract are exaggerated in congenital heart disease, and thereby provide the substrate for phase 2 reentry, ventricular tachycardia, and sudden cardiac death.

Controversy exists as to the most suitable diagnostic tests for prediction of arrhythmias and sudden death in tetralogy of Fallot patients. The resting ECG, exercise stress ECG, ambulatory ECG monitoring, and invasive electrophysiology studies have each been used in the attempt to predict life-threatening arrhythmias or sudden cardiac death.[33–36] Future studies may allow for the assessment of multiple electrical and genetic-based markers in patients with conotruncal defects, and will hopefully determine predictive indicators of ventricular vulnerability and sudden cardiac death.

Cytogenetic analysis can be routinely obtained for chromosomal microdeletion analysis, with greater sensitivity compared with standard karyotyping. A specific chromosome 22q11 microdeletion in the critical DiGeorge region is identified in approximately 15% of patients with tetralogy of Fallot.[37,38] In an unselected retrospective analysis, referrals for FISH analysis were made on 74 patients in the neonatal intensive care unit. Of these, 52 (70%) had congenital heart disease, including 23% with tetralogy of Fallot, 9% with persistent truncus arteriosus, 6% with a single ventricle anatomy, 6% with double-outlet right ventricle, 6% with atrioventricular canal defects, 6% with pulmonic stenosis, and 6% with an atrial septal defect. The patients without congenital heart disease were referred due to the presence of cleft palate, facial dysmorphism, dysplastic kidneys, multiple congenital abnormalities, or fetal alcohol syndrome. Only 5 of 74 (6.7%) of the samples were classified positive by FISH analysis for chromosome 22q11 microdeletions, and none of the patients without congenital heart disease were determined to have an abnormal FISH test. Expansion to other conotruncal developmental defects and further correlation with specific chromosomal microdeletions may identify prognostic genetic indicators of future arrhythmia development, and may allow for presymptomatic identification of at-risk individuals.

The Muscular Dystrophies

Duchenne's Muscular Dystrophy

Duchenne's muscular dystrophy is a relatively common disorder (1 out of every 3500 live-born males) with an X-linked inheritance pattern. Approximately one third of cases are due to new sporadic mutations. The disease is characterized by focal but widespread muscle degeneration. Death is due to ventricular arrhythmias, cardiomyopathy, or respiratory failure/infection. The causative dystrophin gene has been localized to the short arm of the human X chromosome (Xp21), and has been successfully isolated and cloned in multiple species.[39] This gene is very large, which may account for the relatively high number of new clinical mutations. The dystrophin protein only accounts for roughly 0.002% of total myocyte protein in both skeletal and cardiac muscle. Whether the cardiomyopathy is a direct result of the abnormal protein content in the heart, of preferential concentration or effect in the conduction system, or of generalized muscle failure has not yet been fully defined.

Becker's Muscular Dystrophy

Becker's muscular dystrophy is much less common (1 in 35,000 live-born males) than Duchenne's muscular dystrophy, but it has a similar autosomal recessive inheritance pattern and is due to defective dystrophin production. The clinical course is typically less severe, with less probability of sudden cardiac death from ventricular arrhythmias. However, some mutations, such as a dystrophin gene G-to-T transversion at the terminal end of exon13, can lead to cardiac involvement preceding skeletal myopathy.[40] Additionally, patients with Becker's muscular dystrophy may present with bundle branch reentry tachycardia, as seen more prevalently in other forms of dilated cardiomyopathy.[41]

Myotonic Dystrophy

Myotonic muscular dystrophy is the most common adult-onset muscular dystrophy, with an incidence of greater than 1 in 7500. The disease affects all muscle subtypes, including smooth, skeletal, and cardiac muscles, and leads to varying degrees of myotonia, skeletal wasting, and cardiac muscle and conduction system disease. The cardiac symptoms relate to progressive atrioventricular block and bradycardia. Myotonic dystrophy is inherited in an autosomal dominant fashion with variable expression and is due to repetitive expansion of a trinucleotide repeat sequence mutation in a protein kinase gene (DMPK), localized on chromosome 19.[42] A murine model of myotonic dystrophy has been designed by targeted disruption of the DMPK gene.[43] The DMPK-deficient mice display abnormalities in skeletal muscle with a progressive skeletal myopathy. In vivo electrophysiological studies via epicardial and endocardial pacing/recording in homozygous mutant mice and age-matched wildtype controls were performed. On ECG, a prolonged PR interval was seen in all mutants compared with wildtype mice, analogous to first-degree atrioventricular block in humans. On electrophysiological testing, some of the mice with the DMPK-targeted disruption had second- and third-degree atrioventricular block during atrial pacing. There were no inducible tachyarrhythmias with programmed atrial or ventricular stimulation, indicating that DMPK-deficient mutant mice have distinct cardiac electrophysiological abnormalities of atrioventricular conduction.[44] This mouse model of myotonic dystrophy may prove useful for the study of pharmacologic and gene therapy approaches to cardiovascular problems seen in the inherited muscular dystrophies.

Emery-Dreifuss Muscular Dystrophy

This is a rare X-linked recessive disorder, noted for preferential cardiac conduction system abnormalities. The patients typically have severe cardiomyopathy and high-grade atrioventricular block. Survival requires permanent pacing in childhood for prevention of progressive (and sometimes sudden) atrioventricular block. No gene has been identified to date for Emery-Dreifuss muscular dystrophy and, therefore, there are no murine models of this rare disease and no effective therapy for the myopathy.

Connexin Defect Disorders

The connexin family, which is responsible for intermyocyte electrical communication, is made up of several gap junction protein members.[45] The connexin isoforms are distributed differently in the atrium compared with the ventricle and the specialized conduction tissue. Disorders of gap junction proteins may lead to distinct forms of cardiac conduction abnormalities, which are dependent on the spatial concentration of the individual connexin protein subtypes.[46] Developmental changes in connexin spatial relationships occur that may alter the functional requirements of the immature heart.[47] Targeted mutagenesis of connexin43, a prevalent isoform, causes homozygous mice to die as neonates from right ventricular outflow tract obstruction.[48] The heterozygote mutant mice survive, without obvious structural heart anomalies. Some studies have suggested that connexin43 mutations are responsible for some cases of heterotaxy syndrome, a form of complex congenital heart and visceral abnormalities, while others have not found that association.[49,50] The heterozygous connexin43 mice have prolongation of the QRS duration but no other abnormalities on ECG or during invasive electrophysiological testing.[51,52] This finding is the ECG correlate of prolonged intraventricular conduction times, consistent with an increased spatial density of the connexin43 isoform in ventricular muscle, and in contrast with atrial muscle and specialized conduction tissue. Long-term pacing has been shown to alter connexin isoform distribution in a goat model of atrial fibrillation,[53] suggesting an important role for gap junctions in arrhythmogenesis.

Summary

Many forms of structural heart disease in children have distinct molecular and genetic foundations. Multiple gene defects appear to be responsible for similar phenotypes of a clinical genetic disease. Specific genotypes may lead to differing severity of phenotype, and differential prognostic risks. There is also variability in phenotype expression, even among identical genotypes within a family, complicating the risk stratification picture.

Genetically manipulated animals are important models for the study of inherited human diseases associated with abnormal cardiac conduction and electrophysiology. The examples illustrated in this chapter highlight studies of in vivo murine electrophysiology in pediatric structural genetic diseases. The development of a mouse model analogous to a human clinical cardiac electrophysiological study allows several types of electrophysiological investigation in transgenic animals. Specific disease models can be studied to discern the relationship between single gene defects and their detailed electrophysiological phenotype in the intact, living animal. Genetically engineered mice harboring mutations in genes encoding proteins highly expressed in myocytes may be shown to have illuminative electrophysiological phenotypes. Furthermore, mutations in individual ion channel genes will allow the in vivo study of channel function and phenotype.

Molecular genetics may be of value in specific diagnostic testing, determining risk stratification, and gene-specific therapy approaches. Although not yet commercially available, the determination of specific gene disorders will become a powerful new tool in the evaluation of cardiac diseases with genetic bases. These tests may become the gold-standard diagnostic test for certain difficult-to-diagnose disease entities such as borderline long QT syndrome and relatively asymptomatic hypertrophic cardiomyopathy. Hopefully, specific pharmacologic treatments and gene replacement procedures can be designed, based on the specific mutations, allowing for effective designer gene therapy.

References

1. Paigen K. A miracle enough: The power of mice. *Nat Med* 1995;1:215–220.
2. Lin MC, Rockman RA, Chien KR. Heart and lung disease in engineered mice. *Nat Med* 1995;1:749–751.
3. Berul CI, Aronovitz MJ, Wang PJ, et al. In vivo cardiac electrophysiology studies in the mouse. *Circulation* 1996;94:2641–2648.
4. Seidman CE, Seidman JG. Gene mutations that cause familial hypertrophic cardiomyopathy. In Haber E (ed): *Molecular Cardiovascular Medicine*. New York: Scientific American Press; 1995:193–210.
5. Watkins H, McKenna W, Thierfelder L, et al. Mutations in the genes for cardiac troponin T and α-tropomyosin in hypertrophic cardiomyopathy. *N Engl J Med* 1995;332:1058–1064.
6. Thierfelder L, Watkins H, MacRae C, et al. Mutations in α-tropomyosin and in cardiac troponin T cause hypertrophic cardiomyopathy. *Cell* 1994;77:701–712.
7. Fananapazir L, Chang AC, Epstein SE, et al. Prognostic determinants in hypertrophic cardiomyopathy: Prospective evaluation of a therapeutic strategy based on clinical, Holter, hemodynamic, and electrophysiological findings. *Circulation* 1992;86:730–740.
8. Epstein ND, Cohn GM, Cyran F, et al. Differences in clinical expression of hypertrophic cardiomyopathy associated with two distinct mutations in β-myosin heavy chain gene. *Circulation* 1992;86:345–352.
9. Wigle ED, Rakowski H, Kimball BP, et al. Hypertrophic cardiomyopathy: Clinical spectrum and treatment. *Circulation* 1995;92:1680–1692.
10. Fananapazir L, Epstein SE. Hemodynamic and electrophysiologic evaluation of patients with hypertrophic cardiomyopathy surviving cardiac arrest. *Am J Cardiol* 1991;67:280–287.
11. Maron BJ, Fananapazir L. Sudden cardiac death in hypertrophic cardiomyopathy. *Circulation* 1992;85:I57-I63.
12. Watson RM, Schwartz JL, Maron BJ, et al. Inducible polymorphic ventricular tachycardia and ventricular fibrillation in a subgroup of patients with hypertrophic cardiomyopathy at risk for sudden death. *J Am Coll Cardiol* 1987;10:761–774.

13. Solomon SD, Wolff S, Watkins H, et al. Left ventricular hypertrophy and morphology in familial hypertrophic cardiomyopathy associated with mutations of the β-myosin heavy chain gene. *J Am Coll Cardiol* 1993;22: 498–505.

14. Spirito P, Rapezzi C, Autore C, et al. Prognosis of asymptomatic patients with hypertrophic cardiomyopathy and nonsustained ventricular tachycardia. *Circulation* 1994;90:2743–2747.

15. McKenna WJ, Sadoul N, Slade AKB, et al. The prognostic significance of nonsustained ventricular tachycardia in hypertrophic cardiomyopathy. *Circulation* 1994;90:3115–3117.

16. Watkins H, Rosenzweig A, Hwang D, et al. Characteristics and prognostic implications of myosin missense mutations in familial hypertrophic cardiomyopathy. *N Engl J Med* 1992;326:1108–1114.

17. Geisterfer-Lowrance A, Christe M, Conner D, et al. A mouse model of familial hypertrophic cardiomyopathy. *Science* 1996;272:731–734.

18. Berul CI, Christe ME, Aronovitz MJ, et al. Electrophysiological abnormalities and arrhythmias in α-MHC mutant familial hypertrophic cardiomyopathy mice. *J Clin Invest* 1997;99:274–280.

19. Berul CI, Christe ME, Aronovitz MJ, et al. Familial hypertrophic cardiomyopathy mice display gender differences in electrophysiological abnormalities. *J Intervent Card Electrophysiol* 1998;2:7–14.

20. Durand JB, Abchee AB, Roberts R. Molecular and clinical aspects of inherited cardiomyopathies. *Ann Med* 1995;27:311–317.

21. Michels VV, Moll PP, Miller FA, et al. The frequency of familial dilated cardiomyopathy in a series of patients with idiopathic dilated cardiomyopathy. *N Engl J Med* 1992;326:77–82.

22. Olson TM, Keating MT. Mapping a cardiomyopathy locus to chromosome 3p. *J Clin Invest* 1996;97:528–532.

23. Durand JB, Bachinski LL, Beling LC, et al. Localization of a gene responsible for familial dilated cardiomyopathy to chromosome 1q32. *Circulation* 1995;92:3387–3389.

24. Ozawa T. Mitochondrial DNA mutations in myocardial disease. *Eur Heart J* 1995;16:10–14.

25. Remes AM, Hassinen IE, Ikaheimo MJ, et al. Mitochondrial DNA deletions in dilated cardiomyopathy. *J Am Coll Cardiol* 1994;23:935–942.

26. Milasin J, Muntoni F, Severini GM, et al. A point mutation in the 5' splice site of the dystrophin gene first intron responsible for X-linked dilated cardiomyopathy. *Human Mol Genet* 1996;5:73–79.

27. Gedeon AK, Wilson MJ, Colley AC, et al. X-linked fatal infantile cardiomyopathy maps to Xq28 and is possibly allelic to Barth syndrome. *J Med Genet* 1995;32:383–388.

28. Arber S, Hunter JJ, Ross J, et al. MPL-deficient mice exhibit a disruption of cardiac cytoarchitectural organization, dilated cardiomyopathy, and heart failure. *Cell* 1997;88:393–398.

29. Rampazzo A, Nava A, Erne P, et al. A new locus for arrhythmogenic right ventricular cardiomyopathy (ARVD2) maps to chromosome 1q42–q43. *Human Mol Genet* 1995;4:2151–2154.

30. Severini GM, Krajinovic M, Pinamonti B. A new locus for arrhythmogenic right ventricular dysplasia on the long arm of chromosome 14. *Genomics* 1996;31:193–200.

31. Coonar AS, Protonotarios N, Tsatsopoulou A, et al. Gene for arrhythmogenic right ventricular cardiomyopathy with diffuse nonepidermolytic

palmoplantar keratoderma and wooly hair (Naxos disease) maps to 17q21. *Circulation* 1998;97:2049–2058.

32. Wappner RS, Brandt IK. Inborn errors of metabolism. In Oski FA, DeAngelis CD, Feigin RD, Warshaw JB (eds): *Principles and Practice of Pediatrics.* Philadelphia: J.B. Lippincott; 1990:123–124.

33. Deanfield JE, McKenna WJ, Hallidie-Smith KA. Detection of late arrhythmia and conduction disturbance after correction of tetralogy of Fallot. *Br Heart J* 1980;44:248–253.

34. Gillette PC, Yeoman MA, Mullins CE, et al. Sudden death after repair of tetralogy of Fallot: Electrocardiographic and electrophysiologic abnormalities. *Circulation* 1977;56:566–571.

35. Walsh EP, Rochenmacher S, Keane JF, et al. Late results in patients with tetralogy of Fallot repaired during infancy. *Circulation* 1988;77:1062–1067.

36. Berul, CI, Hill SL, Geggel RG, et al. Electrocardiographic markers of late sudden death risk in postoperative tetralogy of Fallot children. *J Cardiovasc Electrophysiol* 1997;8:1349–1356.

37. Goldmuntz E, Driscoll DA, Budarf ML, et al. Microdeletions of chromosomal region 22q11 in patients with conotruncal cardiac defects. *J Med Genet* 1993;30:807–812.

38. Amati F, Mari A, Diglio MC, et al. 22q11 deletions in isolated and syndromic patients with tetralogy of Fallot. *Human Genet* 1995;95:479–482.

39. Gussoni E, Blau HM, Kunkel LM. The fate of individual myoblasts after transplantation into muscles of DMD patients. *Nat Med* 1997;3:970–977.

40. Yu Y, Yamabe H, Fujita J, et al. Cardiac involvement in a family with Becker muscular dystrophy. *Intern Med* 1995;34:919–923.

41. Negri SM, Cowan MD. Becker muscular dystrophy with bundle branch reentry ventricular tachycardia. *J Cardiovasc Electrophysiol* 1998;9:652–654.

42. Housman DE, Shaw DJ. Expansion of an unstable DNA region and phenotypic variation in myotonic dystrophy. *Nature* 1992;355:545–546.

43. Reddy S, Smith DBJ, Rich MM, et al. Mice lacking the myotonic dystrophy protein kinase develop a late-onset progressive myopathy. *Nat Genet* 1996;13:325–335.

44. Berul CI, Reddy S, Aronovitz MJ, et al. Atrioventricular conduction abnormalities in a mouse model of myotonic dystrophy. *PACE* 1997;20:1101.

45. Saffitz JE, Davis LM, Darrow BJ, et al. The molecular basis of anisotrophy: Role of gap junctions. *J Cardiovasc Electrophysiol* 1995;6:498–510.

46. Davis LM, Kanter HL, Beyer EC, et al. Distinct gap junction protein phenotypes in cardiac tissues with disparate conduction properties. *J Am Coll Cardiol* 1994;24:1124–1132.

47. Peters NS, Severs NJ, Rothery SM, et al. Spatiotemporal relation between gap junctions and fascia adherens junctions during postnatal development of human ventricular myocardium. *Circulation* 1994;90:713–725.

48. Reaume AG, deSousa PA, Kulkarni S, et al. Cardiac malformation in neonatal mice lacking connexin43. *Science* 1995;267:1831–1834.

49. Britz-Cunningham SH, Shah MM, Zuppan CW, et al. Mutations of the connexin43 gap junction gene in patients with heart malformations and defects of laterality. *N Engl J Med* 1995;332:1323–1329.

50. Gebbia M, Towbin JA, Casey B. Failure to detect connexin43 mutations in 38 cases of sporadic and familial heterotaxy. *Circulation* 1996;94:1909–1912.

51. Thomas SA, Schuessler RB, Beardslee MA, et al. Disparate effects of deficient expression of connexin43 in atrial and ventricular myocardium. *Circulation* 1998;97:686–691.

52. Berul CI, Thomas SA, Aronovitz MJ, et al. Ventricular conduction abnormalities in heterozygote connexin43 mutant mice. *Circulation* 1997;96:I-673.
53. Van der Velden HMW, van Kempen MJA, Wijffels MCEF, et al. Altered pattern of connexin40 distribution in persistent atrial fibrillation in the goat. *J Cardiovasc Electrophysiol* 1998;9:596–607.

Chapter 9

Long QT Syndrome:
Genetic Aspects

Jeffrey A. Towbin, MD

Disease Classification

The long QT syndromes (LQTSs) are disorders of repolarization identified by the electrocardiographic abnormalities of prolongation of the QT interval corrected for heart rate, relative bradycardia, T wave abnormalities, and episodic ventricular tachyarrhythmias, particularly torsades de pointes.[1] LQTS can occur as an inherited disorder or a sporadic disorder, or it may be acquired. The clinical presentation is similar in all forms of LQTS, but minor variations should be noted. Two inherited forms of LQTS have been described thus far, and include the Romano-Ward syndrome[2,3] and the Jervell and Lange-Nielsen syndrome.[4]

The Romano-Ward syndrome is the most common of the inherited forms of LQTS and appears to be transmitted as an autosomal dominant trait.[1-3] In this disorder, gene carriers are expected to be clinically affected, and have a 50% likelihood of passing the disease-causing gene to their offspring. Individuals with Romano-Ward syndrome have the pure clinical syndrome of prolonged QT interval on electrocardiogram (ECG) with the associated symptom complex of syncope, sudden death, and, in some patients, seizures.[5,6] Occasionally, other noncardiac abnormalities such as diabetes mellitus,[7,8] asthma,[9] or syndactyly[10] may also occur. LQTS may also be involved in some cases of sudden infant death syndrome (SIDS).[11-13]

The Jervell and Lange-Nielsen syndrome is a relatively uncommon inherited form of LQTS with apparent autosomal recessive transmis-

From: Quan L, Franklin WH (eds). *Ventricular Fibrillation: A Pediatric Problem.* Armonk, NY: Futura Publishing Company, Inc.; ©2000.

Dr. Towbin is funded by NIH grants from the National Heart, Lung, and Blood Institute (NHLBI RO1–HL33843–06; R01–HL51618–06) and the Texas Children's Hospital Foundation Chair in Pediatric Cardiac Research.

sion. Affected patients have a clinical presentation identical to that of those with Romano-Ward syndrome, but they also have associated sensorineural deafness.[4,14,15] Individuals with Jervell and Lange-Nielsen syndrome usually have longer QT intervals as compared with individuals with Romano-Ward syndrome, and they also have a more malignant course.

Mapping of LQTS Genes in Romano-Ward Syndrome

The first gene for autosomal dominant LQTS was mapped by Keating et al[16] to chromosome 11p15.5 (*LQT1*) using genome-wide linkage analysis in a large Utah family. Soon afterwards, Keating et al[17] reported consistent linkage of several other LQTS families linked to chro-

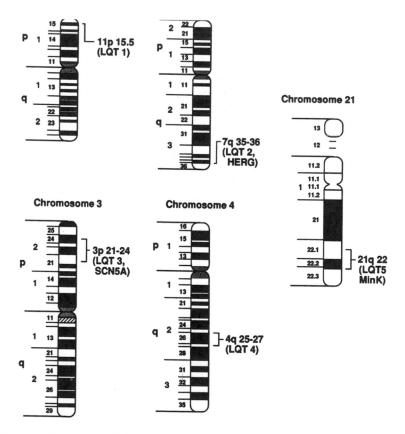

Figure 1. Ideograms of chromosomes 11, 7, 3, 4, and 21 showing approximate locations of *LQT1 (KVLQT1), LQT2 (HERG), LQT3 (SCN5A), LQT4,* and *LQT5 (minK)*, respectively.

mosome 11p15.5. However, LQTS locus heterogeneity was subsequently reported[18-21] and confirmed by the mapping of the second LQTS locus to chromosome 7q35–36 (*LQT2*), and the third LQTS locus to chromosome 3p21–24 (*LQT3*).[22] Schott et al[23] mapped the fourth LQTS locus to chromosome 4q25–27 (*LQT4*), while a fifth gene, *minK*, which is located on chromosome 21q22, was speculated to be *LQT5* (Figure 1).[24,25] Several other families with autosomal dominant LQTS are not linked to any known LQTS loci, indicating the existence of additional LQTS-causing genes.

Gene Identification in Romano-Ward Syndrome

Cardiac Potassium Channel Gene
KVLQT1 and *LQT1*

The positional cloning method was used to identify the *LQT1* gene *KVLQT1*, a novel potassium channel gene with six membrane-spanning segments.[26] *KVLQT1* is widely expressed in human tissues including heart, kidney, lung, placenta, and pancreas, but not in skeletal muscle, liver, or brain. In the original report, 11 different types of *KVLQT1* mutations (one three base-pair deletion and ten missense mutations) were identified in 16 LQTS families, establishing *KVLQT1* as *LQT1*. The alanine residue at position 212 of *KVLQT1* was mutated in seven families, identifying this site as a mutation "hot spot." To date, more than 30 families with *KVLQT1* mutations have been described, and the alanine residue at position 212 has been reportedly mutated ten times (33%).

Analysis of the predicted amino acid sequence of *KVLQT1* suggests that it encodes a potassium channel subunit with a conserved potassium-selective pore-signature sequence flanked by six membrane-spanning segments (Figure 2).[26] Recent electrophysiological characterization of the *KVLQT1* protein in various heterologous systems confirmed that *KVLQT1* is a voltage-gated potassium channel protein.[23,24] *minK (IsK)*, or *KCNE1*, encodes a short protein with a mere 130 amino acids and has only one transmembrane-spanning segment.[27] It does not have any sequence or structural homologies to any other cloned channels. However, when *minK* and *KVLQT1* were coexpressed in either mammalian cell lines or *Xenopus* oocytes, a potassium current was formed that is similar to the slowly activating potassium current (I_{Ks}) in cardiac myocytes.[24,25] Immunoprecipitation experiments also confirmed the physical interaction between *KVLQT1* and *minK*.[24] Thus, *KVLQT1* interacts with *minK* to form the cardiac slowly activating delayed rectifier I_{Ks} current (Figure 2). Combination of normal and mutant *KVLQT1* subunits was found to form abnormal I_{Ks} channels and,

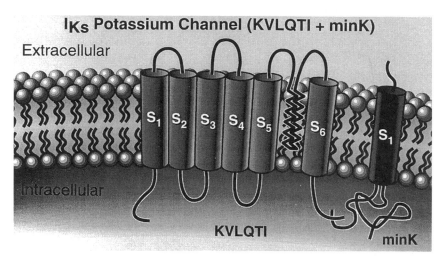

Figure 2. The molecular architecture of the cardiac I_{Ks} potassium channel encoded by *KVLQT1* and *minK*.

hence, LQTS-associated mutations of *KVLQT1* are believed to act through a dominant-negative mechanism (the mutant form of *KVLQT1* interferes with the function of the normal wildtype form through a "poison pill" type of mechanism) or a loss-of-function mechanism (only the mutant form loses activity).

Since mutations in *KVLQT1* cause chromosome 11-linked LQTS (*LQT1*), mutations in *minK* were also expected to cause LQTS (*LQT5*). Recently, mutations in *minK* have been identified (see section on LQT5).[28]

Cardiac Potassium Channel Gene

Both *LQT2* and *LQT3* (described below) were identified by the positional candidate gene approach. The candidate gene approach relies on a mechanistic hypothesis based on knowledge of the physiology of the disease of interest. Since LQTS is associated with prolongation of the QT interval on ECGs, an indication of abnormal repolarization, genes encoding ion channels or proteins modulating channel function were considered candidates for LQTS. After the initial localization of *LQT2*, a candidate gene called *HERG*, a cardiac potassium channel gene with six transmembrane segments (Figure 3), was characterized[29,30] and linkage analysis was performed. Curran et al[31] demonstrated linkage of *HERG* to the *LQT2* locus on chromosome 7q35–36, and six LQTS-associated mutations were identified in *HERG*, including three missense mutations (N470D, A561V, G628S), two intragenic deletions

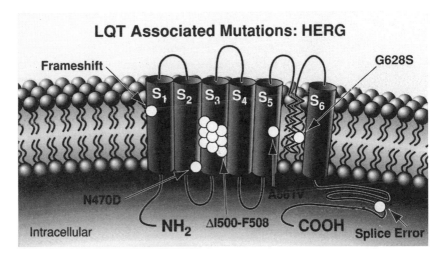

Figure 3. The molecular architecture of the cardiac I_{Kr} potassium channel encoded by *HERG*. Mutations are noted.

(ΔI500–F508, Δ1261a), and a splicing mutation. Later, Schulze-Bahr et al[32] reported a single base pair deletion (ΔT1671) and a stop codon change mutation (T611stop) in *HERG*. Dausse et al[33] reported a missense mutation A561T, and Benson et al[34] also reported an I593R mutation in *HERG*, all confirming that *HERG* is the *LQT2*-causing gene when mutated.

HERG, the human ether-a-go-go-related gene, was initially isolated by Warmke and Ganetzky,[30] who screened a human hippocampal cDNA library with a mouse homolog of a *Drosophila* potassium channel gene, ether-a-go-go (the gene, ether-a-go-go, was named because of the peculiar hopping movement seen in mutant flies when placed in ether).[29] Later, it was found that *HERG* is highly expressed in the heart.[31] Electrophysiological and biophysical characterization of expressed *HERG* in *Xenopus* oocytes established that *HERG* encodes the rapidly activating delayed rectifier potassium current (I_{Kr}).[35,36] Electrophysiological studies of five LQTS-associated mutations showed that they act through either a loss-of-function mechanism or a dominant-negative mechanism.[37] Recently, McDonald et al[38] demonstrated that the complexing of *HERG* with *minK* is needed to regulate the I_{Kr} potassium current.

Cardiac Sodium Channel Gene *SCN5A* and *LQT3*

The positional candidate gene approach was also used to establish that the gene responsible for chromosome 3-linked LQTS (*LQT3*) is the cardiac sodium channel gene *SCN5A*.[39,40] *SCN5A* is highly expressed in human myocardium but not in skeletal muscle, brain, liver, or uterus.[41,42] It encodes a protein of 2016 amino acids with a putative structure that consists of four homologous domains (DI–DIV), each of which contains six membrane-spanning segments (S1–S6) (Figure 4).[39–41] Linkage studies with *LQT3* families and *SCN5A* initially demonstrated linkage to the *LQT3* locus on chromosome 3p21–24,[40,41] and three types of mutations, one 9-bp intragenic deletion ($\Delta K_{1505}P_{1506}Q_{1507}$) and two missense mutations ($R_{1644}H$ and $N_{1325}S$) were also identified in six LQTS families.[41,42] All three mutations were expressed in *Xenopus* oocytes and it was found that all mutations generated a late phase of inactivation-resistant, mexiletine- and tetrodotoxin-sensitive whole-cell currents through multiple mechanisms.[43,44] Two of the three mutations showed dispersed reopening after the initial transient, but the other mutation showed both dispersed reopening and long-lasting bursts.[44] These results suggested that *SCN5A* mutations act through a gain-of-function mechanism (the mutant channel functions normally but with altered properties such as delayed inactivation) and that the mechanism of chromosome 3-linked LQTS is persistent, noninactivated sodium current in the plateau phase of the action potential. Recently, mutations in *SCN5A* were identified in patients with Brugada syndrome and idiopathic ventricular fibrillation.[45] These mutations result in more rapid recovery from inactivation of the mutant channels or loss of function, causing the Brugada syndrome-type phenotype.[45]

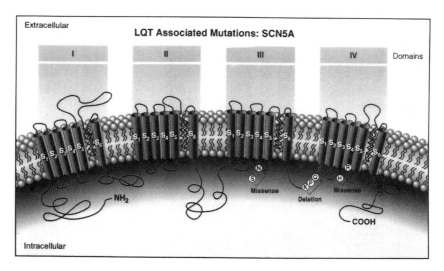

Figure 4. The molecular architecture of the cardiac I_{Na} sodium channel encoded by *SCN5A*. Mutations are identified.

Cardiac Potassium Channel Gene *minK* and *LQT5*

minK (*IsK*), or *KCNE1*, encodes a short protein consisting of 130 amino acids, and has only one transmembrane-spanning segment (Figure 2).[27] It does not have any sequence or structural homologies to any other cloned channel. When expressed in *Xenopus* oocytes, it produces potassium current that closely resembles the slowly activating delayed rectifier potassium current I_{Ks} in cardiac cells.[46,47] The fact that the *minK* clone was only expressed in *Xenopus* oocytes and not in mammalian cell lines raised the question of whether *minK* is a human channel protein. With the cloning of *KVLQT1* and coexpression of *KVLQT1* and *minK* in both mammalian cell lines and *Xenopus* oocytes, the molecular secret to the mystery was revealed: *KVLQT1* interacts with *minK* to form the cardiac slowly activating delayed rectifier I_{Ks} current.[24,25] *minK* alone cannot form a functional channel but induces the I_{Ks} current by interacting with endogenous *KVLQT1* protein in *Xenopus* oocytes and in mammalian cells. Immunoprecipitation experiments also demonstrated the physical interaction between *KVLQT1* and *minK*.[24] McDonald et al[38] showed than *minK* complexes with *HERG* to regulate the I_{Kr} potassium current as well. Since mutations in *KVLQT1* cause chromosome 11-linked LQTS and *HERG* mutations cause *LQT2*, mutations in *minK* alone were expected to cause LQTS. Recently Splawski et al[28] identified mutations in two families with LQTS. In both cases, they identified missense mutations (S74L, D76N) that reduced I_{Ks} by shifting the voltage dependence of activation and accelerating channel deactivation. The functional consequences of these mutations include delayed cardiac repolarization and, hence, an increased risk of arrhythmias.

Genetics and Physiology of Autosomal Recessive LQTS (Jervell and Lange-Nielsen Syndrome)

Recently, Neyroud et al[48] reported the first molecular abnormality in patients with Jervell and Lange-Nielsen syndrome when they reported on two families in which three children were affected by Jervell and Lange-Nielsen syndrome and in whom a novel homozygous deletion-insertion mutation of *KVLQT1* in three patients was found. A deletion of 7 bp (CAGTACT) and an insertion of 8 bp (GTTGAGAT) at the same location led to premature termination at the C-terminal end of the *KVLQT1* protein. More recently, Splawski et al[49] also identified a homozygous insertion of a single nucleotide (guanosine), which caused a frame shift in the coding sequence after the second putative transmembrane domain of the *KVLQT1* protein.

Together, these data strongly suggest that at least one form of Jervell and Lange-Nielsen syndrome is caused by homozygous mutations in *KVLQT1*.

It is interesting to note that heterozygous mutations in *KVLQT1* cause Romano-Ward syndrome (LQTS only), but homozygous mutations in *KVLQT1* cause Jervell and Lange-Nielsen syndrome (LQTS and deafness). The likely explanation is that although heterozygous *KVLQT1* mutations act by a dominant-negative mechanism, some functional *KVLQT1* potassium channels still exist in the stria vascularis of the inner ear. Therefore, congenital deafness is averted in patients with heterozygous *KVLQT1* mutations. For patients with homozygous *KVLQT1* mutations, no functional *KVLQT1* potassium channels can be formed. It has been shown by in situ hybridization that *KVLQT1* is expressed in the inner ear,[48] suggesting that homozygous *KVLQT1* mutations can cause the dysfunction of potassium secretion in the inner ear and lead to deafness.

Schulze-Bahr et al[50] have also shown that mutations in *minK* result in Jervell and Lange-Nielsen syndrome. Hence, abnormal I_{Ks} current, whether it occurs due to homozygous mutations in *KVLQT1* or in *minK*, results in LQTS and deafness.

Genetic Testing

Currently, three LQTS-causing genes have been identified with more than 50 mutations described to date. This genetic heterogeneity makes genetic testing more difficult than if a single gene defect were responsible for the disease. However, under certain conditions, genetic testing can be performed. In large families in which linkage analysis may be performed, identification of the gene of interest (if the linkage is to one of the known genes) can be discerned rapidly and screening of mutations undertaken. Once a mutation is identified in one affected family member (usually the proband), the remaining family members can be quickly screened for this mutation. In small families or sporadic cases, mutation screening for all known genes must be initiated. Usually *KVLQT1* (*LQT1*) mutations are screened initially, since this appears to be the most common disease-causing gene.[51] If no mutation is uncovered in *KVLQT1*, *HERG* and *SCN5A* are then analyzed. If no mutation is found in any of these three genes, one cannot conclude that the subject does not have LQTS, since other disease-causing genes remain to be discovered and because only portions of the gene sequences of *KVLQT* and *HERG* are currently known.

Summary

During the past decade, breakthroughs in the clinical and molecular genetic understanding of the LQTSs have occurred. Much, however, remains to be learned. Collaborative interactions between clinicians and basic scientists have facilitated many of the new findings, and continued close working relationships should provide the incentive necessary to continue this growth in knowledge. It is hoped that the dawn of the 21st century will bring with it better diagnostic and therapeutic capabilities for this potentially devastating disease.

References

1. Schwartz PJ, Locati EH, Napolitano C, et al. The long QT syndrome. In Zipes DP, Jalife J (eds): *Cardiac Electrophysiology: From Cell to Bedside*. Philadelphia: W.B. Saunders Co.; 1996:788–811.
2. Romano C, Gemme G, Pongiglione R. Antmie cardiache rare in eta pediatrica. *Clin Pediatr* 1963;45:656–683.
3. Ward OC. A new familial cardiac syndrome in children. *J Ir Med Assoc* 1964;54:103–106.
4. Jervell A, Lange-Nielsen F. Congenital deaf-mutism, function heart disease with prolongation of the Q-T interval and sudden death. *Am Heart J* 1957;54:59–68.
5. Ratshin RA, Hunt D, Russell RO Jr, et al. QT-interval prolongation, paroxysmal ventricular arrhythmias, and convulsive syncope. *Ann Intern Med* 1971;75:19–24.
6. Singer PA, Crampton RS, Bass NH. Familial Q-T prolongation syndrome: Convulsive seizures and paroxysmal ventricular fibrillation. *Arch Neurol* 1974;31:64–66.
7. Bellavere F, Ferri M, Guarini L, et al. Prolonged QT period in diabetic autonomic neuropathy: A possible role in sudden cardiac death. *Br Heart J* 1988;59:379–383.
8. Ewing DJ, Boland O, Neilson JMM, et al. Autonomic neuropathy, QT interval lengthening, and unexpected deaths in male diabetic patients. *Diabetologia* 1991;34:182–185.
9. Weintraub RG, Gow RM, Wilkinson JL. The congenital long QT syndromes in children. *J Am Coll Cardiol* 1990;16:674–680.
10. Marks ML, Trippel DL, Keating MT. Long QT syndrome associated with syndactyly identified in females. *Am J Cardiol* 1976;10:744–745.
11. Schwartz PJ, Segantini A. Cardiac innervation, neonatal electrocardiography and SIDS. A key for a novel preventive strategy? *Ann N Y Acad Sci* 1988;533:210–220.
12. Schwartz PJ, Stramba-Badiale M, Segantini A, et al. Prolongation of the QT interval and the sudden infant death syndrome. *N Engl J Med* 1998; 338:1709–1714.
13. Towbin JA, Friedman RA. Prolongation of the long QT syndrome and sudden infant death syndrome. *N Engl J Med* 1998;338:1760–1761.
14. Jervell A. Surdocardiac and related syndromes in children. *Adv Intern Med* 1971;17:425–438.

15. James TN. Congenital deafness and cardiac arrhythmias. *Am J Cardiol* 1967;19:627–643.
16. Keating MT, Atkinson D, Dunn C, et al. Linkage of a cardiac arrhythmia, the long QT syndrome, and the Harvey ras-1 gene. *Science* 1991;252: 704–706.
17. Keating MT, Atkinson D, Dunn C, et al. Consistent linkage of the long QT syndrome to the Harvey ras-1 locus on chromosome 11. *Am J Hum Genet* 1991;49:1335–1339.
18. Towbin JA, Pagotto L, Siu B, et al. Romano-Ward long QT syndrome (RWLQTS): Evidence of genetic heterogeneity. *Pediatr Res* 1992;31:23A. Abstract.
19. Benhorin J, Kalman YM, Madina A, et al. Evidence of genetic heterogeneity in the long QT syndrome. *Science* 1993;260:1960–1962.
20. Curran ME, Atkinson D, Timothy K, et al. Locus heterogeneity of autosomal dominant long QT syndrome. *J Clin Invest* 1993;92:799–803.
21. Towbin JA, Li H, Taggart T, et al. Evidence of genetic heterogeneity in Romano-Ward long QT syndrome: Analysis of 23 families. *Circulation* 1994;90:2635–2644.
22. Jiang C, Atkinson D, Towbin JA, et al. Two long QT syndrome loci map to chromosome 3 and 7 with evidence for further heterogeneity. *Nat Genet* 1994;8:141–147.
23. Schott J, Charpentier F, Peltier S, et al. Mapping of a gene for long QT syndrome to chromosome 4q25–27. *Am J Hum Genet* 1995;57:1114–1122.
24. Barhanin J, Lesage F, Guillemare E, et al. KVLQT1 and IsK (minK) proteins associate to form the I_{ks} cardiac potassium current. *Nature* 1996; 384:78–80.
25. Sanguinetti MC, Curran ME, Zou A, et al. Coassembly of KvLQT1 and minK (IsK) proteins to form cardiac I_{ks} potassium channel. *Nature* 1996; 384:80–83.
26. Wang Q, Curran ME, Splawski I, et al. Positional cloning of a novel potassium channel gene: KVLQT1 mutations cause cardiac arrhythmias. *Nat Genet* 1996;12:17–23.
27. Lai LP, Deng CL, Moss AJ, et al. Polymorphism of the gene encoding a human minimal potassium ion channel (minK). *Gene* 1994;151:339–340.
28. Splawski I, Tristani-Firouzi M, Lehmann MH, et al. Mutations in the *hminK* gene cause long QT syndrome and suppress I_{Ks} function. *Nat Genet* 1997;17:338–340.
29. Bruggeman A, Pardo LA, Struhmer W, et al. Ether-a-go-go encodes a voltage-gated channel permeable to K^+ and Ca^{2+} and modulated by cAMP. *Nature* 1993;365:445–448.
30. Warmke JE, Ganetzky B. A family of potassium channel genes related to Eag in *Drosophila* and mammals. *Proc Natl Acad Sci U S A* 1994;91:3438–3442.
31. Curran ME, Splawski I, Timothy KW, et al. A molecular basis for cardiac arrhythmia: HERG mutations cause long QT syndrome. *Cell* 1995;80: 795–803.
32. Schulze-Bahr E, Haverkamp W, Funke H. The long-QT syndrome. *N Engl J Med* 1995;333:1783–1784.
33. Dausse E, Berthet M, Denjoy I, et al. A mutation in HERG associated with notched T waves in long QT syndrome. *J Mol Cell Cardiol* 1996;28:1609–1613.
34. Benson DW, MacRae CA, Vesely MR, et al. Missense mutation in the pore

region of HERG causes familiar long QT syndrome. *Circulation* 1996;93: 1791–1795.

35. Sanguinetti MC, Jiang C, Curran ME, et al. A mechanistic link between an inherited and an acquired cardiac arrhythmia: HERG encodes the I_{Kr} potassium channel. *Cell* 1995;81:299–307.

36. Trudeau MC, Warmke J, Ganetzky B, et al. HERG, a human inward recti fier in the voltage-gated potassium channel family. *Science* 1995;269:92–95.

37. Sanguinetti MC, Curran ME, Spector PS, et al. Spectrum of HERG K$^+$- channel dysfunction in an inherited cardiac arrhythmia. *Proc Natl Acad Sci U S A* 1996;93:2208–2212.

38. McDonald TV, Yu Z, Ming Z, et al. A minK-HERG complex regulates the cardiac potassium current I_{Kr}. *Nature* 1997;388:289–292.

39. Gellens M, George AL, Chen L, et al. Primary structure and functional expression of the human cardiac tetrodotoxin-insensitive voltage-dependent sodium channel. *Proc Natl Acad Sci U S A* 1992;89:54–558.

40. George AL, Varkony TA, Drakin HA, et al. Assignment of the human heart tetrodotoxin-resistant voltage-gated Na channel α-subunit gene (SCN5A) to band 3p21. *Cytogenet Cell Genet* 1995;68:67–70.

41. Wang Q, Shen J, Splawski I, et al. SCN5A mutations associated with an inherited cardiac arrhythmia, long QT syndrome. *Cell* 1995;80:805–811.

42. Wang Q, Shen J, Li Z, et al. Cardiac sodium channel mutations in patients with long QT syndrome, an inherited cardiac arrhythmia. *Hum Mol Genet* 1995;4:1603–1607.

43. Bennett PB, Yazawa K, Makita N, et al. Molecular mechanism for an inherited cardiac arrhythmia. *Nature* 1995;376:683–685.

44. Dumain R, Wang Q, Keating MT, et al. Multiple mechanisms of sodium channel-linked long QT syndrome. *Circ Res* 1996;78:916–924.

45. Chen Q, Kirsch GE, Zhang D, et al. Genetic basis and molecular mechanism for idiopathic ventricular fibrillation. *Nature* 1998;392:293–296.

46. Arena JP, Kass RS. Block of heart potassium channels by clofilium and its tertiary analogs: Relationship between drug structure and type of channel blocked. *Mol Pharmacol* 1988;34:60–66.

47. Honore E, Attali B, Heurteaux C, et al. Cloning, expression, pharmacology and regulation of a delayed rectifier K$^+$ channel in mouse heart. *EMBO J* 1991;10:2805–2811.

48. Neyroud N, Tesson F, Denjoy I, et al. A novel mutation on the potassium channel gene KVLQT1 causes the Jervell and Lange-Nielsen cardioauditory syndrome. *Nat Genet* 1997;15:186–189.

49. Splawski I, Timothy KW, Vincent GM, et al. Brief report: Molecular basis of the long-QT syndrome associated with deafness. *N Engl J Med* 1997; 336:1562–1567.

50. Schulze-Bahr E, Wang Q, Wedekind H, et al. KCNE1 mutations cause Jervell and Lange-Nielsen syndrome. *Nat Genet* 1997;17:267–268.

51. Li H, Schwartz P, Locati E, et al. Chromosome 11-linked long QT syndrome (LQT1) is the most common form of long QT syndrome. *Pediatrics* 1996;98:534.

Chapter 10

Ventricular Fibrillation in the Postoperative Cardiac Patient

George F. Van Hare, MD

Fortunately, ventricular fibrillation (VF) is a rare event in post-operative pediatric cardiac patients, and very few well documented cases exist. Other arrhythmias, such as atrioventricular block, sinus node dysfunction, and atrial flutter, are much more common. However, while sudden death in the postoperative cardiac patient is unusual, it has been reported persistently since the introduction of complete repair for congenital heart defects such as tetralogy of Fallot and transposition of the great arteries.[1] While few reports of recordings of the electrophysiological mechanism of sudden death following congenital heart disease repair are available, those few reports support the notion that VF plays a role, either as a primary event or, more likely, as the final common pathway following rhythms such as ventricular tachycardia (VT) or atrial flutter. At the same time, there are many patients who have either atrial flutter or VT following congenital heart disease repair who nevertheless tolerate these rhythms quite well without adverse consequences. Other factors, then, must contribute to the occurrence of VF. Such factors are known in some cases and simply hypothesized in others, and may be divided into those which operate early, ie, during or immediately following cardiac surgery, and those which operate later, ie, months or years after surgery. In view of the recent availability of reliable implantable transvenous defibrillation systems of small size,[2] it is critically important that a strategy is developed for the identification of patients who may be at risk for VF following surgical repair of congenital heart defects.

From: Quan L, Franklin WH (eds). *Ventricular Fibrillation: A Pediatric Problem.* Armonk, NY: Futura Publishing Company, Inc.; ©2000.

Initiation of VF

In the postoperative period, VF may be initiated by several mechanisms. First and probably most commonly, a patient may develop a fast, poorly tolerated regular tachyarrhythmia and experience degeneration into VF. While such a scenario is most likely with VT, it is possible for the initiating arrhythmia to be a supraventricular tachyarrhythmia, such as atrial flutter or atrial fibrillation with rapid atrioventricular conduction. Similarly, inadvertent rapid ventricular pacing may lead to VF. For this reason, temporary pacemakers capable of high-rate (>180 bpm) pacing must never be connected to epicardial ventricular pacing wires.

The "R on T" phenomenon is, in fact, rare in children. However, it is possible to induce VF with a critically timed premature ventricular contraction (PVC) of sufficient magnitude, particularly in a patient with a vulnerable myocardium. For this reason, when connecting a temporary ventricular pacemaker, one must always assess pacemaker sensing function, as ventricular undersensing is one mechanism of inadvertent delivery of such a critically timed PVC. All electrical interfaces to the patient, such as devices with skin electrodes and especially those with a direct connection to the myocardium (eg, pacing wires), must be protected from accidental contact with line current. Biomedical instrumentation devices may generate leakage current due to capacitive coupling combined with a ground fault, and such leakage current can, if delivered directly to the myocardium, induce VF. For these reasons, all such devices must be carefully checked and periodically rechecked for leakage current.

There are other possible causes of VF in patients with pacemakers. First, the entity termed "pacemaker runaway" in the past has been reported in patients with pacemakers.[3] Although now quite rare, prior to 1970 the incidence of pacemaker runaway was 2% to 4%, and it carried a mortality risk of 30% to 40%. This phenomenon was usually due to loss of the hermetic seal on the pulse generator, most often resulting from overtightening of the set screws. Extremely rapid cardiac pacing that could not be terminated by magnet application or reprogramming would result, and patients required emergent pacemaker removal. Now, the only appreciable risk of pacemaker runaway is related to the use of magnetic resonance imaging, which had been reported to occur due to the intense radiofrequency exposure of the pulse generator.[4] Second, patients who have antitachycardia pacemakers implanted, usually for atrial flutter, can experience acceleration of atrial flutter to atrial fibrillation due to antitachycardia pacing.[5] If atrial fibrillation is associated with more rapid atrioventricular conduction, such patients are at risk for the development of VF.

Finally, myocardial cooling can induce VF. This is often observed early in the cardiac operation, when the patient undergoes cooling on cardiopulmonary bypass.[6] In addition, the fibrillation threshold is dramatically lowered with cooling, making VF more likely. While surface cooling is a successful therapeutic strategy in patients with incessant postoperative junctional ectopic tachycardia,[7] overcooling should be avoided.

Early Postoperative VF

Several general classes of patients who can be considered to be at risk for early postoperative VF can be identified.

Coronary Ischemia

It has been well known for many years that VF can occur in adults during the acute ischemia that occurs during myocardial infarction. While atherosclerotic coronary artery disease is quite rare in children, coronary anomalies do occur with various forms of congenital heart disease, may become significant in the immediate postoperative period. In patients with transposition of the great vessels, the arterial switch procedure involves transplantation of the coronary arteries to the neoaorta. Most commonly with variations in coronary artery origin, but also occasionally with normally arising coronaries, the anastomosis may kink one or both coronary arteries, which leads to ischemia that may manifest immediately or shortly after surgery, leading to VF.[8,9] Similarly, patients with anomalous origin of the left main coronary artery from the pulmonary root, and those with origin of the left main coronary from the right coronary sinus, usually undergo transplantation of the coronary artery to the correct origin, and therefore are also at risk. Patients with tetralogy of Fallot often have associated coronary anomalies, the most prominent being origin of the left anterior descending coronary artery from the right coronary artery, which then crosses the right ventricular outflow tract.[10] While this anomaly is usually identified prior to or during surgery, inadvertent damage to this vessel will lead to ischemia. Patients with pulmonary atresia and intact ventricular septum may develop coronary sinusoids connecting the right ventricular chamber with the coronary arterial circulation, and this may be associated with loss of the normal connection of the coronaries to the aorta.[11] In such patients, surgical decompression of the right ventricle leads to catastrophic cardiac ischemia and, often, intractable VF. Patients with hypoplastic left heart syndrome and aortic valve atresia usually have a very small ascending aorta, which supplies the coronaries retrogradely. In such patients, completion of the first stage of the Norwood operation may distort this small vessel and limit coronary perfusion.[12] Finally, any patient undergoing cardiopulmonary bypass and open heart surgery is at risk for coronary air embolus, usually to the right coronary artery, due to insufficient de-airing at the conclusion of the intracardiac repair. Unexpected VF in the immediate postoperative period in a patient without preexisting coronary anomalies should raise the possibility of coronary air embolus.

Ventricular Hypertrophy

Ventricular hypertrophy is associated with both sudden death and the problem of VF.[13] The mechanism of VF in such patients may involve limitation of subendocardial coronary perfusion, particularly if there is arterial diastolic hypotension in the immediate postoperative period. The increase in risk of VF is most likely quite modest, but it is possible to identify several patient populations for whom there is some concern. Patients with severe aortic stenosis or pulmonic stenosis, particularly those with suprasystemic right ventricular pressures, may be at increased risk. In tetralogy of Fallot, right ventricular hypertrophy as well as a ventriculotomy are created as part of the repair. Similarly, in patients with severe obstructive hypertrophic cardiomyopathy, surgery involves extensive myomectomy, and hypertrophy may be well out of proportion to the degree of obstruction.

Poor Ventricular Function

A low ejection fraction is a major risk factor for sudden death in the adult population.[13] Clearly, poor ventricular function influences the survivability of a patient undergoing major cardiac surgery. Cardiac dysfunction may be due to idiopathic dilated cardiomyopathy or due to myocarditis, chronic incessant tachycardia, or toxins such as alcohol. Cardiopulmonary bypass carries with it a significant risk of postoperative cardiac dysfunction, depending upon the quality of myocardial preservation techniques used by the surgeon. This postoperative cardiac dysfunction, when superimposed on a preexisting cardiomyopathy, may lead to postoperative VF.

Electrolyte Abnormalities

Many forms of electrolyte imbalance may lead to VF in the immediate postoperative period. Of note are extreme hyperkalemia, especially at levels greater than 9 mEq/L, or hypokalemia, especially that associated with hypocalcemia or digoxin toxicity.

Drug-Induced Ventricular Arrhythmias

Various pharmacologic agents may lead to ventricular arrhythmias and VF in the immediate postoperative period. As noted above, digoxin may be associated with VF, although it would be quite unusual in a child in the absence of a massive overdose. Class IA antiarrhythmic agents such as procainamide or quinidine, as well as Class IC agents such as flecainide, may lead to torsades de pointes and ultimately VF, particularly if there are other risk factors present; these risk factors may include electrolyte abnormalities or ventricular dysfunction.[14] Catecholamine infusions may be arrhythmogenic, particularly if large doses of agents such as epinephrine and isoproterenol are used. The latter, if used in high doses, may cause subendocardial ischemia due to the combination of low arterial diastolic pressure, tachycardia with limited diastolic coronary perfusion time, and increased myocardial oxygen demand. Finally, the inhaled anesthetic agent halothane may cause cardiac arrest, particularly if used in conjunction with catecholamines, as halothane is thought to sensitize the myocardium to the effects of catecholamines.[15]

Late Postoperative VF

Unlike the situation during the immediate postoperative period, in which episodes of VF are observed by cardiac monitoring, for late postoperative patients there are very few instances in which the episode of sudden death or aborted sudden death has been recorded, and, therefore, the exact electrophysiological mechanism of sudden death is not proven in many cases. The recordings from the few cases reported, however, as well as some additional information available from patients who have undergone implantation of implantable cardioverter-defibrillators (ICDs), suggest that VF plays a prominent role in such patients. Some information can be gleaned as well from pediatric patients who have survived an episode of cardiac arrest and have gone on to have implantation of an ICD. For example, in 1990 Kron et al[16] reported on 40 young patients who underwent implantation of an ICD, and identified only three who had had repaired congenital heart disease. Subsequently, Silka et al[2] reported the experience with 125 young patients in the US who had undergone ICD implantation, noting that 22 (17.6%) were patients who had repaired congenital heart disease. Of these 22, nine had a Mustard procedure for transposition of the great vessels, 5 had repaired tetralogy of Fallot, and 5 were status post surgery for aortic valve stenosis.

Atrial Flutter and Atrial Repair of Congenital Heart Disease

In 1985, Garson et al[17] reported the national experience with 380 young patients who presented with atrial flutter. Notably, fully 73% of these patients had previously undergone repair or palliation of congenital heart disease. Furthermore, there was a 10% incidence of sudden death in this group. While most of these patients who died suddenly did not have electrocardiographic recordings at the time of death, for several there was documentation of atrial flutter as the initiating factor for VF. The incidence of sudden death was highest in those with complex repaired congenital heart defects such as the Mustard procedure for transposition of the great vessels and the Fontan procedure for various forms of single ventricle and tricuspid atresia. The incidence was also higher in those for whom an antiarrhythmic agent could not be found that controlled the episodes of atrial flutter.

Silka et al[2] report a case that documents the relationship of atrial flutter to VF in a postoperative patient. A 9-year-old patient who had previously undergone repair of partially anomalous pulmonary venous return had an episode of documented VF while playing at school. Following implantation of an ICD, electrocardiographic recording of an episode showed progression from atrial tachycardia with 2:1 conduction to 1:1 conduction and thereafter to VF.

Acceleration of Atrial Flutter by Antitachycardia Pacing

Rhodes et al[5] report their experience with antitachycardia pacing in a series of 18 postoperative patients with intraatrial reentry (atrial flutter), two of whom died suddenly. One patient who died was wearing a Holter monitor during the episode, and this clearly documented the onset of atrial flutter, several attempts by the pacemaker to terminate the episode by atrial burst pacing, acceleration to atrial fibrillation with rapid ventricular rate, and finally, VF. This experience has, to some extent, called into the question the utility and safety of antitachycardia pacing as the primary therapeutic strategy for late postoperative atrial flutter. Certainly, the experience suggests that, at the very least, patients undergoing implantation of antitachycardia pacemakers have concomitant treatment with an agent that will limit atrioventricular function in the event of an atrial tachyarrhythmia.

Postoperative Tetralogy of Fallot

From the very beginning of the experience with complete repair of tetralogy of Fallot, sudden death late after repair has been noted.[1,18,19] One important early report (by Garson et al[20]) estimated the incidence of sudden death at 3.4%, but also noted an incidence of 30% among postoperative repaired tetralogy of Fallot patients with extremely frequent PVCs. Subsequent studies have set the true incidence somewhat lower, closer to 1.4% when multiple large studies are collated.[21] The shift to a lower incidence is partly explained by a more recent trend toward repair at a younger age, which most likely reduces the risk of sudden death. In a large study of a cohort of patients undergoing corrective surgery for tetralogy of Fallot, in Toronto, Nollert et al[22] found that the incidence of sudden death was 0.24% per year for the first 25 years following repair, but increased significantly, to 0.91% per year, in patients followed beyond 25 years.[22] The risk therefore increases in older patients, and may reflect the effect of other risk factors that accumulates over time.

Other risk factors for sudden death have been reported. Poor right ventricular hemodynamics are often seen in patients who have VT and have survived a VF arrest. Garson et al[20] report that a right ventricular systolic pressure greater than 60 mm Hg or a right ventricular end-diastolic pressure greater than 8 mm Hg increase the risk of sudden death.[20] Severe pulmonic regurgitation, as assessed echocardiographically in a study by Zahka et al,[23] was found to be the most important risk factor for sudden death. Pulmonary regurgitation primarily raises the end-diastolic pressure, and this was more important in this study than residual ventricular obstruction. Finally, several reports note the association of a markedly prolonged QRS duration with an elevated risk of sudden death in patients with tetralogy of Fallot.[24-26] Gatzoulis et al[24] note that the critical value is 180 milliseconds, and that patients with QRS durations greater than 180 milliseconds are at a significantly increased risk of sudden death. The mechanism by which QRS prolongation increases the risk of sudden death is unclear. One may speculate that it is a direct result of disordered ventricular activation and, therefore, disordered repolarization.[26,27] Alternatively, a prolonged QRS duration may simply be a marker for a more important risk factor such as extreme right ventricular dilation or extensive right ventricular outflow tract myomectomy.

Unfortunately, despite a great deal of early enthusiasm for the use of electrophysiological studies in postoperative patients, such studies have not been shown to be particularly helpful in the management of the condition and in the prevention of sudden death in this patient population. In a national study by Chandar et al,[28] of 359 postoperative patients with tetralogy of Fallot, all of whom underwent invasive electrophysiologic study, VT was inducible in 17%, none of whom went on to have sudden death. Late sudden death occurred in 5 of the 359 (1.4%), of whom none had a positive electrophysiological study.

Conclusions

Sudden death following surgery for congenital heart disease continues to be a problem for pediatric cardiologists and, of course, their patients. Large cooperative studies are beginning to identify patient subgroups who may be at risk of sudden death and, hopefully, careful prospective trials will begin to answer the question of how to prevent this catastrophic complication of otherwise successful surgery for congenital heart disease.

References

1. Quattlebaum TG, Varghese PJ, Neill CA, et al. Sudden death among postoperative patients with tetralogy of Fallot. A follow-up study of 243 patients for an average of twelve years. *Circulation* 1976;54:289–293.
2. Silka MJ, Kron J, Dunnigan A, et al. Sudden cardiac death and the use of implantable cardioverter-defibrillators in pediatric patients. The Pediatric Electrophysiology Society. *Circulation* 1993;87:800–807.
3. Mickley H, Andersen C, Nielsen LH. Runaway pacemaker: A still existing complication and therapeutic guidelines. *Clin Cardiol* 1989;12:412–414.
4. Fontaine JM, Mohamed FB, Gottlieb C, et al. Rapid ventricular pacing in a pacemaker patient undergoing magnetic resonance imaging [In Process Citation]. *PACE* 1998;21:1336–1339.
5. Rhodes LA, Walsh EP, Gamble WJ, et al. Benefits and potential risks of atrial antitachycardia pacing after repair of congenital heart disease. *PACE* 1995;18:1005–1016.
6. Mortensen E, Berntsen R, Tveita T, et al. Changes in ventricular fibrillation threshold during acute hypothermia. A model for future studies. *J Basic Clin Physiol Pharmacol* 1993;4:313–319.
7. Bash SE, Shah JJ, Albers WH, et al. Hypothermia for the treatment of postsurgical greatly accelerated junctional ectopic tachycardia. *J Am Coll Cardiol* 1987;10:1095–1099.
8. Mayer JE Jr, Sanders SP, Jonas RA, et al. Coronary artery pattern and outcome of arterial switch operation for transposition of the great arteries. *Circulation* 1990;82:IV139-IV145.
9. Tamisier D, Ouaknine R, Pouard P, et al. Neonatal arterial switch operation: Coronary artery patterns and coronary events. *Eur J Cardiothorac Surg* 1997;11:810–817.
10. Carvalho JS, Silva CM, Rigby ML, et al. Angiographic diagnosis of anomalous coronary artery in tetralogy of Fallot. *Br Heart J* 1993;70:75–78.

11. Freedom RM, Wilson G, Trusler GA, et al. Pulmonary atresia and intact ventricular septum. *Scand J Thorac Cardiovasc Surg* 1983;17:1–28.
12. Bartram U, Grunenfelder J, Van Praagh R. Causes of death after the modified Norwood procedure: A study of 122 postmortem cases. *Ann Thorac Surg* 1997;64:1795–1802.
13. Stevenson WG, Sweeney MO. Arrhythmias and sudden death in heart failure. *Jpn Circ J* 1997;61:727–740.
14. Fish FA, Gillette PC, Benson DW Jr. Proarrhythmia, cardiac arrest and death in young patients receiving encainide and flecainide. The Pediatric Electrophysiology Group [see comments]. *J Am Coll Cardiol* 1991;18: 356–365.
15. Katz RL, Bigger JT Jr. Cardiac arrhythmias during anesthesia and operation. *Anesthesiology* 1970;33:193–213.
16. Kron J, Oliver RP, Norsted S, et al. The automatic implantable cardioverter-defibrillator in young patients. *J Am Coll Cardiol* 1990;16:896–902.
17. Garson AJ, Bink BM, Hesslein PS, et al. Atrial flutter in the young: A collaborative study of 380 cases. *J Am Coll Cardiol* 1985;6:871–878.
18. Marin-Garcia J, Moller JH. Sudden death after operative repair of tetralogy of Fallot. *Br Heart J* 1977;39:1380–1385.
19. Gillette PC, Yeoman MA, Mullins CE, et al. Sudden death after repair of tetralogy of Fallot. Electrocardiographic and electrophysiologic abnormalities. *Circulation* 1977;56:566–571.
20. Garson A Jr, Randall DC, Gillette PC, et al. Prevention of sudden death after repair of tetralogy of Fallot: Treatment of ventricular arrhythmias. *J Am Coll Cardiol* 1985;6:221–227.
21. Wren C. Late postoperative arrhythmias. In Wren C, Campbell RWF (eds): *Paediatric Cardiac Arrhythmias*. Oxford: Oxford University Press; 1996:238–259.
22. Nollert G, Fischlein T, Bouterwek S, et al. Long-term survival in patients with repair of tetralogy of Fallot: 36-year follow-up of 490 survivors of the first year after surgical repair [see comments]. *J Am Coll Cardiol* 1997; 30:1374–1383.
23. Zahka KG, Horneffer PJ, Rowe SA, et al. Long-term valvular function after total repair of tetralogy of Fallot. Relation to ventricular arrhythmias. *Circulation* 1988;78:III14-III19.
24. Gatzoulis MA, Till JA, Somerville J, et al. Mechanoelectrical interaction in tetralogy of Fallot. QRS prolongation relates to right ventricular size and predicts malignant ventricular arrhythmias and sudden death [see comments]. *Circulation* 1995;92:231–237.
25. Balaji S, Lau YR, Case CL, et al. QRS prolongation is associated with inducible ventricular tachycardia after repair of tetralogy of Fallot. *Am J Cardiol* 1997;80:160–163.
26. Gatzoulis MA, Till JA, Redington AN. Depolarization-repolarization inhomogeneity after repair of tetralogy of Fallot. The substrate for malignant ventricular tachycardia? *Circulation* 1997;95:401- 404.
27. Berul CI, Sweeten TL, Dubin AM, et al. Use of the rate-corrected JT interval for prediction of repolarization abnormalities in children. *Am J Cardiol* 1994;74:1254–1257.
28. Chandar JS, Wolff GS, Garson AJ, et al. Ventricular arrhythmias in postoperative tetralogy of Fallot. *Am J Cardiol* 1990;65:655–661.

Section V

Treatment of Pediatric Ventricular Fibrillation

Chapter 11

Ion Channels
and Ventricular Fibrillation

Glenn T. Wetzel, MD, PhD

Introduction

Over the past decade, knowledge of the genetics, structure, and physiology of cardiac sarcolemmal ion channels has grown exponentially as a result of molecular approaches to identifying, cloning, and expressing wildtype and mutant ion channel genes. Perhaps the ultimate achievement of this approach, in regards to ventricular fibrillation (VF), is exemplified by the identification of specific ion channel defects associated with the long QT syndrome and familial VF.[1] However, the precise relationship between ion channel function and clinical VF remains an enigma. As a result, the treatment of VF has depended on a strictly empirical clinical approach. Further progress in the identification of risk factors and the treatment of VF is likely to be accelerated by using approaches specifically directed by a detailed understanding of the mechanisms that produce and sustain VF. The present understanding of the relationships between ion channel function and VF is not sufficient to provide significant insight into the mechanisms involved in the initiation and maintenance of VF to assist with clinical care of pediatric patients. Accordingly, the goal of this chapter is to introduce the reader to recent advances and new concepts in cardiac cellular electrophysiology that may provide the framework for future therapeutic approaches to VF in pediatric patients.

From: Quan L, Franklin WH (eds). *Ventricular Fibrillation: A Pediatric Problem.* Armonk, NY: Futura Publishing Company, Inc.; ©2000.

Supported in part by the American Heart Association, Greater Los Angeles Affiliate, Grant 829 GI, the National Institutes of Health, Grant HL-02723, the Laubisch Fund, the Variety Club, and the J.H. Nicholson Endowment.

A Paradigm For VF

In seeking to develop a detailed understanding of the mechanism of VF, it is critical to consider the various levels of physiology that are involved in VF. Figure 1 presents a paradigm for VF that emphasizes the hierarchical nature of the mechanisms involved in the generation of VF. Clinical and laboratory observations have led to the elucidation of many risk factors for the development of VF.[2-4] These risk factors can be loosely categorized as congenital (eg, congenital heart disease), acquired (hypertrophy or drug side effect), or functional (R on T phenomenon) risk factors. Each of these risk factors appears to exert its influence at a subcellular organizational level by mediating changes in the function of any one of a series of sarcolemmal ion channels. At the cellular level, the summation of the individual ion channel and ion pump activities results in the development of the action potential. Since the ionic current passing through many of these channels is voltage sensitive, the cardiac action potential exerts a feedback effect on ion channel function. At the tissue level, propagation of action potential depolarizations from cell to cell can be characterized in terms of conduction velocity and refractoriness of the tissue. Finally, the interactions between these propagating waves with anatomic factors at the organ level (areas of inhomogeneous, absent, or slowed conduction resulting from histologic and metabolic factors) results in reentry and VF. This paradigm demon-

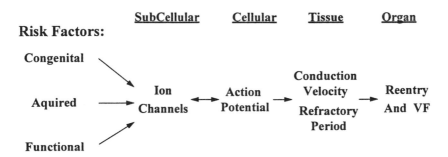

Figure 1. A paradigm for ventricular fibrillation (VF). VF can be considered the clinical manifestation of a series of processes that occur at several physiological levels. The known risk factors for VF generally have their effect at the subcellular level by modifying ion channel function. However, the initiation and maintenance of VF is dependent on the interactions between electrophysiological processes at each of these levels.

strates the multiple steps separating the effects of the risk factors on the ion channels and the final clinically observed response of VF. However, in order to move beyond an empirical approach for treating VF, a very precise understanding of the relationships between each of these factors must be developed.

Models of the Cardiac Action Potential

In 1994, Luo and Rudy[5] published a mathematical model for ionic currents in cardiac ventricular myocytes that incorporated consideration of dynamic changes in intracellular ionic concentrations and ionic fluxes, particularly those involving intracellular Ca^{2+}. They demonstrated that such a model can be used to simulate the generation of the cardiac action potential, including such arrhythmogenic phenomena as afterdepolarizations and triggered activity. Their model includes the interactions of 15 distinct ionic currents, pumps, and exchangers involved in the generation of the action potential and Ca^{2+} homeostasis in the cell. To add to the complexity of the model, each of these ionic fluxes has its own time- and voltage-dependent characteristics. Furthermore, many of these ionic fluxes exhibit significant age-dependent changes in expression.[6] Finally, the parameters that characterize these ionic fluxes each exhibit complex regulation by multiple factors in the local cell environment (ionic concentrations, chemical mediators such as cyclic adenosine monophosphate, adenosine triphosphate [ATP], pH and G-proteins, etc.).

The Luo-Rudy model used the known characteristics of many of these ionic currents to generate a mathematical model of the action potential and to describe the individual currents that play a major role in its formation. Figure 2 is reproduced from the work of Luo and Rudy,[5] and shows an action potential and the time course of each of the major currents involved in generating the cardiac action potential. This result demonstrates that despite the previously described complexity of the factors involved in the generation of the action potential, knowledge of the characteristics of the individual ion channels has developed to such an extent that it is now possible to predict the effects of specific modifications of ion channel function on the action potential. However, the application of these models of the action potential to VF is limited by the lack of a clear understanding of the relationships between action potential characteristics and the tissue conduction properties that initiate VF.

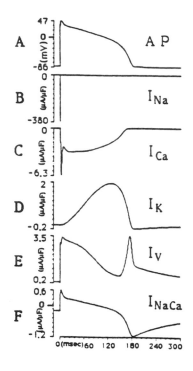

Figure 2. Major ionic currents that determine the shape of the action potential. A. Luo and Rudy used a mathematical model of the major ionic currents in a cardiac ventricular myocyte to calculate the configuration of the action potential (AP). B through F. The traces indicate the amplitude and time course of the fast Na+ current (I_{Na}; B), the L-type Ca2+ current (I_{Ca}; C), the repolarizing K+ current (I_K; D), the total time-independent current (I_V; E), and the Na+-Ca2+ exchange current (I_{NaCa}; F). Modified from Reference 5, with permission.

Ion Channels as Risk Factors for Ventricular Arrhythmias

Despite the previously described difficulties involved in attempts to model VF based on known ion channel characteristics, several recent reports provide examples of specific situations in which there is a clear link between ionic channel function and ventricular arrhythmias.

The long QT syndrome is probably the most widely studied example of defects in ion channel function resulting in malignant ventricular arrhythmias. The long QT syndrome is a disorder of cardiac repolarization associated with prolongation of the electrocardiographic QT interval, a specific and unusual form of ventricular arrhythmia called torsades de pointes, and a high incidence of syncope and sudden cardiac death. Specific genetic defects have been identified in familial cases of the long QT syndrome, including mutations in three potassium channel genes (*KVLQT1, HERG*, and *minK*) and a sodium channel gene (*SCN5A*). Other variants of the long QT syndrome are known to exist and are expected to also involve defects in ion channel function that result in prolongation of the action potential.[7] The electrophysiological consequences of mutations in these genes has been studied extensively.[7] Each of the reported mutations results in a weakening of the net repolarizing current during the plateau of the action potential. Prolongation of the action potential results in a prolongation of the QT interval on recordings of the surface electrocardiogram (ECG) and early afterdepolarizations on recording of cardiac monophasic action potentials. However, despite this recent advance in the determination of the genetic etiology of the long QT syndrome, the specific mechanisms by which these ion channel defects result in clinically significant arrhythmias have not been established.

A second example of ion channel defects resulting in VF is provided by a recent study of a familial form of VF associated with characteristic ECG findings (right bundle branch block and ST segment elevation in the anterior precordial leads).[8] Three new mutations of the gene for the *SCN5A* Na$^+$ channel are described in three families. One of these mutations has been found to shorten the time constant of recovery from inactivation of the Na$^+$ current. Another mutation produces an in-frame stop codon that terminates the synthesis of the sodium channel at the pore region of domain III and appears to result in a nonfunctional channel. The functional consequences of the third mutant have not been described.

The association with each of these mutations with ECG changes and clinically significant arrhythmias seems well established. However, the precise mechanism by which these mutants effect action potential morphology and increase the prevalence of specific malignant arrhythmias is not clear. For example, some mutations associated with the long QT syndrome result in an *increase* in delayed depolarizing currents (prolongation of inward *SCN5A* Na$^+$ current in *LQT3*). In contrast, one of the mutations in *SCN5A* associated with VF is expected to result in a *decrease* in inward Na$^+$ current. The differences in phenotype between these two diseases may be readily explained by the opposing effects of these mutants on the *SCN5A* channel. However, the reported mutant in *SCN5A* described above results in a shortening of the time constant of recovery of the Na$^+$ channel from inactivation. This mutation might be expected to exhibit an *increase* in Na$^+$ current, but its phenotype is that of idiopathic VF rather than the long QT syndrome.

Another example of the role of ion channels in VF is that of intracellular calcium overload. Specifically, in the case of digoxin toxicity, it is known that by inhibiting the sodium-potassium ATPase, digoxin toxicity results in a decrease in intracellular potassium and an increase in intracellular sodium. Increased intracellular Na^+ then results in an increase in intracellular calcium as a result of the inhibition of sodium-calcium exchange. Finally, calcium overload is associated with initiating and sustaining VF, activating calcium-sensitive ion channels, inducing triggered activity via delayed afterdepolarizations, and increasing tissue metabolic load.

Ion Channels and the Treatment of VF

VF has long been believed to result from multiple simultaneous reentry circuits in the myocardium. Since such complex reentry is dependent on differences in refractoriness between myocytes within the various reentry circuits, one approach to treating VF has been based on an attempt to decrease the dispersal of refractoriness within the heart. This has been done using empirical medical therapy with a wide variety of agents. Recent approaches to medical therapy for arrhythmias have attempted to direct therapy based on the known effects of the medications on ion channel activity, cell membrane receptors, or intracellular signaling.[9] However, little progress has been made in the treatment of VF in the pediatric population, perhaps in part due to the previously described complexity of the relationship between these subcellular components and clinical arrhythmias. Current models of VF do not allow for a complete picture of the role of ion channels in its treatment. Some investigators have suggested that therapy for the long QT syndrome may be able to be tailored to the specific genetic defect or phenotype.[10] However, the safety and effectiveness of such tailored therapy have not been established.

A similar difficulty exists in terms of nonmedical therapy for VF. A growing body of knowledge is being acquired in regard to defibrillation therapy for VF. This is occurring as a result of the increasing use of implantable defibrillator devices in the pediatric population as well as the increased recognition of the prevalence of the long QT syndrome in the differential diagnosis of syncope or seizures. Little is known, however, regarding the role of specific ion channels in defibrillator therapy. Some investigators have recently advocated the use of biphasic defibrillator discharges, and such an approach may have a theoretical basis. A biphasic waveform may result in an initial repolarization of the cell membrane potential that is expected to enhance cardiac sodium channel recovery from inactivation. The subsequent depolarization phase would then result in the activation (opening) of the sodium channels and stimulate a synchronous action potential throughout the heart.[11]

New Concepts

Recent reports have described recordings of VF from a two-dimensional array of electrodes in direct contact with the ventricular epicardium. These studies suggest that VF is the result of multiple, interacting spiral waves randomly propagating through the myocardium.[12] Comparable studies have been performed in a mathematical model of the heart using a two-dimensional array of virtual cells. In these computer models, each virtual cell exhibits electrophysiological characteristics derived from the Luo-Rudy model of the action potential in a single cell. Interestingly, the mathematical model exhibits many of the findings described for VF in tissue preparations.[13] Premature "stimuli" introduced during the repolarization phase of the action potential can induce a spiral wave. This spiral wave may continue as a stable "ventricular tachycardia" (see Figure 4, panel E). However, when different parameters are used for the action potential model, the spiral wave begins to break up spontaneously and degenerates to a pattern of multiple smaller waves (see Figure 4, panel D) that are very similar in appearance to the recordings of VF described above.[13] The similarities between these models suggest that computer models may represent a useful way of studying VF.

The degeneration of ventricular tachycardia to VF that occurs in the computer model is also commonly observed in clinical and laboratory models of VF in intact heart. Figure 3 depicts the ECG of a patient

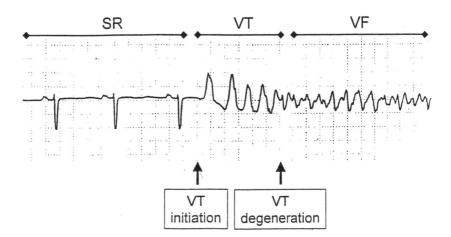

Figure 3. Degeneration of ventricular tachycardia (VT) into ventricular fibrillation (VF). This electrocardiographic strip demonstrates the typical initiation of VF as the result of degeneration of VT. Reprinted from Reference 14, with permission.

who developed VF. The patient is initially in sinus rhythm but then develops a short run of ventricular tachycardia. The ventricular tachycardia can then be seen to degenerate into VF. The observation that VF is frequently the result of degeneration of ventricular tachycardia may be an important clue to understanding the basic mechanisms underlying VF.

VF has generally been considered to be the result of a random combination of multiple localized reentry wavefronts of electrical depolarization throughout the myocardium. However, the computer model can also produce this apparently random pattern of wave, even though there is no randomness to the computer program! That is, each state of the model is completely determined by the previous state of the model. Repeated trials of the model yield identical results unless the initial conditions are changed. Investigators recently attempted to determine whether VF is actually a random process.[13] These reports indicate that VF in intact canine heart, in isolated ventricular septal preparations, or in simulated two-dimensional sheets of cardiac tissue is not random but exhibits quasiperiodicity.[13] This kind of underlying order in the face of an apparently random process has been studied by a mathematical approach termed chaos theory.

Chaos theory has demonstrated that apparently random behavior can be produced by a system exhibiting three or more independent oscillations. Interestingly, multiple levels of oscillations in heart rate have been observed in cardiac preparations immediately prior to the initiation of VF.[13] Thus, mathematical chaos theory may provide a means of explaining how the initiation and maintenance of VF results from oscillation of known physiological processes in human heart.

One such oscillation is the periodicity of spiral wave reentry. Spiral wave reentry is an inherent property of excitable media, as indicated by the computer-generated spiral waves described above. Other oscillatory processes inherent in the generation of an action potential include action potential duration (APD) restitution and tissue conduction velocity restitution.

APD restitution is a way of describing the changes in APD during premature beats. For example, if a premature beat occurs at shorter and shorter diastolic intervals, the APD is decreased (Figure 4, panel A). If APD is plotted as a function of diastolic interval, an APD curve is generated (Figure 4, panel B). Similarly, conduction velocity restitution is derived from a plot of the conduction velocity as a function of diastolic interval. These relationships have important clinical significance, since an increase in the steepness of the APD restitution curve has been associated with the onset of VF.[14] This clinical observation is also demonstrable using a computer model of the heart. With use of a two-dimensional Luo-Rudy model of the heart, APD and conduction

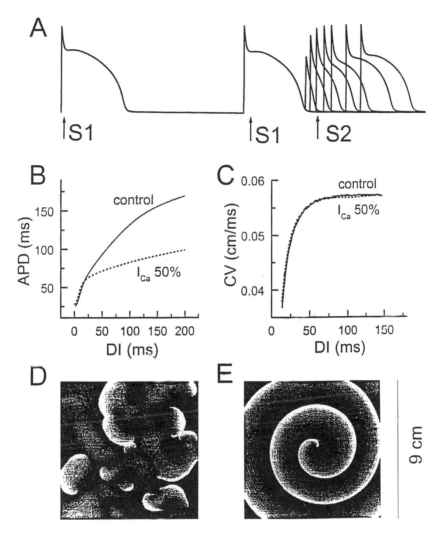

Figure 4. Effects of Ca^{2+} channel blockade in the Luo-Rudy model. A. The introduction of premature stimuli (S2) during a paced rhythm (S1-S1) in a modified version of the Luo-Rudy model of a ventricular myocyte results in a progressive shortening of the action potential duration (APD) as the diastolic interval is decreased. B. An APD restitution curve is obtained by plotting APD as a function of the diastolic interval (DI). Inhibition of the calculated Ca^{2+} current (I_{Ca}) by 50% during the action potential reduces the slope of the APD restitution curve for diastolic intervals greater than 25 ms. C. Inhibition of I_{Ca} by 50% has no effect on conduction velocity (CV) restitution. D and E. Spiral wave reentry is initiated in a two-dimensional model of simulated cardiac tissue. After 5 seconds under control conditions, the spiral wave has degenerated into multiple wavelets similar to those recorded from clinical examples of VF (D). When I_{Ca} is inhibited by 50%, the spiral wave remains intact (E). Reprinted from Reference 14, with permission.

velocity restitution are determined under baseline conditions and when voltage-gated Ca^{2+} channel current has been decreased by 50% (Figure 4, panels B and C). Under control conditions, a premature stimulus initiates a spiral wave which rapidly degenerates into multiple wavefronts resembling fibrillation (Figure 4, panel D). Inhibition of inward Ca^{2+} current by 50% decreases the slope of the APD restitution curve but does not affect conduction velocity restitution. When the slope of the APD restitution curve is decreased, the premature stimulus initiates a stable spiral wave which does not degenerate into fibrillation (Figure 4, panel E). Suppression of the intracellular Ca^{2+} transient by use of intracellular Ca^{2+} buffers does not affect the slope of the APD restitution curve. Comparable results have been reported for recordings of APD in a preparation of isolated ventricular myocytes.[15] These results suggest that specific clinical interventions, such as using calcium channel blockers to decrease the slope of the action potential restitution curve, may have predictable antifibrillatory effects.

Summary

Future advances in antifibrillatory therapy are likely to depend heavily on the development and validation of detailed models of VF at the cellular, tissue, and organ levels. Computer models, spiral waves, chaos theory, and restitution curves may all play important roles in the development of such a detailed model of VF. Such a model may provide a rational approach to manipulation of ion channels to specifically treat patients at risk for VF. From a clinical perspective, such a rational approach will also likely involve clinical trials of drugs specifically directed for the treatment of VF. As specific antifibrillatory therapy is developed for adult patients, additional factors will need to be considered for pediatric patients. Since the ability to sustain a spiral wave is dependent on the amount of tissue involved, heart size may become an important consideration in antifibrillatory therapy in smaller pediatric patients. In addition, the many age-related changes in ionic channel function and metabolism that have been reported may have to be considered in the development of a model of VF specific for pediatric patients.

References

1. Wang Q, Chen Q, Towbin JA. Genetics, molecular mechanisms and management of long QT syndrome. *Ann Med* 1998;30:58–65.
2. Vergara I, Wharton JM. Ventricular tachycardia and fibrillation in normal hearts. *Curr Opin Cardiol* 1998;13:9–19.
3. Mogayzel C, Quan L, Graves J, et al. Out-of-hospital ventricular fibrilla-

tion in children and adolescents: Causes and outcomes. *Ann Emerg Med* 1995;25:484–491.

4. Barinaga M. Tracking down mutations that can stop the heart. *Science* 1998;281:32–34.
5. Luo CH, Rudy Y. A dynamic model of the cardiac ventricular action potential. I. Simulations of ionic currents and concentration changes. *Circ Res* 1994;74:1071–1096.
6. Huynh TV, Chen F, Wetzel GT, et al. Developmental changes in membrane Ca^{2+} and K^+ currents in fetal, neonatal, and adult rabbit ventricular myocytes. *Circ Res* 1992;70:508–515.
7. Wang Q, Shen J, Splawski I, et al. SCN5A mutations associated with an inherited cardiac arrhythmia, long QT syndrome. *Cell* 1995;80:805–811.
8. Chen Q, Kirsch GE, Zhang D, et al. Genetic basis and molecular mechanism for idiopathic ventricular fibrillation. *Nature* 1998;392:293–296.
9. Task Force of the Working Group on Arrhythmias of the European Society of Cardiology. The Sicilian gambit: A new approach to the classification of antiarrhythmic drugs based on their actions on arrhythmogenic mechanisms. *Circulation* 1991;84:1831–1851.
10. Moss AJ. The long QT syndrome revisited: Current understanding and implications for treatment. *PACE* 1997;20:2879–2881. Editorial.
11. Walcott GP, Knisley SB, Zhou X, et al. On the mechanism of ventricular defibrillation. *PACE* 1997;20:422–431.
12. Chen PS, Garfinkel A, Weiss JN, et al. Spirals, chaos, and new mechanisms of wave propagation. *PACE* 1997;20:414–421.
13. Garfinkel A, Chen PS, Walter DO, et al. Quasiperiodicity and chaos in cardiac fibrillation [see comments]. *J Clin Invest* 1997;99:305–314.
14. Weiss JN, Garfinkel A, Karagueuzian HS, et al. Chaos and the transition to ventricular fibrillation: A new approach to antiarrhythmic drug evaluation. *Circulation* 1999;99:2819–2826.
15. Goldhaber JI, Qu Z, Garfinkel A, et al. Determinants of action potential duration restitution in isolated ventricular myocytes. *Circulation* 1997; 96(suppl l):I672.

Chapter 12

Pediatric Defibrillation

Dianne L. Atkins, MD

Introduction

Life-threatening arrhythmias are less common in the pediatric population than in the adult population, and thus the need for emergent defibrillation occurs less frequently in the pediatric population. Differences in body size, body composition, and chest configuration potentially affect optimum defibrillation technique and success rates. Unfortunately, there is a distressing paucity of experimental data concerning appropriate equipment and energy dose for pediatric defibrillation, in marked contrast to the extensive studies documenting efficacy, safety, dose, and proper technique in adult patients.[1–5] Lack of data and infrequency of use have led to a fear of defibrillation in children. As recently as 1985, emergency medical technicians were instructed to withhold defibrillation in children until receiving specific medical authorization.[6]

Transthoracic Impedance

Transthoracic impedance is the major determinant of current flow during defibrillation. Average impedance values in adults range from 50 to 70 Ω.[7] In adults, larger electrode surface area decreases transthoracic impedance and larger chest width increases transthoracic impedance.[4,7] Using a test pulse technique that permits measurement of transthoracic impedance without actually delivering a shock,[8] we measured transthoracic impedance in a pediatric outpatient population.[9] Body weight and body surface area were statistically correlated with transthoracic impedance but the correlations were not sufficiently great to be clinically useful (Table 1). Rather, electrode size was the major de-

From: Quan L, Franklin WH (eds). *Ventricular Fibrillation: A Pediatric Problem.* Armonk, NY: Futura Publishing Company, Inc.; ©2000.

Table 1

Transthoracic Impedance and its Determinants

Determinant and Paddle Size	*r* Value	*p* Value
Weight		
Pediatric	0.52	<0.01
Adult	0.47	<0.05
Body surface area		
Pediatric	0.49	<0.01
Adult	044	<0.05
Interelectrode distance		
Pediatric	0.39	<0.05
Adult	0.23	NS

Reproduced from Reference 9, by permission of *Pediatrics.*

terminant of transthoracic impedance (Figure 1). Standard adult electrodes (surface area: 83 cm^2) halved transthoracic impedance, compared with pediatric electrodes (surface area: 21 cm^2) in infants and
children (57±11 Ω versus 108±24 Ω; $P<0.05$).

We have demonstrated similar relationships during actual shock delivery (Figure 2).[10] Twenty pediatric patients received 55 shocks, 38 delivered with pediatric electrode paddles and 18 with adult electrode pad-

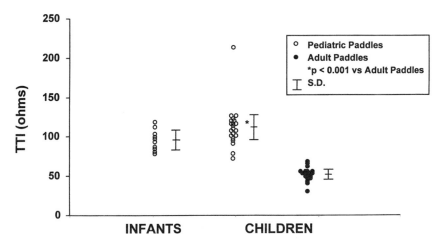

Figure 1. Effect of paddle electrode size on transthoracic impedance (TTI.) Pediatric paddles = 21 cm^2; adult paddles = 83 cm^2; bar indicates mean and
standard deviation. From Atkins DL, Sirna S. Kieso, R, Kerber RE. Pediatric defibrillation: Importance of paddle size in determining transthoracic impedance.
Pediatrics 82:914–918, 1988. Reproduced by permission of *Pediatrics.*

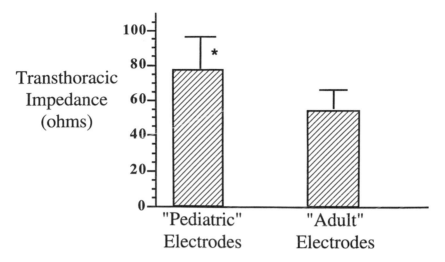

Figure 2. Transthoracic impedance by electrode size. N=55 shocks, 38 with pediatric electrode paddles (21 cm²), 18 with adult electrode paddles (83 cm²). *P<0.0008 compared with adult electrode paddles. From Atkins DL, Kerber, RE. Pediatric defibrillation: Current flow is improved by using "adult" electrode paddles. *Pediatrics* 94:90–93, 1994. Reproduced by permission of *Pediatrics.*

dles. Total energy delivered with the pediatric and adult electrodes did not differ. However, because the transthoracic impedance was significantly lower with the adult electrode paddles, peak current flow was 25% greater with the adult electrode paddles (Figure 3). Although we were unable to demonstrate a difference in shock success based on current flow due to the small number of patients, such a relationship has been demonstrated in adult patients.[11] Adult patients with high impedances had lower success rates when initially given shocks of 100 J, and a clear relationship between shock success and peak current was demonstrated for ventricular fibrillation, atrial fibrillation, and atrial flutter.

Energy Dose

There are no human experimental data to identify the appropriate energy dose for defibrillation. The correct energy dose is one that will maximize defibrillation and minimize myocardial damage and other complications. Consensus and experience of pediatric cardiologists have determined current recommendations of 2 to 4 J/kg. Gutgesell et al[12] reviewed 71 defibrillation attempts in 27 children and found that 91% of shocks delivered within 10 J above or below 2 J/kg successfully defibrillated the patients (Figure 4). Only two patients received dosages

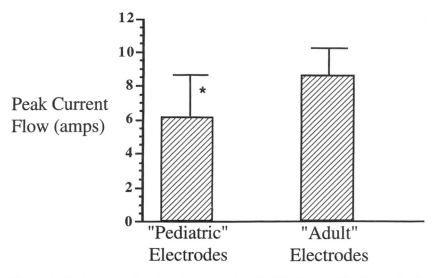

Figure 3. Peak current flow by electrode size. N=55 shocks, 38 with pediatric electrode paddles (21 cm^2), 18 with adult electrode paddles (83 cm^2). *P<0.0002 compared with adults electrode paddles. From Atkins DL, Kerber, RE. Pediatric defibrillation: Current flow is improved by using "adult" electrode paddles. *Pediatrics* 94:90–93, 1994. Reproduced by permission of *Pediatrics.*

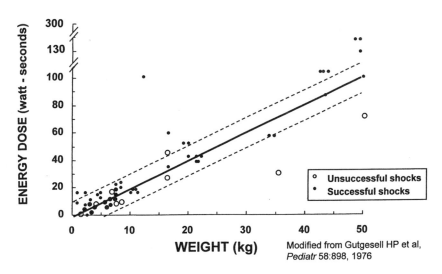

Figure 4. Relationship of energy dose versus body weight during pediatric defibrillation. Solid line represents energy dose of 2 J/kg; area between dotted lines represents 10 J above and below this dose. Modified from Gutgesell HP et al. Energy dose for ventricular defibrillation of children. *Pediatrics* 58:898, 1976.

substantially less than 2 J/kg, and they were not successfully defibrillated. This report, however, concentrated on effectiveness rather than toxicity. Twelve patients received energy dosages greater than 2 J/kg and 11 were effectively defibrillated, although final outcome was not reported. Animal studies have shown that the energy threshold for defibrillation ranged from 0.5 to 10 J/kg, with the energy requirement per kilogram increasing with body weight.[13] Animal studies have also shown that dosages even up to 10 J/kg result in a less than 25% risk of myocardial damage and in no risk of death from the shock alone.[14]

Electrode Size

The American Heart Association recommends that adult electrode pads be 8 to 10 cm in diameter and that "pediatric" electrodes be 4.5 cm. The Association for the Advancement of Medical Instrumentation recommends that the minimum contact area for adult electrodes be 50 cm^2, and 15 cm^2 for pediatric electrodes.[15] There are no human studies to suggest ideal size for infants and children. Patel and Galysh[16] suggested that 5-cm electrodes were appropriate for pediatric use, based on their study in dogs weighing less than 9 kg. Transthoracic impedance, delivered energy, and peak voltage were inversely proportional to diameter, with excessive energy and voltage delivered using electrodes less than 3 cm. By measuring intracardiac voltage gradients as a parameter of intracardiac current, Pagan-Carlo et al[17] demonstrated that there is no simple relationship between body size or habitus to predict an electrode size that would maximize intracardiac current. Since transthoracic impedance in children is lower and similar to adult values with the larger electrodes, the larger electrodes should be used even in young children weighing more than 10 to 15 kg.[9,10]

Self-adhesive electrodes are widely available and are equivalent to hand-held electrodes in adults in terms of transthoracic impedance and shock success.[18] They offer several advantages over the standard hand-held electrodes, including constant position, incorporation of a coupling agent as part of the pad, unimpeded access to the patient, and increased safety to the operator. Although the pads are marketed in a pediatric size, 5.8 cm^2, there are little data to support any one diameter as superior. We have shown that transthoracic impedance is directly related to pad diameter.[19] Pad diameter less than 5.8 cm resulted in impedances that were greater than 97 Ω, which, in adults, predict low rate of defibrillation (Figure 5).[8] Twenty-one of 25 children had transthoracic impedance of less than 97 Ω when pad diameter was 7 cm. If pad diameter was greater than 8 cm, the transthoracic impedance was al-

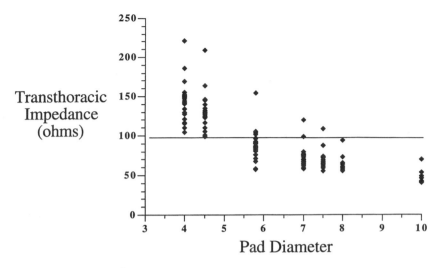

Figure 5. Effect of paddle diameter on transthoracic impedance of self-adhesive electrode pads. Horizontal line indicates a value of 97 Ω, approximately 1 SD about the adult mean transthoracic impedance value. From Samson RA, Atkins DL, Kerber RE. Optimal size of self-adhesive preapplied electrode pads in pediatric defibrillation *Am J Cardiol* 75:544–545, 1995. Reproduced by permission of *Am J Cardiol.*

ways less than 97 Ω. Thus, we recommended a pad diameter of 5.8 cm for infants, and one of at least 7 cm for children.

Electrode Position

The most commonly used position is the apex-anterior position, although the anterior-posterior position may improve current flow. The anterior-posterior position has not received wide clinical acceptance because of the difficulty of placing the posterior electrode. Self-adhesive pads make the anterior-posterior position more reasonable, especially for use during electrophysiological studies. They also allow larger electrodes to be used in young children. Placement over pacemakers and implanted defibrillators must be avoided.

The appropriate electrode position has been difficult to determine experimentally. We found no significant relationship between interelectrode distance and transthoracic impedance when both paddles were placed in an apex-anterior position in infants and children, even when the electrodes were very close (1.5 to 4 cm).[9] Caterine and colleagues[20] have shown that interelectrode distances of less than 2 cm decrease transthoracic impedance in adults, but that current traversing the heart is decreased by approximately 10%.

Defibrillator Design for Pediatric Use

All defibrillators should provide flexibility for pediatric use. The requirements for pediatric use include a broad range of energy selection. Energy levels of 2, 3, 5, 10, 20, 30, 50, and 70 J provide a reasonable range for patients who weigh 1 to 50 kg. Conversion to pediatric electrodes should be simple. In this author's experience, the easiest design is one in which the pediatric electrodes are directly beneath the adult electrodes. If the pediatric electrodes are needed, the adult plates can be removed quickly. This design also improves accessibility and storage. Defibrillators that have entirely separate electrode pediatric paddles and cables potentially increase delay in instituting defibrillation and risk loss of the pediatric attachments.

Complications

Pathologic examination of cardiac specimens after electric countershock has shown mitochondrial disruption,[21–23] contraction-band necrosis,[24] and subepicardial coagulation and necrosis.[21] The extent of damage depends on energy dose,[25] electrode size,[21] and recurrent shocks.[24] Analysis of effects that may be specific to the immature myocardium is limited. In one study, technetium-99m pyrophosphate uptake in piglets was not increased until shocks of 150 J/kg were given.[26] However, when autopsied specimens from children who had received electric countershocks were examined, contraction-band necrosis was present in all and focal hemorrhages and epicardial coagulation were observed in the majority of specimens.[25] These findings were accentuated when catecholamines had been administered during resuscitation efforts. Clearly, the significance of these data is unclear because preexisting conditions and the effects of resuscitation cannot be controlled.

More recent data evaluating potential cardiac damage from direct countershock indicate that myocardial damage is limited. Specific indicators of cardiac damage, cardiac troponin I and T, are either normal or minimally elevated after defibrillation or cardioversion.[27–30] Significant elevations probably indicate myocardial damage unrelated to direct current shock.

Skin erythema and tenderness are often observed after defibrillation. Skin biopsies demonstrate epidermal necrosis and upper dermal perivascular inflammation. The severity of these findings is a function of peak and cumulative shock energy.[31] Skin sloughing is rare.

If the coupling gel is smeared across the chest between the electrodes, a low-impedance pathway over the chest surface develops and current is shunted away from the heart.[20] This problem can be avoided with application of the gel directly to the paddles instead of to the chest. The chest should be wiped off in between shocks.

The risk of thromboembolism is substantial in adults with atrial fibrillation of greater than 23 hours' duration. Most patients receive anticoagulation for several weeks prior to elective cardioversion. Such therapy has not been standard for patients with atrial flutter, as thromboembolic events are thought to be rare. There are, however, increasing reports of embolic events following cardioversion of chronic atrial flutter.[32-34] In an adult population with chronic atrial flutter, 6% had thromboembolic events during atrial flutter or after cardioversion to sinus rhythm.[32] The risk of thromboembolism declined with effective anticoagulation. In pediatric patients with poor ventricular function or significant atrial surgery, anticoagulation should be considered prior to cardioversion.

Indications for Pediatric Defibrillation

Infants and children experience virtually all of the rhythm disorders observed in adults, with differing frequencies, but the indications for defibrillation (or cardioversion) are not different. Children with ventricular fibrillation need immediate defibrillation. Once ventricular fibrillation has been documented, airway and vascular access should be delayed until the child has received three shocks. Wide-complex tachycardias are more likely to be ventricular tachycardia than supraventricular tachycardia, and should be treated as such. Pharmacologic manipulation of a wide-complex tachycardia should be undertaken only when the mechanism of the tachycardia is known, or by a physician who is knowledgeable about complex cardiac rhythms. Cardioversion with appropriate anesthesia is a much safer option for primary care providers.

Supraventricular tachycardias are the most common rhythm abnormalities in children, but life-threatening hemodynamic compromise is uncommon in children with normal hearts. Typically, this rhythm can be terminated with vagal maneuvers or the newer pharmacologic agents, especially adenosine and verapamil for the older child. However, cardioversion is always an acceptable alternative if there is any reluctance to treat pharmacologically. Complex atrial tachyarrhythmias are increasingly recognized in the pediatric population, especially in patients who have undergone extensive atrial surgery for congenital heart disease. Hemodynamic compromise is more common because of the underlying anatomic and physiological abnormalities. The indications for cardioversion are the same as for supraventricular tachycardia. Consideration should be given to anticoagulation and to prevention of severe bradycardia after cardioversion.

Summary

Pediatric defibrillation is an effective, easily administered, and safe treatment. Although energy doses have not been as thoroughly tested for children as for adults, the guidelines published by the American Heart Association have stood the test of time. Physicians and medical personnel must be aware of the indications and appropriate techniques with respect to the age and size of the pediatric patient.

References

1. Aylward PE, Kieso R, Hite P, et al. Defibrillator electrode-chest wall coupling agents: Influence on transthoracic impedance and shock success. *J Am Coll Cardiol* 1985;6:682–686.
2. Dalzell GWN, Adgey AAJ. Determinants of successful transthoracic defibrillation and outcome in ventricular fibrillation. *Br Heart J* 1991;65:311–316.
3. Dalzell GWN, Cunningham SR, Anderson J, et al. Electrode pad size, transthoracic impedance and success of external ventricular defibrillation. *Am J Cardiol* 1989;64:741–744.
4. Kerber RE, Jensen SR, Gascho JA, et al. Determinants of defibrillation: Prospective analysis of 183 patients. *Am J Cardiol* 1983;52:739–745.
5. Weaver WD, Cobb LA, Copass MK, et al. Ventricular defibrillation—a comparative trial using 175-J and 320-J shocks. *N Engl J Med* 1982;307: 1101–1106.
6. Bunting-Blake L, Parker J, Weigel A. Defibrillation procedures. In *Defibrillation. A Manual for the EMT*. Philadelphia: J.B. Lippincott Co.; 1985:85–110.
7. Kerber RE, Grayzel J, Hoyt R, et al. Transthoracic resistance in human defibrillation. Influence of body weight, chest size, serial shocks, paddle size and paddle contact pressure. *Circulation* 1981;63:676–682.
8. Kerber RE, Kouba C, Martins J, et al. Advance prediction of transthoracic impedance in human defibrillation and cardioversion: Importance of impedance in determining the success of low-energy shocks. *Circulation* 1984;70:303–308.
9. Atkins DL, Sirna S, Kieso R, et al. Pediatric defibrillation: Importance of paddle size in determining transthoracic impedance. *Pediatrics* 1988;82:914–918.
10. Atkins DL, Kerber RE. Pediatric defibrillation: Current flow is improved by using "adult" paddle electrodes. *Pediatrics* 1994;94:90–93.
11. Kerber RE, Martins JB, Kienzle MG, et al. Energy, current, and success in defibrillation and cardioversion: Clinical studies using an automated impedance-based method of energy adjustment. *Circulation* 1988;77:1038–1046.
12. Gutgesell HP, Tacker WA, Geddes LA, et al. Energy dose for ventricular defibrillation of children. *Pediatrics* 1976;58:898–901.
13. Geddes LA, Tacker WA, Rosborough JP, et al. Electrical dose for ventricular defibrillation of large and small subjects using precordial electrodes. *J Clin Invest* 1974;53:310.
14. Babbs CF, Tacker WA, VanVleet JF, et al. Therapeutic indices for tran-

schest defibrillator shocks: Effective, damaging, and lethal electrical doses. *Am Heart J* 1980;99:734–738.

15. Geddes LA. Electrodes for transchest and ICD defibrillation and multifunctional electrodes. In Tacker WA Jr (ed): *Defibrillation of the Heart ICDs, AEDs, and Manual.* St. Louis: Mosby-Year Book, Inc.; 1994:82–118.

16. Patel AS, Galysh FT. Experimental studies to design safe external pediatric paddles for a DC defibrillator. *IEEE Trans Biomed Eng* 1972;19:228–232.

17. Pagan-Carlo LA, Birkett CL, Smith RA, et al. Is there an optimal electrode pad size to maximize intracardiac current in transthoracic defibrillation? *PACE* 1997;20:283–292.

18. Kerber RE, Martins JB, Kelly KJ, et al. Self-adhesive preapplied electrode pads for defibrillation and cardioversion. *J Am Coll Cardiol* 1984;3:815–820.

19. Samson RA, Atkins DL, Kerber RE. Optimal size of self-adhesive preapplied electrode pads in pediatric defibrillation. *Am J Cardiol* 1995;75: 544–545.

20. Caterine MR, Yoerger DM, Spencer KT, et al. Effect of electrode position and gel-application technique on predicted transcardiac current during transthoracic defibrillation. *Ann Emerg Med* 1997;29:588–595.

21. Dahl CF, Ewy GA, Warner ED. Myocardial necrosis from direct current countershock: Effect of paddle electrode size and time interval between discharges. *Circulation* 1974;50:956–961.

22. Ewy GA. Cardiac arrest and resuscitation: Defibrillators and defibrillation. *Curr Probl Cardiol* 1978;2:45–47.

23. Karch SB, Billingham ME. Myocardial contraction bands revisited. *Hum Pathol* 1986;17:9–13.

24. Doherty PW, McLaughlin RR, Billingham ME, et al. Cardiac damage produced by direct current countershock applied to the heart. *Am J Cardiol* 1979;43:225–232.

25. Karch SB. Resuscitation-induced myocardial necrosis. Catecholamines and defibrillation. *Am J Forensic Med Pathol* 1987;8:3–8.

26. Gaba DM, Talner NS. Myocardial damage following transthoracic direct current countershock in newborn piglets. *Pediatr Cardiol* 1982;2:281–288.

27. Allan JJ, Feld RD, Russell AA, et al. Cardiac troponin I levels are normal or minimally elevated after transthoracic cardioversion. *J Am Coll Cardiol* 1997;30:1052–1056.

28. Neumayr G, Hagn C, Ganzer H, et al. Plasma levels of troponin T after electric cardioversion of atrial fibrillation and flutter. *Am J Cardiol* 1997;80:1367–1369.

29. Garre L, Alvarez A, Rubio N, et al. Use of cardiac troponin T rapid assay in the diagnosis of a myocardial injury secondary to electrical cardioversion. *Clin Cardiol* 1997;20:619–621.

30. Georges JL, Spentchian M, Caubel C, et al. Time course of troponin T, myoglobulin, and cardiac enzyme release of electrical cardioversion. *Am J Cardiol* 1996;78:825–826.

31. Pagan-Carlo LA, Stone MS, Kerber RE. Nature and determinants of skin "burns" after transthoracic cardioversion. *Am J Cardiol* 1997;79:689–691.

32. Lanzarotti CJ, Olshansky B. Thromboembolism in chronic atrial flutter: Is the risk underestimated? *J Am Coll Cardiol* 1997;30:1506–1511.

33. Mehta D, Baruch L. Thromboembolism following cardioversion of "common" atrial flutter. Risk factors and limitations of transesophageal echocardiography. *Chest* 1996;110:1001–1003.

34. Liaudet L, Kehtari R, Enrico JF. Cerebral thromboembolism after direct current cardioversion for pure atrial flutter. *Intensive Care Med* 1997;23: 196–197.

Chapter 13

Implantable Cardioverter-Defibrillators

Michael J. Silka, MD and Jack Kron, MD

Introduction

Implantable cardioverter-defibrillators (ICDs) represent a category of medical devices which have revolutionized the treatment of patients at risk for sudden cardiac death due to sustained ventricular tachycardia (VT) or ventricular fibrillation (VF). The antiarrhythmic capabilities, implant methods, and clinical indications for these devices have evolved rapidly since their initial human use in 1980.[1] The rapid development of ICDs has been driven by the absolute magnitude of the problem of sudden cardiac death in the adult population, primarily associated with ischemic heart disease.[2] The use of these devices in pediatric patients has primarily occurred as an "epiphenomenon" following the use of ICDs in adult patients.

The current use and benefit of ICDs in pediatric patients has not been subjected to careful analysis due to the limited number of pediatric sudden death survivors at any individual center. The limited data that have been reported have been derived primarily from voluntary clinical registries and manufacturer databases. The purposes of this chapter are to offer a perspective on the epidemiology of arrhythmic sudden death and use of ICDs in the pediatric population, a review of the current available data regarding the clinical use of these devices in pediatric patients and their subsequent outcome, and a consideration of several unanswered questions regarding the evolving indications for the use of defibrillators as they apply to younger patients. A review of the technical aspects of ICD arrhythmia detection and therapy is be-

From: Quan L, Franklin WH (eds). *Ventricular Fibrillation: A Pediatric Problem*, Armonk, NY: Futura Publishing Company, Inc.; ©2000.

yond the scope of this chapter; the reader is referred to several recent reviews of this topic.[3-5]

Sudden Death and ICDs
in Pediatric Patients: Epidemiology

The primary candidate for ICD therapy is the individual who is at risk for sudden cardiac death, defined in most cases following resuscitation from a prior cardiac arrest due to sustained VT or VF.[6] To understand the limited use of ICDs in young patients, one must first consider the incidence of sudden arrhythmic death in the pediatric population compared with that in older age groups. The incidence and mechanisms of sudden death among various age groups was a subject of analysis of the Seattle Heart Watch Program.[7] This 13-year study (1976 to 1989) evaluated all victims of out-of-hospital cardiac arrest in a population of 1 million, of whom 25% were younger than 18 years, 24% were between the ages of 18 and 35 years, and 51% were older than 35 years of age. All causes of cardiac arrest, excluding trauma, were included in this study. Overall, 8054 cardiac arrest victims were identified, including 353 (4%) patients younger than 18 years of age, 252 (3%) in the 18- to 35-year-old group, and 7449 (93%) older than 35 years. However, a tachyarrhythmic cause of cardiac arrest (VT/VF) was identified in only 6% of pediatric victims, compared with 31% in the 18- to 35-year-old group and 46% in those older than 35 years. Thus, in this population of 1 million followed for 13 years, there were only 22 cardiac arrests due to VT or VF among patients younger than 18 years of age, accounting for less than 1% of the total of all sudden arrhythmic deaths (Table 1).

To continue this analysis, if less than 1% of all sudden deaths due to VT/VF occur in patients less than 18 years of age, one would antici-

Table 1

Seattle Heart Watch (1976–1989):
Incidence of Cardiac Arrest per Age

Age (yrs)	Total Population	# Cardiac Arrest Victims	% Arrest Victims with VT/VF	# Arrest Victims with VT/VF
0–17	250,000	353	6%	22
18–35	240,000	252	31%	78
>35	510,000	7449	46%	3427

VF = ventricular fibrillation; VT = ventricular tachycardia.

Table 2

Total Number and Number of ICDs Implanted in Pediatric Patients

Year(s)	Total ICDs	ICDs <13 yrs	ICDs 13–19 yrs
1980–89	8568	17	77
1990–93	32,092	27	200
1994–96	54,130	65	324
1997	28,068	46	205
Totals	122,858	155	806

ICD = implantable cardioverter-defibrillator.

pate a similar percentage of ICD implantations in this age group. In fact, this has been demonstrated consistently by manufacturer databases in which the age at initial ICD implant has been recorded (Table 2). As demonstrated in the cumulative data (bottom row), patients younger than 13 represent 0.1% of all ICD recipients, while those younger than 20 account for 0.6% of all ICD patients. This is consistent with data from the Seattle Heart Watch Program,[7] where of the 3427 cardiac arrest victims found to be in VT/VF, only 22 (0.6%) were in the pediatric age group. Thus, it appears that the relatively limited use of these devices in pediatric patients is a function of the incidence of sudden arrhythmic death in this population. This trend also appears to be maintained as the indications for ICD implantation have evolved from treatment of recurrent sudden death ("secondary prevention") to the use of ICDs for non-life-threatening episodes of sustained VT and "primary prevention," in which ICDs are implanted in patients perceived to be at high risk for malignant ventricular arrhythmias.

Clinical Use of ICDs in Pediatric Patients

Several small series of pediatric ICD patients have been reported in the literature to date, representing approximately 25% of the nearly 1000 patients with ICDs (Table 3).[1,8–15] One pattern that emerges from these reports is that there are three major forms of cardiovascular disease in young patients who have been resuscitated from sudden cardiac arrest and who subsequently receive ICDs. The first are hypertrophic and dilated cardiomyopathies, accounting for the largest proportion of pediatric patients to receive ICDs. Of note, the second patient ever to receive an ICD (termed an Automatic Implantable Defibrillator in the initial report), in 1980, was a 16 year old with a right ven-

Table 3

Summary of Medical Literature Regarding ICDs
in Pediatric Patients

Author[ref]	Year	Cardiomyopathy	Primary Electrical Disease	Congenital Heart Disease
Mirowski et al[1]	1980	1		
Kral et al[8]	1989	1		3
Kaminer et al[9]	1990	4		
Kron et al[10]	1990	15	16	4
Silka et al[11]	1993	66	33	22
Kron et al[12]	1994	7	9	1
Silka et al[13]	1996	12	17	9
Hamilton et al[14]	1996	7	3	
Epstein et al[15]	1998	8	8	20
Total		121	86	59

ICD = implantable cardioverter-defibrillator.

tricular cardiomyopathy.[1] The second largest group comprises patients with primary electrical diseases, either long QT or idiopathic VF. The third group includes patients who have had prior surgical treatment of congenital heart disease.

Hypertrophic Cardiomyopathies

Hypertrophic cardiomyopathies (HCMs) have been often identified in young patients and in athletes who have died suddenly, with sudden death commonly the first manifestation of cardiovascular disease. Criteria to risk-stratify these patients remain uncertain, although patients with a positive family history for sudden death or inducible sustained ventricular arrhythmias appear to be the subgroups at highest risk.[16,17] In general, patient outcome has been favorable among young patients with HCM who have received ICDs following resuscitation from cardiac arrest (Table 4). Primo et al[18] have reported that ICD use may be lower in patients with HCM following cardiac arrest or sustained VT than for other survivors of sudden cardiac death. However, given considerations of the unreliable methods available for risk stratification of these patients and the low peri-implant morbidity, the ICD would appear to be a logical therapy for patients with HCM who have been resuscitated from cardiac arrest or who experience sustained VT.[19,20]

Table 4

Summary of ICDs in Patients with Hypertrophic Cardiomyopathies

Author[ref]	# Patients	Follow-up (mo)	#/% with ICD Rx
Silka et al[11]	44	31±23	25/57%
Tripodi et al[20]	31	33±7	11/32%
Borgreffe et al[19]	14	48±24	6/43%
Hamilton et al[14]	6	<60	4/66%
Primo et al[18]	13	26±18	2/21%

ICD = implantable cardioverter-defibrillator.

Dilated Cardiomyopathies

Patients with dilated cardiomyopathies represent a somewhat heterogeneous group, including those with idiopathic dilated forms, arrhythmogenic right ventricular dysplasia, and ischemic cardiomyopathies due to either congenital or acquired coronary artery anomalies. The significance and optimal treatment of ventricular arrhythmias and syncope in these patients remain controversial.[21] In patients with advanced ventricular dysfunction and sustained ventricular arrhythmias, the primary role of ICD therapy appears to be that of a "bridge" to orthotopic heart transplant.[22] Conversely, for patients with ventricular arrhythmias as the principal manifestation of cardiomyopathy, the ICD may play a primary role; ablation or antiarrhythmic drugs would be reserved for patients with frequent episodes of tachycardia.

Primary Electrical Diseases

Primary electrical diseases consist of the prolonged QT syndromes and idiopathic VF. Of note, in 75% of young patients with these diagnoses who have received ICDs, resuscitated cardiac arrest was the initial manifestation of the heart disease.[23,24] As these are primary electrophysiological disorders, in the absence of structural heart disease or ventricular dysfunction, a good long-term prognosis would be anticipated if arrhythmia control is achieved. For high-risk patients with the long QT syndromes, the ICD has been demonstrated to be an effective therapy. However, the indications for these devices in patients who experience syncope or cardiac arrest in the absence of any other therapy (pharmacologic or pacemaker) continue to be debated.

The use of ICDs in patients who are resuscitated from idiopathic VF appears to be less controversial due to the absence of an identifiable cause of VF and the relatively high risk of a recurrent event (30% at 12-month follow-up and 67% at 40-month follow-up).[18,24] However, for the small number of patients with this diagnosis, particularly the individual patient who remains ICD-therapy-free during long-term follow-up, a reevaluation of this conclusion will be necessary.

Congenital Heart Defects

Patients with congenital heart defects comprise the third major group of young patients to receive an ICD following resuscitation from sudden cardiac arrest. The most common types of congenital heart defects among these patients have been transposition of the great arteries, complex single ventricle, tetralogy of Fallot, and aortic stenosis.[11] The indications for ICD implantation in these patients are similar to those for other forms of heart disease: resuscitated cardiac arrest, sustained VT in the absence of a reversible cause, and syncope with inducible sustained ventricular arrhythmias at electrophysiological testing. Although indications are similar, recent data have suggested that implant thresholds may be significantly higher in this patient group, and that "spurious" ICD discharges in response to atrial tachycardias are a frequent problem.[15] Additionally, venous access continues to be a limiting factor for some patients, due to complex anatomy or to residual intracardiac shunts (Figure 1).

Clinical Use and Patient Outcome Following ICD Implantation

Determination of the benefit of ICD survival remains a complex issue due to the number of different endpoints that have been evaluated: overall patient survival, sudden-death-free survival, ICD shock, and antitachycardia pacing.[25] The use of surrogate endpoints such as *any* ICD therapy may result in an overestimation of ICD benefit, as not all episodes of VT are fatal; conversely, death due to noncardiac etiologies may result in underestimation of ICD efficacy. This is further complicated by the fact that different VT/VF detection criteria may be programmed, limiting the ability to compile data from multiple centers when a large-scale evaluation of ICD therapy in young patients has been attempted.

Regarding patient survival and shock-free survival, data on 125 pediatric patients with ICDs and at least 24 months follow-up were re-

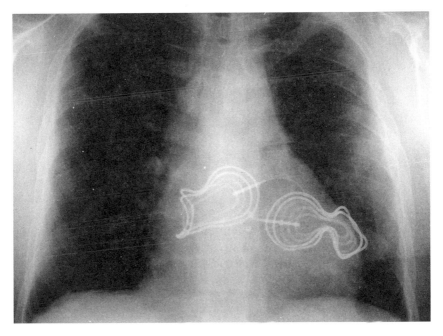

Figure 1. Chest x-ray from a young man, demonstrating an epicardial bipolar defibrillation lead system. This patient had undergone a prior Fontan procedure for tricuspid atresia and was resuscitated from an episode of ventricular fibrillation that occurred during moderate exertion. Due to the absence of transvenous access to the right ventricle, an epicardial lead system was required. Some crumpling of the concentric coil epicardial patches is evident, although this was not associated with change in the defibrillation threshold.

ported by the Pediatric Electrophysiology Society in 1993.[11] At 24 months post ICD implant, the sudden-death-free survival rate for this group was 95%, with an overall survival rate of 93%. Regarding potential ICD benefit, the incidence of at least one ostensibly appropriate shock was 50% at 24-month follow-up. Evaluation of ICD impact on outcome for these patients must be considered with regard to the fact that most (90%) of these patients had been resuscitated from hypotensive VT/VF and most of these devices were capable of "shock-only" therapy. It would seem fair, however, to conclude that in this very high risk population, the ICD provided a significant benefit regarding survival.

Evaluation of the postimplant mortality rates over time demonstrated an early 2% sudden and 3% total mortality within 30 days of implant. A continuing risk of late mortality beyond 2 years of follow-up was also noted, with the incidence of sudden death increasing from 5% to 10% and total mortality increasing from 7% to 15% at 60-month follow-up. This late mortality includes several patients whose devices were not replaced after battery depletion had been identified.

Multivariate analysis of the factors that were associated with cardiac death following ICD implant identified impaired ventricular function as the primary correlate of a poor outcome. Patients with previous ICD shocks also had an incremental risk of late death. However, inducibilty or noninducibilty at programmed stimulation and the types of associated cardiovascular disease were not correlated with outcome.

Evaluation of the use of ICDs by pediatric patients is a complex issue, as device capabilities have evolved along with implant techniques as well as indications for the use of defibrillators. Figure 2 displays the trends for ICD therapies as devices and implantation criteria have evolved. For the first generation of shock-only ICDs, when most patients had been resuscitated from VF, the incidence of appropriate shocks was 25% at 12 months and 50% at 24 months. This compares with second- and third-generation devices with antitachycardia pacing, cardioversion, and defibrillation capabilities, implanted between 1990 and 1993, with which the incidence of device therapy was 50% at 12 months but did not change appreciably thereafter. In the most recent

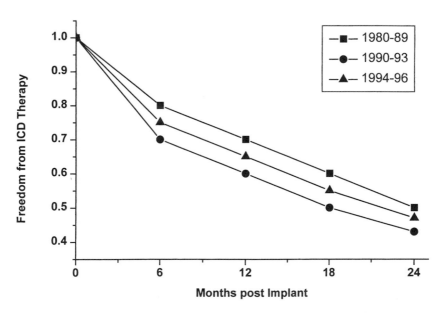

Figure 2. Incidence of device therapy during three sequential series evaluating ICDs in pediatric patients. The intervals 1980 to 1989, 1990 to 1993, and 1994 to 1996 are presented. With third-generation programmable devices, there is a higher incidence of at least one ICD intervention with the first year post implant. However, the rates of device intervention converge at approximately 50% by 24-month follow-up for all generations of devices.

analysis of tiered-therapy transvenous devices, some form of ICD therapy was noted in 40% of patients at 12-month follow-up. However, only 50% of patients in this series had been resuscitated from cardiac arrest. Thus, it would appear that determination of ICD benefit will remain a complex issue, with prevention of sudden cardiac death the primary criterion to evaluate this therapy, rather than any ICD intervention on one hand or patient mortality due to any cause at the other extreme.

The decision to proceed with ICD placement in a pediatric patient must also include consideration of potential alternative therapies as well as of complications of ICDs. Remediable causes of cardiac arrest (Wolff-Parkinson-White syndrome, drug toxicity, etc.) are discussed elsewhere in this volume. Furthermore, pharmacologic therapy, pacemaker implantation, and coronary revascularization may offer potential "cures" for patients with long QT syndromes, complete atrioventricular block, or coronary artery anomalies. One complex and difficult decision process arises when cardiac arrest occurs in a pediatric patient with severe ventricular dysfunction. As discussed previously, the primary correlate of death in pediatric patients following ICD implantation is impaired ventricular function; conversely, given the severe paucity of suitable donors for young patients, the decision to proceed with orthotopic heart transplantation as primary therapy must be made with consideration of the fact that donor procurement time may be several months. Short- and long-term outcomes must also be considered. Table 5 compares the relative survival rates for pediatric patients following ICD implantation with those in patients undergoing heart transplantation.[26]

Discussion of the use of ICDs in young patients must also include

Table 5

Survival in Pediatric Patients (5–16 years of age): ICD versus Heart Transplant

Interval	Sudden Death Free Survival (ICD)	Overall Survival (ICD)	Overall Survival (Transplant)
60 days	98	97	88
1 yr	97	95	80
2 yr	95	90	76
3 yr	93	88	70
4 yr	90	88	67

ICD = implantable cardioverter-defibrillator.

consideration of the potential for complications. By far, the most common complication is inappropriate ICD therapy in response to sinus or atrial tachycardia, estimated to occur in 25% of patients in the first 3 months of follow-up. Biphasic waveforms and reduction in device size have reduced the incidence of problems related to excessive defibrillation threshold or device erosion and infection. One other problem that remains, however, is that of the psychological and lifestyle impacts associated with the presence of the defibrillator.

Several earlier problems associated with ICD use in pediatric patients have been solved with the development of transvenous lead systems. Between 1990 and 1993, 35% of young patients undergoing ICD implantation received transvenous lead systems; this number increased to 75% between 1994 and 1996. It is currently estimated that 45% of generators are placed in a pectoral position and 55% are abdominal. However, a few unique considerations must be made regarding the use of transvenous lead systems in young patients. The first concerns anatomic variants in patients with congenital heart disease. A second issue is the placement and length of transvenous leads and coils designed for adult-sized hearts (Figure 3). Third is the need for lifelong vascular access, as well as the problems of lead failure and extraction.

Indications for ICDs in Pediatric Patients

Guidelines for the implantation of cardiac pacemakers and antiarrhythmia devices were recently revised, and include the use of ICDs in pediatric patients.[6] There is general agreement regarding implantation of these devices following resuscitation from hypotensive VT or VF, or in patients with recurrent syncope or with nonsustained VT and advanced ventricular dysfunction, who have inducible sustained VT or VF during electrophysiological testing. However, some specific considerations must be made for unique conditions that may exist in pediatric patients. For example, if a child with severely impaired ventricular function is resuscitated, should this patient undergo ICD implant, be listed for transplant, or both? A second controversy is cardiac arrest as the initial manifestation of the prolonged QT syndrome—which therapy: ICD, β-blockade, or both? Another uncertainty occurs when cardiac arrest occurs in the patient with congenital heart disease and atrial flutter. Should therapy be directed to the atrial flutter, to ablation of the atrioventricular node, or to VF? Finally, regarding the young patient with idiopathic VF—after years or decades of not using a device, should the ICD be replaced when elective generator replacement is indicated due to decrease in battery voltage?

The indications for use of ICDs as primary prevention are more diffi-

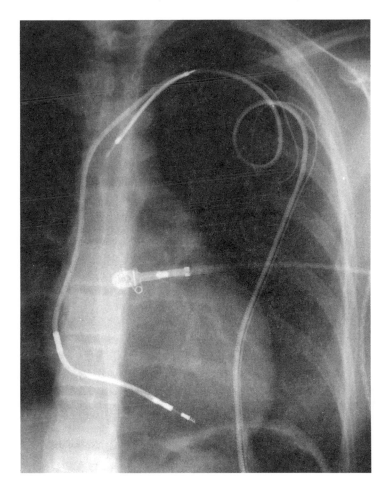

Figure 3. Chest x-ray from a 12 year old with hypertrophic cardiomyopathy and a 2-lead transvenous ICD system. The ventricular lead and coil extends from the right ventricular apex to the acute margin of the heart, where a 90° bend in the coil is evident. Prolapse of the lead system across the tricuspid valve resulted in significant valvar insufficiency. An additional concern in this patient is lead migration and growth, for which a strain relief curve has been placed in the infraclavicular region.

cult. Randomized clinical trials in adults with ischemic heart disease must be used cautiously to guide decisions regarding a young population with diverse forms of heart disease.[27,28] There are currently no data to guide the clinician regarding difficult cases such as families with long QT syndromes or HCM in which an immediate family member has died suddenly.

In summary, the data regarding the use of ICDs in pediatric patients are limited, as this group represents less than 1% of patients experiencing sudden tachyarrhythmic death. It does appear that ICD use and outcome for young patients are comparable to data reported for adults. However, the incidence of device complications, particularly inappropriate therapies, appears higher. Regarding indications, the thoughtful use of ICDs is advocated for secondary prevention of sudden death; however, the indications for ICDs as primary prevention remain undefined.

References

1. Mirowski M, Reid PR, Mower MM, et al. Termination of malignant ventricular arrhythmias with an implanted automatic defibrillator in human beings. *N Engl J Med* 1980;303:322–324.
2. Lown B. Sudden cardiac death: The major challenge confronting contemporary cardiology. *Am J Cardiol* 1979;43(2):313–328.
3. Powell AC, Fuchs T, Finkelstein DM, et al. Influence of implantable cardioverter-defibrillators on the long-term prognosis of survivors of out-of-hospital cardiac arrest. *Circulation* 1993;88:1083–1092.
4. Saksena S, Krol RB, Kaushik RR. Innovations in pulse generators and lead systems: Balancing complexity with clinical benefit and long-term results. *Am Heart J* 1994;127:1010–1021.
5. Sarter BH, Callans DJ, Gottlieb CD, et al. Implantable defibrillator diagnostic storage capabilities: Evolution, current status, and future utilization. *PACE* 1998;21:1287–1298.
6. Gregoratos G, Cheitlin MD, Conill A, et al. ACC/AHA guidelines for implantation of cardiac pacemakers and antiarrhythmia devices: A report of the American College of Cardiology/American Heart Association Task Force on Practice Guidelines (Committee on Pacemaker Implantation). *J Am Coll Cardiol* 1998;31:1175–1209.
7. Safranek DJ, Eisenberg MS, Larsen MP. The epidemiology of cardiac arrest in young adults. *Ann Emerg Med* 1992;21:1102–1106.
8. Kral MA, Spotnitz HM, Hordof A, et al. Automatic implantable cardioverter defibrillator implantation for malignant ventricular arrhythmias associated with congenital heart disease. *Am J Cardiol* 1989;63:118–119.
9. Kaminer SJ, Pickoff AS, Dunnigan A, et al. Cardiomyopathy and the use of implanted cardio-defibrillators in children. *PACE* 1990;13:593–597.
10. Kron J, Oliver RP, Norsted S, et al. The automatic implantable cardioverter-defibrillator in young patients. *J Am Coll Cardiol* 1990;16:896–902.
11. Silka MJ, Kron J, Dunnigan A, et al. Sudden cardiac death and the use of implantable cardioverter-defibrillators in pediatric patients. *Circulation* 1993;87:800–807.
12. Kron J, Silka MJ, Ohm OJ, et al. Preliminary experience with nonthoracotomy implantable cardioverter-defibrillators in young patients. *PACE* 1994;17:26–30.
13. Silka MJ, Kron J, Halperin BD. Current experience with transvenous implantable cardioverter defibrillators systems in patients younger than 21 years of age. *J Am Coll Cardiol* 1996;27(suppl A);397A. Abstract.

14. Hamilton RM, Dorian P, Gow RM, et al. Five-year experience with implantable defibrillators in children. *Am J Cardiol* 1996;77:524–526.
15. Epstein MR, Alexander ME, Saul JP, et al. Implantable cardioverter-defibrillators: Unique features in children and patients with congenital heart disease. *PACE* 1998;21(part II):876. Abstract.
16. McKenna WJ, Camm AJ. Sudden death in hypertrophic cardiomyopathy: Assessment of patients at high risk. *Circulation* 1989;80:1489–1492.
17. Maron BJ, Fananapazir L. Sudden cardiac death in hypertrophic cardiomyopathy. *Circulation* 1992;85(suppl I):I57-I63.
18. Primo J, Geelen P, Brugada J. Hypertrophic cardiomyopathy: Role of the implantable cardioverter-defibrillator. *J Am Coll Cardiol* 1998;31:1081–1085.
19. Borggrefe M, Breithardt G. Is the implantable defibrillator indicated in patients with hypertrophic cardiomyopathy and aborted sudden death? *J Am Coll Cardiol* 1998;31:1086-1088.
20. Tripodi D, McAreavey D, Epstein ND, Fananapazir L. Impact of the implantable defibrillator in hypertrophic cardiomyopathy patients at high risk for sudden death. *J Am Coll Cardiol* 1993;21(suppl A):352A.
21. Packer M. Lack of relation between ventricular arrhythmias and sudden death in patients with chronic heart failure. *Circulation* 1992;85(suppl 1):I50-I56.
22. Haverich A, Troster J, Wahlers T, et al. The automatic implantable cardioverter defibrillator (AICD) as a bridge to heart transplantation. *PACE* 1992;15:701–707.
23. Groh WJ, Silka MJ, Oliver RP, et al. Use of cardioverter-defibrillators in the congenital long QT syndrome. *Am J Cardiol* 1996;78:703–706.
24. Priori SG. Survivors of out-of-hospital cardiac arrest with apparently normal heart: Need for definition and standardized clinical evaluation. *Circulation* 1997;95:265–272.
25. Myerburg RJ, Mitrani R, Interian A Jr, Castellanos A. Interpretation of outcomes of antiarrhythmic clinical trials: Design features and population impact. *Circulation* 1998;97:1514–1521.
26. Hosenpud JD, Bennett LE, Keck BM, et al. The registry of the international society for heart and lung transplantation: 14th official report—1997. *J Heart Lung Transplant* 1997;16:691–712.
27. The Antiarrhythmics versus Implantable Defibrillators (AVID) Investigators. A comparison of antiarrhythmic drug therapy with implantable defibrillators in patients resuscitated from near-fatal ventricular arrhythmias. *N Engl J Med* 1997;337:1576–1583.
28. Moss AJ, Hall WJ, Cannom DS, et al. Improved survival with an implanted defibrillator in patients with coronary disease at high risk for ventricular arrhythmias. *N Engl J Med* 1996;335:1933–1940.

Section VI

Automated External Defibrillators

Chapter 14

Automated External Defibrillators:
Use in the Field

Robert Delagi, MA, NREMT-P

The facts speak for themselves. According to the American Heart Association (AHA), cardiovascular disease accounts for almost 1 million deaths each year in the United States. Almost 500,000 of those deaths can be directly attributed to coronary artery disease. A significant number of these deaths occur outside the hospital with patients presenting in sudden cardiac arrest as their first sign.[1] Many adults suffering out-of-hospital sudden cardiac death present with ventricular fibrillation (VF). The definitive therapy for VF is electrical countershock, commonly called defibrillation. Time to defibrillation is a key element in survivability. Data suggest that a person's chance of survival decreases by approximately 10% for every minute that goes by without defibrillation.[2]

Electric reversal of VF by external electrodes was first described in 1956[3] and was performed by physicians, using bulky equipment, in the hospital setting. In the 1960s, cardiopulmonary resuscitation (CPR) was introduced to sustain ventilation and circulation long enough to bring the defibrillator to the patient's side. This notion has led to the AHA's "Chain-of-Survival" concept, which places early access, early CPR, early defibrillation, and early advanced care as vital links in reducing mortality and morbidity from sudden cardiac arrest.

Prior to the advent of the automated external defibrillator (AED), prehospital defibrillation was limited to advanced emergency medical technicians (AEMTs: paramedics) who are trained to interpret rhythm strips and perform manual defibrillation. It is the basic EMT, however, who represents the largest group of prehospital providers and encounters the largest number of patients.

Advances in technology have resulted in a new breed of defibril-

From: Quan L, Franklin WH (eds). *Ventricular Fibrillation: A Pediatric Problem.* Armonk, NY: Futura Publishing Company, Inc.; ©2000.

lator, the AED. The AED's sophisticated microprocessor evaluates the patient's heart rhythm and decides if it is "shockable" or "nonshockable," based on the amplitude and speed of the electrical activity. The AED has a computer-generated voice, audible tones, and visual signals that prompt the operator to perform critical actions at the appropriate time. These machines, affectionately dubbed "doc-in-a-box," are highly accurate in shocking appropriately, and the chance of human error is far greater than that of mechanical error.

Once turned on, the AED assesses the patient's rhythm and protocol dictates that one of two situations will occur. If the machine detects a shockable rhythm, it charges to the appropriate energy level and delivers the shock or series of stacked shocks. If, however, the machine detects a nonshockable rhythm, the machine prompts the operator to check breathing and pulse—an indication to perform CPR. The machine then reassesses the patient and responds with the appropriate command. Typically, AEDs are programmed to either deliver energy at 200 J, 200 and 300 J, or to prompt the user to perform CPR. Second-generation devices, known as semiautomated external defibrillators, work exactly the same but require the operator to deliver the shock by pressing a button when prompted to do so by the device. Many clinicians feel that this device is much safer to use because the operator must actually deliver the shock, whereas the AED will deliver the shock regardless of the actions of the rescuers who may be in physical contact with the victim.

The advantages of automated defibrillators are that the devices are easy to learn to use, are lightweight, portable, and capable of delivering electrical therapy seconds after the device is applied.

A computer chip allows for real-time recording of the electrocardiographic sequences, and event summary for each patient encounter for record keeping and quality improvement purposes. Due to these combined factors, clinicians and researchers alike have advocated widespread use of the device.

Since VF is the most common and treatable rhythm following sudden cardiac arrest in the adult patient, time is a critical factor. AED training takes a short time, and technological advances allow the skill to be used without an in-depth knowledge of cardiac electrophysiology. The AED has become the standard of care at the basic level in most emergency medical service (EMS) systems. We are currently at the threshold of a concept called public-access defibrillation, in which AEDs are being used by targeted first-responder groups such as security guards in gated communities and casinos, first aid teams in office buildings, family members of patients at higher risk for VF, and flight attendants working for major air carriers. Automated external defibrillation has been proven effective in saving lives and is so easy to use that many states are enacting legislation to allow lay persons with CPR certification access to AED training and authorization to use the devices.

Training usually takes about 6 hours and is given in two sessions. Basic EMTs learn about the chain of survival, receive an introductory-level presentation on the cardiac conduction system, and learn to troubleshoot the equipment and how to integrate other skills into the resuscitation sequence. On-line and off-line medical control options, special resuscitation situations, quality improvement, "did not resuscitate," and operator safety issues are also discussed, and EMTs receive hands-on practice using specialized mannequins and rhythm generators.

Treatment protocols typically are as follows: *shockable rhythm*— three stacked shocks followed by 1 minute of CPR, reassess, three stacked shocks, move to ambulance while performing CPR, reassess, three stacked shocks, transport while performing CPR with a reassessment every few minutes until arrival at the hospital; *nonshockable rhythm*—1 minute of CPR, reassess, 1 minute of CPR, reassess, and after three no-shock advisories, disconnect the AED and perform CPR en route to the hospital.

The pediatric population presents unique and interesting challenges with regard to AED use. The two main issues deal with the underlying etiology of the pediatric arrest and the widely variant energy settings necessary to perform defibrillation at the recommended level of 2 J/kg.[4] Researchers should be encouraged to investigate whether AEDs can be programmed with both adult and pediatric algorithms and whether a modification of this type will affect the overall simplicity of the AED.

Another option may be to develop a pediatric AED. Either way, clinicians will still be faced with the issues surrounding selection of energy ranges required for the pediatric patient.

There are also a host of emotional aspects that surface when dealing with the pediatric arrest. Typically, the EMS provider's feelings are overwhelming while the parents of the patient urge him or her to "get the child to the hospital." This sentiment is not without merit. This author does believe that although defibrillation has been demonstrated time and time again to be the definitive care in adult cardiac arrest, the etiology of the pediatric arrest is far more complex and requires the diagnostic expertise and therapeutic options that can only be found in the hospital setting.

Training EMS providers to use AEDs for children is the easiest task to accomplish. If technology were available to develop an AED for the pediatric patient, incorporation into the current AED training curriculum would have little impact on the format of the course. Electrode placement, use of the device, and standard operating procedures would be essentially the same as they are now. As demonstrated in the adult model, in-depth knowledge of cardiac physiology or arrest etiology would not be necessary.

As in many aspects of healthcare, there are economic implications that may ultimately affect the prehospital approach to the treatment of VF in the pediatric patient. This scenario is no different than many scenarios in which healthcare providers try to balance the desire to provide the highest quality of care with the reality of cost/benefit analysis and the difficult task of trying to place a price tag on a human life. In many locations, EMS providers do not see large numbers of critically ill children, and they see even fewer episodes of cardiac arrest. Pediatric patients who have out-of-hospital cardiac arrest are typically not in VF.

The costs associated with adding a pediatric AED for every adult AED in service, and the addition of battery-support systems and disposable items such as electrodes, may be overly burdensome, and the equipment infrequently utilized. EMS managers will ultimately have to examine the economy of scope by trying to justify the cost when compared with the potential for use.

Ethical considerations will also play a role in the process. Survivability and cerebral performance, quality-of-life issues, termination of resuscitation, and dealing with the death of a child will all have an impact on EMS providers.

While rapid advances in the science surrounding pediatric cardiac arrest and out-of-hospital treatment options occur, EMS providers will remain in the forefront of VF recognition and treatment of all individuals suffering from out-of-hospital cardiac arrest. Indeed, it will be the contribution of EMS providers to the research effort that will identify pediatric VF as a significant clinical problem. It is well established that EMS providers can handle a multitude of emergencies that occur outside the hospital, and given the appropriate tools, they will employ strategies to successfully deal with pediatric VF.

References

1. Dan BB, Southgate MT, Lundberg GD, et al. Guidelines for cardiopulmonary resuscitation and emergency cardiac care—Recommendations of the 1992 National Conference. *JAMA* 1992;268:2172–2183.
2. Eisenberg MS, Bergner L, Hallstrom A, et al. Paramedic programs and out-of-hospital cardiac arrest: Factors associated with successful resuscitation. *Am J Public Health* 1979;69:39–42.
3. Zoll PM, Linenthal AJ, et al. Termination of ventricular fibrillation in man by externally applied countershock. *N Engl J Med* 1956;254:727–732.
4. Cummins RO. Defibrillation. In *Advanced Cardiac Life Support*. Dallas: American Heart Association; 1997–1999;4–6–4–10.

Chapter 15

Pediatric Experience with Automated External Defibrillators

Dianne L. Atkins, MD

Introduction

Automated external defibrillators (AEDs), first described in 1979,[1] are computerized defibrillators that can be operated by minimally trained personnel. Once self-adhesive electrode pads are attached to the patient's chest, the AED analyzes the patient's cardiac rhythm. If a ventricular rhythm is identified, the unit charges to an appropriate energy level and delivers a defibrillating shock. Semiautomated units require the operator to push an additional button before a shock is delivered. The machines provide voice prompts to the operator and the electrocardiogram (ECG) is recorded and stored for subsequent review.

Early defibrillation is a major determinant of successful resuscitation from cardiac arrest. Rapid defibrillation by emergency medical technicians (EMTs) in both urban and rural settings increases the detection of ventricular fibrillation (VF) and, more importantly, results in improved survival rates, from 3% to 4% to as high as 19% to 26%.[2–6] Survival rates increase to 44% when AEDs are used in an urban setting in which there is widespread knowledge of cardiopulmonary resuscitation (CPR) and a rapid-response emergency medical service (EMS) system.[7] The rhythm detection algorithms are at least as accurate as paramedic interpretation of ECGs.[8,9] These encouraging results prompted the American Heart Association (AHA) to include AED training in both basic and advanced cardiac life support training programs for emergency personnel.[10] Furthermore, the

From: Quan L, Franklin WH (eds). *Ventricular Fibrillation: A Pediatric Problem.* Armonk, NY: Futura Publishing Company, Inc.; ©2000.

AHA encourages widespread availability of AEDs in the community[11,12] and is developing guidelines for lay rescuers to use this new technology.

Pediatric experience with AEDs has been limited but appears promising. This chapter discusses four questions as we consider the appropriate use of AEDs in children. First, is there a need for AED use in children based on the epidemiology of sudden death and the frequency of ventricular arrhythmias? Second, what is our current experience with AED use in children? Third, is there a need for equipment modification? Fourth, how can we optimize AED use in children?

Do We Need AEDs for Children Less than 12 Years Old?

The epidemiology of pediatric cardiac arrest is different from that observed in adult populations. The most common rhythms observed in patients 0 to 17 years of age are asystole and pulseless electrical activity (PEA).[13-20] The most common etiologies include sudden infant death syndrome, trauma including drowning, and acute or chronic medical disease. Primary respiratory arrest is more common than primary cardiac arrest, and is the most common cause of cardiac arrest in children less than 5 years old. Successful resuscitation rates are distressingly low (<10%), costs are extremely high,[13] and permanent neurologic sequelae are common. Patients who arrive at the emergency department with a preterminal (asystole, PEA, or idioventricular) rhythm are unlikely to survive or to have a good neurologic outcome.[13,17] These data direct the emphasis on early immediate CPR, calling *fast* (instead of *first*), early intubation, and vascular access for pediatric resuscitation.[21]

However, awareness that VF may account for a significant portion of pediatric arrest has recently increased. Sudden death (not traumatic) in children, especially those greater than 8 years old, is increasingly recognized and may account for 11% of all deaths in children aged 1 to 20 years.[18] In several epidemiological studies of cardiac arrest in children, VF was present in 10% to 22% of those in whom an ECG was obtained.[13-17,19,20] In the most complete study of VF in children, Mogayzel et al[19] report VF as the initial rhythm in 19% of children (>5, <18 years) who experienced out-of-hospital cardiac arrest. The presence of VF was evenly distributed among all categories of arrest: drownings, overdoses, trauma, and medical illnesses, supporting the hypothesis that VF occurs in pediatric arrest and is not rare.

Most importantly, however, is the marked difference in successful resuscitation rates and good neurologic outcomes experienced by victims of VF compared with those with asystole or PEA. Pediatric patients who were successfully defibrillated at the scene had markedly improved survival (38%) and good neurologic outcomes (17%) compared with patients with asystole, 3% and 2%, respectively. Long-term survival of patients with VF reported in the cited studies is 25% to 40%.[13,14,16]

Pediatric Experience

Because of the dramatic success in adults, the AHA's *Advanced Cardiac Life Support* recommends the use of AEDs in children greater than 8 years of age.[22] This recommendation however, is based on supposition of usefulness rather than published data documenting effectiveness and/or lack of toxicity. Published information about AED use in children is extremely limited.[23,24] Hazinski et al[24] demonstrated sensitivity (detecting shockable rhythms) and specificity (detecting nonshockable rhythms) of greater than 90% in 21 hospitalized infants and children less than 8 years old. There were, however, variations in treatment decisions with alternate pad placement, with occasional shock recommendation for nonshockable rhythms. In our study of AED use during cardiac arrest and resuscitation in 18 patients of an average age of 12 years, AEDs had a sensitivity of 88% and a specificity of 100%.[23] During the course of the resuscitations, a total of 67 rhythms were analyzed (including initial rhythm), and consisted of 25 episodes of VF, 32 episodes of asystole/PEA, 6 episodes of sinus bradycardia, and 4 episodes of sinus tachycardia. VF was recognized accurately 22 of 25 times, asystole 32 of 32, sinus bradycardia 6 of 6, and sinus bradycardia 4 of 4. There were no instances of a shock recommendation for a nonshockable rhythm. In the three instances in which VF was not recognized initially (Figure 1), a second analysis was correct and shocks were delivered. In addition, we observed 34% survival in patients with VF and 43% survival in patients who received a defibrillatory shock as opposed to 11% survival with nonshockable rhythms (Figure 2). Multiple AEDs were used by the services and there was no difference in accuracy among the various units.

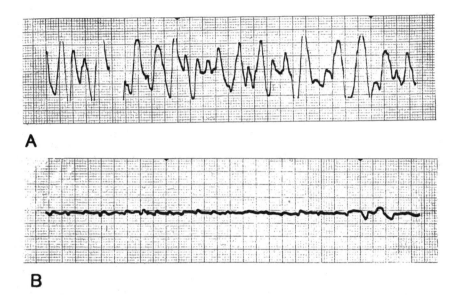

A

B

Figure 1. Ventricular fibrillation (VF) not recognized by automated external defibrillators. A. Ventricular fibrillation in a 15-year-old boy was not recognized and a no shock advisory was provided. A second analysis correctly identified this as VF and a shock was advised. B. Fine VF in a 15-year-old patient, that was not recognized on two separate analyses. Both times an immediate reanalysis recommended defibrillation. Paper speed = 25 mm/s. From Atkins DL, Hartley LL, York DK. Accurate recognition and effective treatment of ventricular fibrillation by automated external defibrillators in adolescents. *Pediatrics* 101:393–397, 1998. Reproduced by permission of *Pediatrics.*

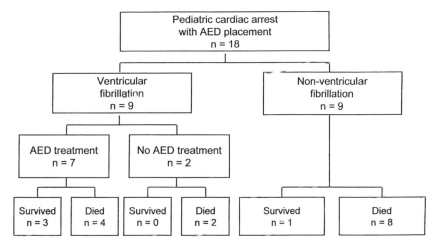

Figure 2. Outcomes of children and adolescents when automated external defibrillators were used during the resuscitation. Of the children who received shocks for ventricular fibrillation, 43% survived to hospital discharge. The one patient who survived a "nonshockable rhythm" had a sinus rhythm during the first analysis. All others had asystole/pulseless electrical activity. From Atkins DL, Hartley LL, York DK. Accurate recognition and effective treatment of ventricular fibrillation by automated external defibrillators in adolescents. *Pediatrics* 101:393–397, 1998. Reproduced by permission of *Pediatrics.*

Equipment Design and Modification

Equipment and design modifications of AEDs may need to be considered for widespread use in children, especially those younger than 8 years. The primary elements that require investigation include the rhythm detection algorithm, the energy dose, and the electrode paddle size and placement.

The accuracy of the rhythm-detecting algorithms for adults has been extensively verified and shown to be as accurate as field ECGs.[8,9] Since heart mass in children is smaller, it is possible that accuracy of rhythm detection will not be as high. The published experience to date is encouraging but very inadequate. In the small number of pediatric patients who have been studied, accuracy rates have been observed that are comparable to those in adults.[23,24] Clearly, larger scale studies must be evaluated, especially of smaller children.

Smaller "pediatric" self-adhesive electrodes are marketed. As with hand-held electrodes, transthoracic impedance is directly related to the diameter of the pad (Figure 3).[25,26] Electrode pads smaller than 5.8 cm in diameter result in transthoracic impedances greater than 97 Ω, which are associated with low shock success in adults.[27] The chests of children

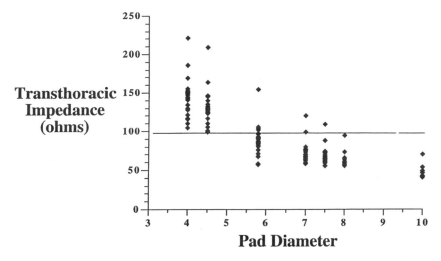

Figure 3. Scattergram of individual transthoracic impedance values grouped by pad diameter. Horizontal line indicates a value of 97 Ω, approximately 1 standard deviation above the adult mean transthoracic impedance value. Reprinted from *Am J Cardiol* 75, Samson RA, Atkins DL, Kerber RE. Optimal size of self-adhesive preapplied electrode pads in pediatric defibrillation, 544–545, 1995, with permission from Excerpta Medica Inc.

older than 8 years can easily accommodate the full-size electrode paddles, which should be used.[10,21] Separate pediatric paddles are not necessary for AED use in children older than 8 years.

A major factor in the evaluation of AED use in children is energy dosage. Fully automated AEDs deliver 200 J, with no capability to alter the dose. Semiautomated units often have a 100-J level, which the operator can set; however, this requires additional training. The fact that the maximum recommended dose for children is 4 J/kg would suggest that patients weighing less than 50 kg would receive energy doses that are higher than those recommended. However, these recommendations have evolved from extremely limited data, which focused on effectiveness rather than toxicity.[28] Animal studies indicate that dosages even up to 10 J/kg result in a less than 25% risk of myocardial damage and no risk of death from the shock alone (Figure 4).[29] Thus, with current equipment design, children weighing as little as 20 kg (an average 5 year old) potentially could be safely defibrillated with 200 J. New designs in waveform delivery permit delivery with lower energy levels (maximum 150 J) and still successfully defibrillate.[30–32] Additional machine design variations may be developed that permit delivery of smaller energies without compromising the simplicity of current AEDs.[33]

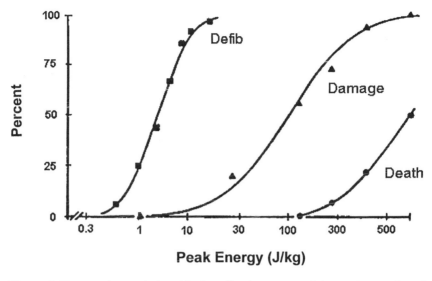

Figure 4. Energy dose relationship for effectiveness, toxicity, and mortality of transchest damped sine wave defibrillator shock given to dogs. From Babbs CF, Tacker WA, VanVleet JF, et al. Therapeutic indices for transchest defibrillator shocks: Effective, damaging, and lethal electrical doses. *Am Heart J* 1980;734–738. Reproduced by permission of *Am Heart J.*

Optimizing AED Use

Because of the high frequency of respiratory arrest and asystole in children, emphasis has been placed on effective ventilation and oxygenation. Thus, intubation and establishment of vascular access receive high priority in pediatric algorithms (Figure 5). Rhythm assessment, despite its importance, receives less emphasis. The prevalence of VF may be underestimated in published reports because pediatric patients do not routinely receive early or rapid rhythm assessment. However, regardless of age, VF deteriorates to asystole within 6 to 10 minutes.[22,34] Once VF has been documented in a child, the AHA pediatric pulseless algorithm is unclear as to whether defibrillation should be performed before or after intubation and vascular access. This is unfortunate because the probability of successful defibrillation decreases with time, and the effective treatment for VF is electrical countershock. If VF is detected and rapidly treated, long-term outcomes may improve. As we consider revisions to pediatric protocols, we should consider whether the algorithm for VF in children should be comparable to that for adults. Thus, if VF is detected, the child would receive three shocks before other interventions are undertaken. Changes in recommendations should be made only after consideration of the relative

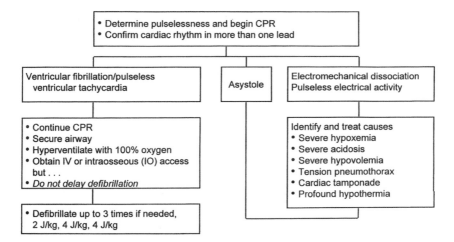

Figure 5. Decision tree for pediatric pulseless arrest. Timing of defibrillation is not definite and may be delayed until after the airway is secured and vascular access is obtained. Modified from *Pediatric Advanced Life Support.* American Heart Association; 1997:7–10.

frequency of VF, the success rates of cardiac arrest, the safety of defibrillation, especially with AEDs, and the adequacy of any design changes of the defibrillators.

References

1. Diack AW, Welborn WS, Rullman RG, et al. An automatic cardiac resuscitator for emergency treatment of cardiac arrest. *Med Instrum* 1979;13:78–83.
2. Eisenberg MS, Copass MK, Hallstrom AP, et al. Treatment of out-of-hospital cardiac arrests with rapid defibrillation by emergency medical technicians. *N Engl J Med* 1980;302:1379–1383.
3. Vukov LF, White RD, Bachman JW, et al. New perspectives on rural EMT defibrillation. *Ann Emerg Med* 1988;17:318–321.
4. Bachman JW, McDonald GS, O'Brien PC. A study of out-of-hospital cardiac arrests in northeastern Minnesota. *JAMA* 1986;256:477–483.
5. Olson DW, La Rochelle J, Fark D, et al. EMT-defibrillation: The Wisconsin experience. *Ann Emerg Med* 1989;18:806–811.
6. Stults KR, Brown DD, Schug VL, et al. Prehospital defibrillation performed by emergency medical technicians in rural communities. *N Engl J Med* 1984;310:219–223.
7. Weaver WD, Hill D, Fahrenbruch CE, et al. Use of the automatic external defibrillator in the management of out-of-hospital cardiac arrest. *N Engl J Med* 1988;319:661–666.
8. Cummins RO, Stults KR, Haggar B, et al. A new rhythm library for testing automatic external defibrillators: Performance of three devices. *J Am Coll Cardiol* 1988;11:597–602.

9. Cummins RO, Eisenberg M, Bergner L, et al. Sensitivity, accuracy and safety of an automatic external defibrillator. *Lancet* 1984;2:318–320.
10. Emergency Cardiac Care Committee and Subcommittees AHA. Guidelines for cardiopulmonary resuscitation and emergency cardiac care. IV: Pediatric advanced life support. *JAMA* 1992;268:2262–2275.
11. Weisfeldt ML, Kerber RE, McGoldrick RP, et al. American Heart Association Report on the Public Access Defibrillation Conference—December 8–10, 1994. *Circulation* 1995;92:2740–2747.
12. Weisfeldt ML, Kerber RE, McGoldrick RP, et al. Public access defibrillation: A statement for healthcare professionals from the American Heart Association Task Force on Automatic External Defibrillation. *Circulation* 1995;92:2763.
13. Ronco R, King W, Donley DK, et al. Outcome and cost at a children's hospital following resuscitation for out-of-hospital cardiopulmonary arrest. *Arch Pediatr Adolesc Med* 1995;149:210–214.
14. Eisenberg M, Bergner L, Hallstrom A. Epidemiology of cardiac arrest and resuscitation in children. *Ann Emerg Med* 1983;12:672–674.
15. Walsh CK, Krongard E. Terminal cardiac electrical activity in pediatric patients. *Am J Cardiol* 1983;51:559–561.
16. Safranek DJ, Eisenberg MS, Larsen MP. The epidemiology of cardiac arrest in young adults. *Ann Emerg Med* 1992;21:1102–1106.
17. Hickey RW, Cohen DM, Strausbaugh S, et al. Pediatric patients requiring CPR in the prehospital setting. *Ann Emerg Med* 1995;25:495–501.
18. Wren C, O'Sullivan JJ, Wright C. Sudden death in children and adolescents—A population based study. *PACE* 1997;20:1051. Abstract.
19. Mogayzel C, Quan L, Graves JR, et al. Out-of-hospital ventricular fibrillation in children and adolescents: Causes and outcome. *Ann Emerg Med* 1995;25:484–491.
20. Appleton GO, Cummins RO, Larson MP, et al. CPR and the single rescuer: At what age should you "call first" rather than "call fast?" *Ann Emerg Med* 1995;25:492–494.
21. American Heart Association. *Pediatric Advanced Life Support.* Dallas: American Heart Association; 1997:1–1–11–11.
22. American Heart Association. Defibrillation. In Cummins RO (ed): *Advanced Cardiac Life Support.* Dallas: American Heart Association; 1997:4–1–4–22.
23. Atkins DL, Hartley LL, York DK. Accurate recognition and effective treatment of ventricular fibrillation by automated external defibrillators in adolescents. *Pediatrics* 1998;101:393–397.
24. Hazinski MF, Walker C, Smith J, Deshpande J. Specificity of automatic external defibrillator (AED) rhythm analysis in pediatric tachyarrhythmias. *Circulation* 1997;96:I561. Abstract.
25. Atkins DL, Kerber RE. Pediatric defibrillation: Current flow is improved by using "adult" paddle electrodes. *Pediatrics* 1994;94:90–93.
26. Samson RA, Atkins DL, Kerber RE. Optimal size of self-adhesive preapplied electrode pads in pediatric defibrillation. *Am J Cardiol* 1995;75:544–545.
27. Kerber RE, Kouba C, Martins J, et al. Advance prediction of transthoracic impedance in human defibrillation and cardioversion: Importance of impedance in determining the success of low-energy shocks. *Circulation* 1984;70:303–308.
28. Gutgesell HP, Tacker WA, Geddes LA, et al. Energy dose for ventricular defibrillation of children. *Pediatrics* 1976;58:898–901.

29. Babbs CF, Tacker WA, VanVleet JF, et al. Therapeutic indices for tran-schest defibrillator shocks: Effective, damaging, and lethal electrical doses. *Am Heart J* 1980;99:734–738.
30. White R. Early out-of-hospital experience with an impedance-compen-sating low-energy biphasic waveform automatic external defibrillator. *J Interv Card Electrophysiol* 1997;1:203–208.
31. Poole JE, White RD, Kanz KG, et al. Low-energy impedance-compensat-ing biphasic waveforms terminate ventricular fibrillation at high rates in victims of out-of-hospital cardiac arrest. LIFE investigators. *J Cardiovasc Electrophysiol* 1997;8:1373–1385.
32. Cummins RO, Hazinski MF, Kerber RE, et al. Low-energy biphasic wave-form defibrillation: Evidence-based review applied to emergency cardio-vascular care guidelines. *Circulation* 1998;97:1654–1667.
33. Morgan CB, Gliner BE, Jorgenson, DB. *Energy Attenuation for Pediatric Ap-plication of AEDs*. Presented at Ventricular Fibrillation: A Pediatric Prob-lem. Seattle: July, 1998. Abstract.
34. Eisenberg MS, Horwood BT, Cummins RO, et al. Cardiac arrest and re-suscitation: A tale of 29 cities. *Ann Emerg Med* 1990;19:179–186.

Chapter 16

Present Automated External Defibrillators:

Technology and Limitations for Use in the Pediatric Population

Ronald E. Stickney

Introduction

Early defibrillation is the most critical treatment for victims of sudden cardiac arrest with ventricular fibrillation (VF). Deployment of automated external defibrillators (AEDs) is accelerating due the lower cost of AEDs (approximately $3000 in 1998), education and training (the American Heart Association's Heartsaver AED course), and legislation (authorizing nontraditional first responders to defibrillate with protection from liability). While rare, sudden cardiac arrest does occur in the pediatric population. It would be desirable if the growing numbers of AEDs could be used for pediatric victims of sudden cardiac arrest, but use of AEDs is recommended only for patients aged 8 years or older.[1]

This chapter explores the following questions:

- Can present AEDs be used on patients less than 8 years old?
- If not, can present AEDs be easily adapted for such use?

When considering use of AEDs on pediatric patients, three issues arise:

- Electrodes
- Electrocardiogram (ECG) analysis
- Electrical dosage

From: Quan L, Franklin WH (eds). *Ventricular Fibrillation: A Pediatric Problem.* Armonk, NY: Futura Publishing Company, Inc.; ©2000.

Electrodes

"Adult" defibrillation paddles are recommended for use on children weighing at least 10 kg (the average weight for a 1-year-old child).[2,3] Since they have approximately the same conductive area as paddles, "adult" defibrillation electrodes are recommended for children who weigh at least 10 kg.

For patients who weigh less than 10 kg, pediatric defibrillation electrodes are available (eg, Pediatric QUIK-COMBO™ pacing/defibrillation/ECG electrodes [Medtronic Physio-Control, Redmond, WA]).

ECG Analysis

Most if not all ECG analysis algorithms for AEDs were developed and tested using adult ECG samples. A recent retrospective analysis of the use of AEDs on patients less than 18 years old in Iowa identified use on 16 such patients, all ages 11 to 15 years old.[4] Accuracy of the shock advisory algorithms in the AEDs (various models by Medtronic Physio-Control and Laerdal [Stavanger, Norway]) for pediatric patients was found to be similar to accuracy in adults. Sensitivity for VF was 88% and specificity (accuracy for asystole and pulseless electrical activity) was 100%. While the sample size is small, the results suggest that accuracy is adequate for adolescents. Accuracy for younger patients, however, remains unproven.

In a current study at Vanderbilt University Medical Center, investigators are collecting pediatric ECGs through defibrillation electrodes for testing Medtronic Physio-Control AEDs.[5] Various nonshockable rhythms have been collected, including sinus tachycardias, other supraventricular tachycardias, and conduction blocks. ECGs are being recorded in both the sternum-apex and anterior-posterior lead positions. Data collection is continuing, and results from preliminary testing of AEDs are encouraging.

Most AEDs claim to shock ventricular tachycardia, and different thresholds are used for heart rate. Rate thresholds of 120, 150, and 180 per minute are common. Models with thresholds of 120 or 150 per minute claim to shock wide-complex tachycardia, but are designed to reach a no-shock decision for narrow-complex (typically supraventricular) tachycardia.

Shock advisory algorithms in AEDs may very well be shown to be adequate for pediatric patients of all ages. If testing does show that improvement is needed for accurate diagnosis of pediatric rhythms, incremental changes to the ECG analysis algorithms will probably achieve the desired improvements. For instance, raising the heart rate thresholds for ventricular tachycardia would be an easy modification to make to an algorithm.

Electrical Dosage

The issue of electrical dosage for pediatric patients is not as easily addressed as the issues of electrodes and ECG analysis. The recommended dosage is 2 J/kg for the first shock, increasing to 4 J/kg for subsequent shocks.[1,6] For a 1-year-old, 10-kg patient, this translates to 20 and 40 J—well below the energy delivered by the AEDs most often purchased today. Damage probably correlates better with current density rather than shock energy. A recent enzyme study suggests minimal cardiac damage from shocks up to 360 J in adults being treated for atrial fibrillation.[7] It is possible that pediatric patients can tolerate substantially more than 4 J/kg, which would allow today's AEDs to be used on patients younger than 8 years. The maximum safe dosage for defibrillation of children has not been determined.

Biphasic defibrillation waveforms hold promise for allowing use of AEDs on smaller children. Lower shock energy can be used. In addition, biphasic waveforms afford less risk of damage at relatively high energy levels.[8–10] These two factors may allow for the use of AEDs with biphasic waveforms on even younger children. The minimum and maximum biphasic energy levels for defibrillation of children have not been determined.

Possible Device Modifications

To allow defibrillation of children by using lower-than-standard energy levels, an AED design could be modified by adding a pediatric switch. Alternatively, defibrillation electrode sets could be designed to dissipate some of the shock energy, thus reducing the energy delivered to the patient.

These potential modifications raise several questions:

- Would a single pediatric energy level suffice for the range of pediatric patients?
- Does the benefit of a pediatric switch outweigh the risk of user error?
- Does the benefit of an energy-reducing pediatric electrode set outweigh the added cost (two sets of electrodes with the AED) and complexity, with risk of using the wrong electrodes?
- Is the demand for pediatric use of AEDs great enough to justify the development cost and added cost to the AED owner?

Conclusions

Three issues pertain to use of AEDs on the pediatric population: electrodes, ECG analysis, and electrical dosage. "Adult" defibrillation electrodes are recommended for use on patients weighing as little as 10 kg (1 year old), and pediatric defibrillation electrodes are available for smaller patients down to neonates. Early results from a current study[5] suggest that existing shock advisory algorithms may have adequate specificity when presented with a variety of nonshockable rhythms from patients of all pediatric ages. A recently published study[4] found acceptable diagnosis of ECG rhythms from adolescents. The shock energy delivered by today's AEDs is recommended for defibrillation of patients as young as 8 years old. Studies are needed to show that energy levels of today's AEDs are safe for even younger patients, especially with biphasic defibrillation. Modified AEDs or electrode sets could allow lower energy for pediatric patients.

References

1. Chameides L, Hazinski MF (eds): *Textbook of Pediatric Advanced Life Support*. Dallas: American Heart Association; 1997:7–13.
2. Atkins DL, Sirna S, Kieso R, et al. Pediatric defibrillation: Importance of paddle size in determining transthoracic impedance. *Pediatrics* 1988;82: 914–918.
3. Atkins DL, Kerber RE. Pediatric defibrillation: Current flow is improved by using "adult" paddle electrodes. *Pediatrics* 1994;94:90–93.
4. Atkins DL, Hartley LL, York DK. Accurate recognition and effective treatment of ventricular fibrillation by automated external defibrillators in adolescents. *Pediatrics* 1998;101:393–397.
5. Hazinski MF, Walker C, Smith J, Deshpande J. Specificity of automatic external defibrillator (AED) rhythm analysis in pediatric tachyarrhythmias. *Circulation* 1997;96:I561. Abstract.
6. Gutgesell HP, Tacker WA, Geddes LA, et al. Energy dose for ventricular defibrillation of children. *Pediatrics* 1976;58:898–901.
7. Grubb NR, Cuthbert D, Cawood P, et al. Effect of DC shock on serum levels of total creatine kinase, MB-creatine kinase mass and troponin T. *Resuscitation* 1998;36:193–199.
8. Negovsky VA, Smerdov AA, Tabak VY, et al. Criteria of efficiency and safety of the defibrillating impulse. *Resuscitation* 1980;8:53–67.
9. Reddy RK, Gleva MJ, Gliner BE, et al. Biphasic transthoracic defibrillation causes fewer ECG ST-segment changes after shock. *Ann Emerg Med* 1997;30:127–134.
10. Chapman FW, El-Abbady TZ, Walcott GP, et al. Dysfunction following transthoracic defibrillation shocks in dogs. *PACE* 1997;20:1128. Abstract.

Chapter 17

Transthoracic Defibrillation:
Waveforms and Damage

Richard E. Kerber, MD

Introduction

The purpose of this chapter is twofold: first, it reviews the various waveforms used for transthoracic defibrillation, emphasizing comparative efficacy. Second, is reviews the manifestations of direct current shock damage, discussing damage mechanisms and cardioprotective strategies.

Waveforms for Transthoracic Defibrillation

The waveforms used for transthoracic defibrillation fall into three categories: monophasic (damped sine wave, truncated exponential), biphasic (including Gurvich and "sawtooth" waveforms), and multipulse multipathway.

Monophasic Waveforms

The damped sinusoidal waveform is the most widely used waveform for transthoracic defibrillation (Figure 1). Variations of this waveform are referred to as "Lown," "Edmark," and "Pantridge." In adults, the energy recommendations for this waveform (initial shock of 200 J, repeating at 200/300 J and 360 J if necessary) are well established, based on long clinical experience.[1,2] For the adult with an average transtho-

From: Quan L, Franklin WH (eds). *Ventricular Fibrillation: A Pediatric Problem.* Armonk, NY: Futura Publishing Company, Inc.; ©2000.

Supported in part by NHLBI Grant #HL53284 and in part by a grant from the Laerdal Foundation for Medical Research.

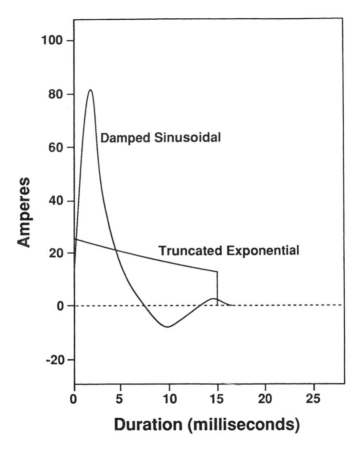

Figure 1. Damped sinusoidal and truncated exponential waveforms for defibrillation. Reproduced from Reference 7, with permission.

racic impedance (70 to 80Ω), a 200-J initial shock will generate a peak current of approximately 30 amperes, an appropriate range for defibrillation.[2] A weight-based electrical dose of 2 J/kg is recommended for children,[1] although this is based on limited data.[3]

Truncated exponential waveforms are effective; however there are relatively few published clinical data available.[4,5] When transthoracic impedance is high, the duration of this shock waveform increases, and this may cause loss of effectiveness when the duration exceeds 35 to 40 milliseconds.[6] In a retrospective study of witnessed prehospital cardiac arrests treated by emergency medical services, Behr et al[7] found that truncated exponential waveform shocks terminated ventricular fibrillation (VF) less often than damped sinusoidal shocks, although there was no significant difference in patient survival.

Biphasic Waveforms

Waveforms consisting of a positive truncated exponential waveform followed immediately by a negative (ie, reversed polarity) truncated exponential waveform were found to be superior for internal (endocardial) defibrillation and are now used uniformly in implantable cardioverter-defibrillators. These waveforms were recently investigated for transthoracic defibrillation. Animal studies have shown that at equal energies, biphasic waveforms terminate VF at a higher rate than do damped sinusoidal waveforms.[8,9] They may be particularly advantageous after long-duration VF,[10] and may be more likely than damped sinusoidal waveforms to restore a perfusing rhythm when combined with cardiopulmonary resuscitation during prolonged VF.[11] Initial human studies, performed in the in-hospital setting of the electrophysiology laboratory or operating room, yielded similar results (Figure 2).[12] Biphasic waveform defibrillators have been approved for clinical use. One biphasic waveform defibrillator delivers a fixed-dose 150-J biphasic shock, and has an impedance-compensating feature, whereby the duration and tilt of the waveform are adjusted by the unit in the first 2 milliseconds of the shock, based on the transthoracic impedance measured by the defibrillator. The total waveform duration varies from 5 to 20 ms. Initial out-of-hospital experience with the first 100 patients has been reported by White[13] and by Poole et al[14]; in these patients, the first and all-shock success rates were very high, 89% and 87%, respectively, and no patient failed to defibrillate after receiving up to three shocks. The range of transthoracic impedance was large, 36 to 171Ω, suggesting the effectiveness of the impedance-compensating approach. However, these were not randomized, prospective studies.

The Gurvich biphasic waveform is essentially a damped sinusoidal waveform with a marked undershoot, which results in a reversed-polarity second phase. This waveform was used in defibrillators in Russia. Although it can defibrillate effectively,[15] it is electrically inefficient and is unlikely to see widespread use.

A sawtooth waveform has been investigated in animals.[16] This waveform features a momentary increase in voltage near the end of the first phase that increases the average current achieved during the first phase and also increases the net change in voltage at the moment of polarity reversal (Figure 3). Both of these increases may contribute to enhanced defibrillation effectiveness.

Multipulse Multipathway Waveforms

Myocytes are directionally sensitive to electrical fields; in a saline bath, a myocyte suspended perpendicular to an electrical field requires

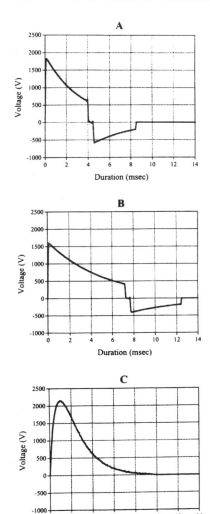

Figure 2. Biphasic waveforms (A and B) and a damped sinusoidal waveform (C) used in initial human studies of biphasic defibrillation. Reproduced from Reference 12, with permission of the American Heart Association.

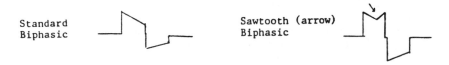

Figure 3. A "sawtooth" biphasic waveform; the voltage is increased at the end of the positive pulse, just prior to polarity reversal.

substantially more energy to depolarize than a myocyte oriented parallel to the field.[17] In the mammalian heart, myocytes are variably oriented. Thus, any single pathway shock may encounter some myocytes that may be unfavorably oriented and may therefore not be depolarized by a shock; this may be a source of failure to terminate VF. The rapid administration of a series of overlapping truncated exponential pulses from a set of electrodes encircling the chest creates a rapidly moving electrical vector that traverses a 360° arc around the thorax (Figure 4). Animal studies have suggested that such waveforms achieve defibrillation at a higher rate than do biphasic shocks of equivalent energy.[18] However, the requirement for multiple electrodes would be a disadvantage in clinical use.

Several important questions must be answered with particular regard to biphasic waveforms. As noted, one biphasic waveform defibrillator approved for clinical use has only one available energy level (150 J). Initial experience indicates that this is a highly efficient waveform at 150 J.[13,14] Is 150 J sufficient? Are there patients who will fail to defibrillate with 150-J biphasic shocks but who would defibrillate if a higher "backup" energy was available? Or, is a heart that fails to defibrillate upon receiving a 150-J biphasic shock so damaged that higher energy biphasic shocks (200 J? 300 to 360 J?) will be similarly ineffective?

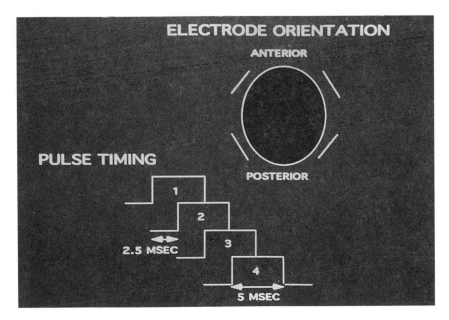

Figure 4. Multipulse multipathway defibrillation. A series of overlapping pulses are administered from electrodes encircling the chest, creating an electrical vector that rapidly traverses a 360° arc around the thorax.

The answer to this question will emerge from further prehospital experience.

A second issue that must be addressed is the role of biphasic waveforms in the defibrillation of neonates and children. As is discussed subsequently, direct current shock damage is related to the energy dose used; 150 J, the sole biphasic energy dose presently available, is excessive for children. In fact, there are no data available at present to identify the optimal energy range for pediatric biphasic waveform defibrillation. This is a fertile area for research.

Direct Current Shock Damage

Tissue damage from direct current shocks given for emergency defibrillation of VF, or for the elective termination of atrial arrhythmias, takes many forms. The erythematous rings commonly seen on the skin after defibrillation (Figure 5), outlining the electrode shape, are in fact first-degree burns, related to the energy used.[19] Direct current shocks can cause derangements of electrical rhythm; unsynchronized shocks given for atrial arrhythmias can induce VF, and high-energy shocks that terminate VF may induce heart block or pulseless electrical activity.[20] Myocardial damage can be demonstrated morphologically on gross inspection (Figure 6) and on microscopic evaluation.[21] Damage is indicated by enzyme release and by positive technetium pyrophos-

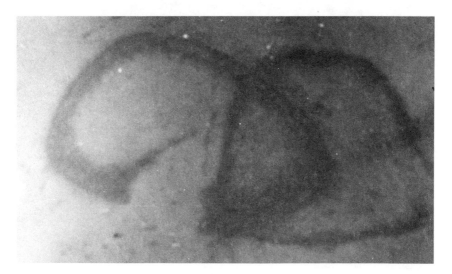

Figure 5. Erythematous rings on the skin outline the electrodes used for defibrillation. Skin biopsies show these to be first-degree burns, caused by preferential current flow at the electrode edges.

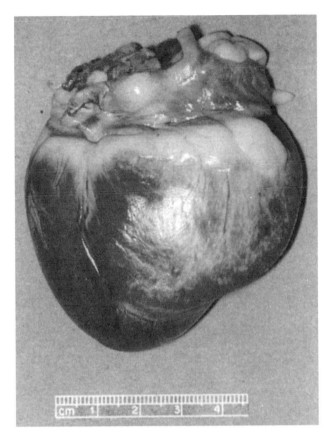

Figure 6. Gross morphologic damage (white areas on left ventricular epicardium) after a single high-energy (16 A/kg) transthoracic shock. Reproduced from Reference 21, with permission of Mosby-YearBook, Inc., St. Louis, MO.

phate scintigrams.[21] Jones and Milne[22] used postshock recovery of beating cultured chick embryo myocytes to demonstrate the comparative toxicity of different defibrillation waveforms; asymmetric biphasic waveforms reduced postshock dysfunction in these models. Experiments using sonomicrometers after epicardial shocks[23] show regional contraction abnormalities (dyskinesis) (Figure 7); global depression of ventricular contractility has also been reported.[24]

What are the mechanisms of shock-induced damage? Intramyocardial temperature rises have been demonstrated.[25] Mitochondrial damage occurs.[26] Free radicals, known to be cardiotoxic, are generated by direct current shocks, a phenomenon related to peak shock energy; free radical scavengers blunt this effect.[27] Electroporation, cell membrane injury, occurs after shocks and may also be a damage mechanism.[28]

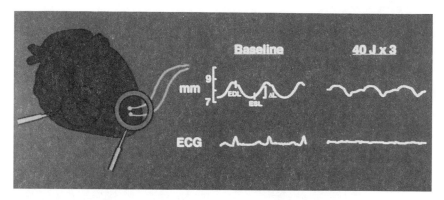

Figure 7. Regional myocardial dyskinesis (systolic bulging) demonstrated by sonomicrometers after three 40-J epicardial shocks from electrode paddles placed over the sonomicrometers. EDL = end-diastolic length; ESL = end-systolic length; ΔL = systolic contraction.

Can shock-induced damage be prevented or reduced? Minimizing the peak and cumulative electrical energy dose is a clearly effective strategy; most indices of damage are dose-related. Clinically used drugs with free radical scavenging properties—for example, angiotensin-converting enzyme inhibitors—may be cardioprotective if administered *before* a shock (eg, in elective cardioversion).[29] New electrodes that achieve a more homogeneous current flow, reducing the tendency of current to preferentially flow at the electrode edge, reduce skin injury.[30]

What questions remain? Experimental studies suggest that biphasic waveforms are associated with less damage than damped sinusoidal waveforms, but the clinical importance and manifestations of this effect are as yet unknown. We do not know if there is an energy or current threshold in humans, above which damage will always occur. Finally, a common electrocardiographic change after direct current shocks is ST segment elevation or depression. Whether this truly represents damage[31] (and can be used as a clinical indicator of damage), or rather is an innocuous membrane effect, is not clear. In the animal laboratory, marked ST changes after shock commonly occur and are transient, and may not in themselves indicate damage (Figure 8).

In conclusion, there are many effective defibrillation waveforms: biphasic waveforms seem likely to replace the damped sinusoidal waveform, which has been the standard for almost 40 years. Defibrillation damage is a direct toxic effect of the electrical current; the most reliable protection is use of the lowest effective energy for defibrillation.

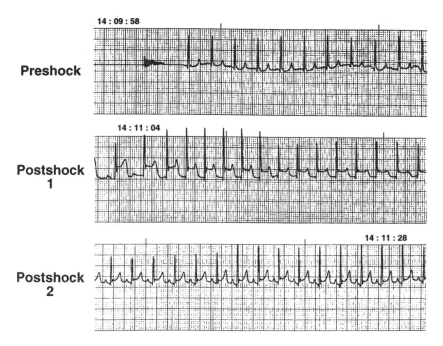

14 : 09 : 58

Preshock

14 : 11 : 04

Postshock 1

14 : 11 : 28

Postshock 2

Figure 8. Electrocardiographic ST segment elevation after direct current epicardial shocks, that rapidly returns to baseline. Whether these changes represent damage or merely a membrane effect is not yet established.

References

1. Emergency Cardiac Care Committee and Subcommittees. American Heart Association Guidelines for Cardiopulmonary Resuscitation and Emergency Cardiac Care. *JAMA* 1992;268:2172–2295.
2. Kerber RE, Martins JB, Kienzle MG, et al. Energy, current and success in defibrillation and cardioversion: Clinical studies using an automated impedance-based method of energy adjustment. *Circulation* 1988;77: 1038–1046.
3. Gutgesell HP, Tacker WA, Geddes LA, et al. Energy dose for ventricular defibrillation of children. *Pediatrics* 1976;58:898–901.
4. Anderson GJ, Suelzer J. The efficacy of trapezoidal waveforms for ventricular defibrillation. *Chest* 1976;70:298–300.
5. Tacker W. Clinical efficacy of a truncated exponential decay defibrillator. *J Electrocardiol* 1976;9:273–274.
6. Schuder JC, Rahmoeller GA, Stoekle H. Transthoracic ventricular defibrillation with triangular and trapezoidal waveforms. *Circ Res* 1966;19: 689–694.
7. Behr JC, Hartley LL, York DK, et al. Truncated exponential vs. damped sinusoidal waveform shocks for transthoracic defibrillation. *Am J Cardiol* 1996;78:1242–1245.
8. Schuder JC, McDaniel WC, Stoeckle H. Defibrillation of 100 kg calves with

asymmetrical, bidirectional rectangular pulses. *Cardiovasc Res* 1984;18: 419–426.

9. Gliner BE, Lyster TE, Dillon SM, et al. Transthoracic defibrillation of swine with monophasic and biphasic waveforms. *Circulation* 1995;92:1634–1643.

10. Jones JC, Swartz JF, Jones RE, et al. Increasing fibrillation duration enhances relative asymmetrical biphasic vs. monophasic defibrillator waveform efficacy. *Circ Res* 1990;67:376–384.

11. Garcia LA, DeJong SC, Kerber RE. Influence of cardiopulmonary resuscitation on resumption of a perfusing rhythm after defibrillation: Biphasic vs. damped sinusoidal waveforms. *J Am Coll Cardiol* 1998;31:403A. Abstract.

12. Bardy GH, Marchlinsky FE, Sharma AD, et al. Multicenter comparison of truncated biphasic shocks and standard damped sinusoidal monophasic shocks for transthoracic ventricular defibrillation. *Circulation* 1996;94: 2507–2514.

13. White R. Early out-of-hospital experience with an impedance-compensating low energy biphasic waveform automatic external defibrillator. *J Interv Card Electrophysiol* 1997;1:203–208.

14. Poole JE, White RD, Kanz KG, et al. Low-energy impedance-compensating biphasic waveforms terminate ventricular fibrillation at high rates in victims of out-of-hospital cardiac arrest. *J Cardiovasc Electrophysiol* 1997; 8:1373–1385.

15. Greene HL, DiMarco JP, Kudenchek PJ, et al. Comparison of monophasic and biphasic defibrillating pulse waveforms for transthoracic cardioversion. *Am J Cardiol* 1995;75:1135–1139.

16. Yamanouchi Y, Brewer JE, Mouray KA, et al. Sawtooth first phase biphasic defibrillation waveform: A comparison with standard waveform in clinical devices. *J Cardiovasc Electrophysiol* 1997;8:517–528.

17. Tung L, Silz N, Mulligan MR. Influence of electrical axis of stimulation on excitation of cardiac muscle cells. *Circ Res* 1991;69:722–730.

18. Kerber RE, Spencer KT, Kallok MJ, et al. Overlapping sequential pulses: A new waveform for transthoracic defibrillation. *Circulation* 1994;89: 2369–2379.

19. Pagan-Carlo LA, Stone MS, Kerber RE. Nature and determinants of skin burns after transthoracic cardioversion. *Am J Cardiol* 1997;79:689–692.

20. Weaver WD, Cobb L, Copass M. Ventricular defibrillation: A comparative trial using 175 J and 330 J shocks. *N Engl J Med* 1982;307:1101–1106.

21. VanVleet JF, Tacker WA. Cardiac damage from transchest and ICD defibrillator shocks. In Tacker WA (ed): *Defibrillation of the Heart. ICD's, AED's and Manual.* St. Louis: Mosby-YearBook; 1994:259–298.

22. Jones JL, Milne KB. Dysfunction and safety factor strength-duration curves for biphasic defibrillator waveforms. *Am J Physiol* 1994;226: H263–H271.

23. Kerber RE, Martins JB, Gascho J, et al. Effect of direct current countershocks on regional myocardial contractility and perfusion. Experimental studies. *Circulation* 1981;63:323–332.

24. Xie J, Weil MH, Sun S, et al. High-energy defibrillation increases the severity of post-resuscitation myocardial dysfunction. *Circulation* 1997;96:683–688.

25. Doherty PW, McLaughlin PR, Billingham M, et al. Cardiac damage produced by direct current countershocks applied to the heart. *Am J Cardiol* 1979;43:225–232.

26. Trouton PG, Allen JD, Yong LK, et al. Metabolic changes and mitochondrial dysfunction early following transthoracic countershocks in dogs. *PACE* 1989;12:1827–1834.
27. Caterine MR, Spencer KT, Pagan-Carlo LA, et al. Direct current shocks to the heart generate free radicals: An electron paramagnetic resonance study. *J Am Coll Cardiol* 1996;28:1598–1609.
28. Tung L. Electrical injury to heart muscle cells. In Lee RC, Cravacho EG, Burke JF (eds): *Electrical Trauma: The Pathophysiology, Manifestations and Clinical Management.* New York: Cambridge University Press; 1992: 361–400.
29. Caterine MR, Spencer KT, Smith RS. Antioxidant enzymes attenuate free radical generation after direct current countershocks. *J Am Coll Cardiol* 1995;25:210A. Abstract.
30. Garcia LA, Pagan-Carlo LG, Stone MS, et al. Increasing electrode perimeter impedance to modify the "edge effect" reduces skin burns after transthoracic countershocks. *Circulation* 1997;96:I560.
31. Reddy RK, Gleva MJ, Gliner BE, et al. Biphasic transthoracic defibrillation causes fewer ECG ST-segment changes after shock. *Ann Emerg Med* 1997; 30:127–134.

Chapter 18

Automated External Defibrillators in Children:
Food and Drug Administration Issues

Carole C. Carey, RN, BSEE, MEng
and Thomas J. Callahan, PhD

Sudden cardiac arrest in the adult population is one of the leading causes of death in the United States, claiming the lives of more than 350,000 Americans each year. The primary cause of cardiac arrest is heart disease. Although the rhythm disorders of adults are also seen in children, life-threatening ventricular fibrillation (VF) and ventricular tachycardia (VT) are uncommon. The origin of the dysrhythmia in the pediatric population is often supraventricular. Children also manifest more rapid ventricular rates than adults. In those cardiac arrests that are primarily cardiac in origin, the definitive therapy is electrical countershock.[1-4]

The device that is used to deliver an electrical current to the heart to interrupt cardiac arrhythmias, especially VF, is called a defibrillator. The term "defibrillator" is used to describe both the implantable cardioverter-defibrillator and the external defibrillator, in which the energy is delivered transthoracically with use of external paddles or pregelled disposable electrodes. This discussion will be limited to external defibrillators.

Many external defibrillators are designed for manual operation with selectable energy level settings that typically range from 2 J to 360 J. The operator selects the energy levels appropriate for either cardioversion or defibrillation, initiates "charging of the capacitors," and then triggers the defibrillator switches to deliver the shock. Manual external defibrillators often include a display of the patient's electrocardiogram (ECG). They can also be equipped with sterile internal paddles

From: Quan L, Franklin WH (eds). *Ventricular Fibrillation: A Pediatric Problem.* Armonk, NY: Futura Publishing Company, Inc.; ©2000.

for emergency use in open-chest surgical procedures. Other optional accessories include pediatric sized paddles and disposable electrodes. Some have special circuitry to provide external transcutaneous pacing. Generally, they are used in clinical settings within the hospital, with some models also configured for the prehospital environment.

For the out-of-hospital resuscitation of adults, an automated or "advisory" external defibrillator (AED) has become the standard defibrillation device. Unlike manual external defibrillators, AEDs are designed with an arrhythmia detection algorithm that automates the detection and interpretation of those cardiac arrhythmias (VF/VT) that require defibrillation. A fully automated AED charges and delivers the shocks when a treatable arrhythmia is detected. Most AEDs are only semiautomated in that they indicate to the user (through visual and/or voice prompts) that a prescribed shock should be delivered. Depending on the medical protocol followed, the device is pre-set to deliver a sequence of increasing shock levels (eg, 200 J, 200 to 300 J, 360 J). Others require that the operator activate the arrhythmia-recognition capability after the electrodes are placed on the patient.

The incorporation of automatic arrhythmia detection is the most significant recent advance in external defibrillator design, making it possible for many more "first responders" to be qualified AED users. There are a large amount of data and extensive clinical experience in prehospital defibrillation that support the safety and effectiveness of AED use in adult patients. However, AED effectiveness for children has never been scientifically tested. The recommendations from the American Heart Association (AHA) discussed later in this chapter appear to be based on consensus and, to some degree, on conjecture. This discussion therefore focuses on the issues pertaining to the promotion of AEDs for use in children.

Introduction to Medical Device Regulations

To the extent that the Food and Drug Administration (FDA) has the statutory authority to regulate the sale of medical devices in the United States, the controversy and unresolved issues posed by pediatric AED use in children is problematic for the FDA. Before analyzing regulatory issues surrounding prehospital defibrillation by AEDs in children, it is necessary to have a basic understanding of medical device law.

The Medical Device Amendments to the Federal Food, Drug, & Cosmetic (FD&C) Act enacted on May 28, 1976 gave the FDA specific authority to regulate medical devices.[5] The FDA must interpret the provisions of the law and make the specific rules that appear in Title 21 of the Code of Federal Regulations (21 CFR). Additional regulatory authority was given to the agency by the Safe Medical Devices Act (SMDA) of 1990 and also by the Medical Device Amendments of 1992. The FDA Modernization Act (FDAMA) of 1997 further amended the FD&C Act to streamline the process of bringing safe and effective medical devices to the US market. The FDA's Office of Device Evaluation (ODE),[1] an office within the Center of Devices and Radiological Health (CDRH),[2] has the responsibility of assuring that medical devices that are introduced to the market are reasonably safe and effective when used in accordance with the product labeling.

Regulatory Classification of Medical Devices

First, the FDA must consider the regulatory history of a device and determine its *preamendment status* (ie, prior to May 28, 1976). Table 1 provides some definitions of common phrases used in medical device review.

Another important consideration is *classification*. In the United States, the device class determines the extent and level of regulatory control imposed on a medical device before it can be legally marketed. Table 2 defines three levels of regulatory control, based on device class, that provide reasonable assurance of safety and effectiveness of each device. The Federal FD&C Act requires the FDA to classify all devices intended for human use into three regulatory categories, namely Class I (*General Controls*), Class II (*Special Controls*), and Class III (*Premarket Approval*). Subsequent to the enactment of the Medical Devices Act in 1976, panels of experts devoted to a medical specialty were established to provide advice and guidance to the FDA. After receiving panel recommendations, the FDA determined which class appeared most appropriate, then published the proposed classification (by notice) in the Federal Register and requested public comment. This procedure provides a mechanism for the public to help determine the best classification for each device. The FDA then responded to the public comments, and classified the device by regulation (Final Rule).

Figure 1 illustrates the market access routes for medical devices in general. It provides an overview of the path that allows device manufacturers to continue the distribution of products that were legally marketed before May 28, 1976. Likewise, the regulatory pathways for new devices developed after the 1976 enactment date are shown.

---

[1]Office Director, Susan Alpert, PhD, MD

[2]Center Director, D. Bruce Burlington, MD

Table 1

Regulatory Device Terms and Rules

Preamendment ("old") devices	Devices in commercial distribution before May 28, 1976. FDA must have a regulatory process to call for PMAs for preamendment Class III devices (see Table 2).
Postamendment ("new") devices	Devices that were first commercially distributed after May 28, 1976. Manufacturers of class III postamendment devices that are not substantially equivalent to preamendment class III devices must obtain PMA before marketing their device.
Premarket notification (or 510[k])	A statutory section in the FD&C Act that requires a person to submit at least 90 days before he intends to market a device for the first time or a device in distribution but is significantly modified in design and use.
510(k) device	A Class I, II, or III device that was cleared for market through a premarket notification process. They include nonexempt Class I, Class II devices, and Class III device in which no effective date has been established of the requirement for premarket approval.
Substantially equivalent (or SE) device	A postamendment device that is found substantially equivalent to a predicate device.
Predicate device	A legally marketed device.
Premarket approval (or PMA) device	Class III devices that are subject to the premarket approval requirements of Section 515 of the FD&C Act.
QSR	Quality system regulation (formerly known as GMP or good manufacturing practices).

FDA = Food and Drug Administration; FD&C = Food, Drug, and Cosmetic.

Table 2

Three Levels of Regulatory Control Based on Device Class

Class I, *"General Controls"*	These are devices needing the lowest level of regulation. They may include establishment registration (manufacturing site), device listing, premarket notification, and good manufacturing practices. Some devices are exempt.
Class II, *"Special Controls*	(Previously associated with "performance standards") These are devices in which sufficient information exists to allow the use of "special controls." In addition to general controls, special controls may include mandatory performance standards, labeling, patient registries, guidelines, and other appropriate controls to protect public health.
Class III, *"Premarket Approval"*	These are devices that potentially pose the greatest hazard to patients and include implantable and life-sustaining or life-supporting devices. Class III devices may require PMA application approval, premarket notification, or both.

PMA = premarket approval.

External Defibrillator Classification and Regulatory Status

External defibrillators are categorized into two separate classes, Class II and Class III. External manual defibrillators as described in 21 CFR 870.5300 are preamendment devices.[6] The FDA classified low-energy, manual direct current defibrillators as Class II, and high-energy defibrillators as Class III. The generic type of Class II, low-energy, manual defibrillators has a maximum output of less than 360 J of energy. Low-energy outputs are typically used in pediatric defibrillation or in cardiac surgery. A separate regulation requiring premarket approval of the high-energy direct current defibrillators (maximum output >360 J) has been promulgated and published in the Federal Register [61FR 50706, Sept. 27, 1996].

Only the preamendment manual external defibrillator was classified. Although there was an AED device that was legally marketed prior to the device amendments (discussed below), the AED has not yet been through the panel classification process. The FDA will continue

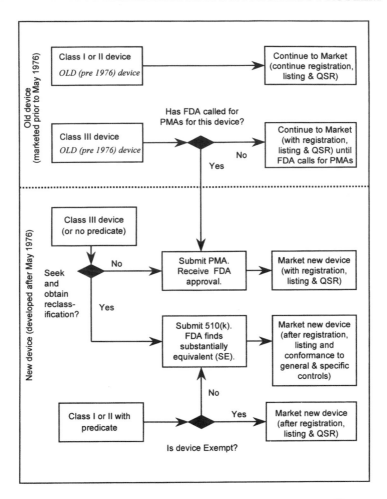

Figure 1. Flow chart of market access routes for medical devices. The top section is for "old" devices distributed prior to May 28, 1976. The bottom section represents the "new" devices distributed after the May 28, 1976 enactment date.

the device classification activities until all devices are classified. However, at present, because the AED is a preamendment device, manufacturers of AEDs are required only to submit a premarket notification to the FDA, and to wait for a premarket clearance letter under the 510(k) provision before beginning commercial distribution in the US. The manufacturer is required only to demonstrate "substantial equivalence" to a *predicate* device. The new device is then subject to the same requirements as the predicate. In a future issue of the Federal Register, the FDA will issue a notice of a panel meeting that will discuss the classification of AEDs.

AED Device History and Configuration

The FDA traced one AED that was in commercial distribution prior to the May 28, 1976 enactment date, that qualified as the "grandfather" AED.[7] It was designed as a fully automated transesophageal defibrillator, and identified as the "HEART AID Model 60 Cardiac Resuscitator" (Cardiac Rescusitatation Corporation, Portland, OR). As an AED, the device automatically analyzed the ECG signal input acquired from a tongue electrode (oropharyngeal airway) and an external chest electrode pad applied to the lower chest (epigastric region). The decision algorithm to treat was quite simple. If a heart rate greater than 200 bpm was detected and there was no apparent breathing in the airway, the defibrillator automatically charged and delivered a shock. Access to this device was by prescription only. However, it could also be used in a home setting by trained family members, but for adult patients only.

Subsequent to the enactment of the medical device amendments, other types of AEDs were introduced into the marketplace. All of the devices incorporated arrhythmia analysis algorithms capable of analyzing the ECG for the presence of VT/VF, followed by defibrillation therapy. As AEDs continued to undergo technological development and gain out-of-hospital field experience, their features and functions also changed. A notable difference between the preamendment "HEART AID Model 60" and postamendment AED devices is the ECG defibrillation pathway. In today's defibrillators, the electrode configuration is transthoracic (anterior/lateral or anterior/posterior), and senses impedance between the two adhesive electrodes. Another modification is the defibrillation shock delivery mechanism. Most AEDs require that the operator command the shock on the "advice" of the machine (semiautomated). Defibrillation technology is continuously being improved, particularly with new output waveforms that have biphasic pulses that are effective and use less energy. Conventional AEDs have monophasic output pulse waveforms that are identical to those used in the standard types of manual external defibrillators.

Areas of Unresolved Issues

Although there have been many technological advances in defibrillator design, including improvements in automatic rhythm recognition, waveforms with lower energy, miniaturization, ease of use, and other features that allow AEDs to expand the pool of users beyond the trained emergency medical service (EMS) personnel, no AED has been optimized for use in the pediatric population. All current AEDs are primarily designed and *"intended for use"* in adults.

The FDA, in taking any regulatory position, relies on the available and credible sources of safety and effectiveness information such as bench tests, animal studies, data from premarket clinical investigations, postmarket field trials, adverse events reports, and peer-reviewed published literature. As we examine the issues pertaining to the use of current AEDs in children, we consider several elements that are critical in our analysis. They may include information on the device history and experience, design and engineering considerations, and labeling claims (eg, indications/contraindications for use, warnings, the intended users, and the intended use environment). Literature review of safety and effectiveness information (published and unpublished) as well as input from the clinical community also play important factors in our evaluation of safety and effectiveness. Risks and benefits are carefully weighed.

AED Use Contraindicated for Pediatrics

There is no predicate AED device labeled for pediatric use that was in commercial distribution during the preamendment era. The use of the HEART AID Model 60 for infants and children was clearly contraindicated. However, when considering the importance of early diagnosis and aggressive treatment of cardiac insufficiency and of avoiding cardiac arrest (the key to improving survival without neurologic deficit), the definition of "child" sometimes becomes blurred. Nonetheless, the FDA believes that labeling an AED for use in pediatric patients (a new intended population) will require scientific evidence that provides a reasonable assurance of safety and effectiveness for its intended population. At present, external defibrillation energies for pediatric use are administered using manual defibrillators, not AEDs. The dose to be administered can vary considerably and, in practice, may depend on the experience of the physician and the available defibrillator. Clinicians use a general guideline of 2 J/kg, based on the 1976 study, *Energy Dose for Ventricular Defibrillation of Children*.[8] These investigators also suggest that the maximum defibrillation shock in children weighing less than 50 kg is 4 J/kg. Considering that most AEDs have a minimum energy level of 200 J, it would appear that they have excessive outputs for patients who weigh less than 50 kg.

A Paradigm Shift in AED Labeling: Weight-Based or Aged-Based?

In the postamendment era, AED labeling has also contraindicated pediatric use. Furthermore, a clarification statement restricts the use of

AEDs based on weight. For example, the user's manual of a typical AED device states that the device is not intended for use on patients who have a body weight of less than 90 lbs (40 to 41 kg). What is the basis of the weight guideline? The statement is based on published pediatric protocols developed by the AHA and the American Academy of Pediatrics.[9–11] The guideline may also be a part of resuscitation protocols used by EMS services. At some, the AHA's guidance (Textbook of Advanced Cardiac Life Support, *Safe Automated Defibrillation*) has shifted from a weight-based limit to a margin based on age: "*For children older than 8 years, follow the standard operating procedures. This recommendation reflects the sense that the opportunity to defibrillate a child in VF should not be missed despite the fact that AED experience in pediatric resuscitation is severely limited.*"[12] With the change in this recommendation, AED labeling has also been modified to reflect the AHA's new criteria.

Can AEDs be Optimized for Pediatric Use?

The therapeutic goal of the AED is the restoration of heartbeat for the suspected victims of cardiac arrest in whom the cardiac arrest is to be verified by the AED. If AEDs are to be used by unskilled, minimally trained individuals, the reliability of these devices for pediatric use cannot be determined because these devices are not designed or tested for correct interpretation of pediatric ECG rhythms. In addition, a corollary to the accurate recognition of VT/VF is that the AED must administer the appropriate dosage required to treat VT/VF in children. Dosage is an essential consideration of any therapy prescription, including the accurate quantification of the appropriate energy level in children.

It would be perilous to make recommendations without scientific data that conclusively establish the safety and effectiveness of AED use in children. Valid scientific evidence is needed to demonstrate that an AED can: 1) perform the crucial diagnostic function of correctly identifying treatable rhythms, and 2) administer the best prescriptive pediatric defibrillation dosage. The standard for dosage of electrical shock for children has yet to be confirmed.

AED effectiveness for children has not been evaluated despite the recommendations from the AHA. The origin of the weight-based automated external defibrillation concept is the study conducted in 1976 by Gutgesell and colleagues.[8] Does this single in-hospital study provide sufficient scientific documentation for designing safe and effective AEDs that are to be used for out-of-hospital pediatric resuscitation? How should we consider AHA's recommended criteria of "more than 8 years old"? Are we sure that anyone older than 8 years should be considered an "adult for purposes of defibrillation"? Why is "8" the magic number? Should use of AEDs for pediatric defibrillation be limited to personnel qualified in advanced pediatric life support, or can we include less trained individuals who potentially may be the citizens at large?

Animal studies and clinical data are sparse. However, a recently published study[13] is very encouraging. The authors of this study conclude that AED use may be effective for children, as it is for adults. The study involved a retrospective cohort of children under 16 years of age (5 to 15 years; mean 12.1 ± 3.7) who underwent out-of-hospital resuscitation and on whom an AED was used during resuscitation.

The Need for Additional Research

The FDA functions as a data-based organization that relies on scientific studies to assure that devices are safe and effective for use in the intended population. To date, sufficient data have not been submitted to the agency to support the labeling of AEDs for use in children. The traditional mechanisms to collect clinical data to support the safety and effectiveness of a new medical device or a medical device with a new intended use (eg, a new patient population) is the Investigational Device Exemption. Consistent with long-standing CDRH policy, the FDAMA now requires that persons who intend to investigate the safety and effectiveness of a Class III device must have an opportunity to submit an investigational plan for FDA review. Prior to submitting the formal plan, the sponsor and the agency convene for the purpose of reaching an agreement regarding that plan. The data obtained from the agreed upon study are then usually submitted as part of an application for premarket approval.

The agency has created a number of mechanisms to encourage and facilitate development of devices; these may be applicable and beneficial to the evaluation of AEDs in children. In 1996, the FDA amended the informed consent rules to provide a narrow exception to the requirements for obtaining and documenting informed human consent from each human subject, or his or her legally authorized representative, prior to initiation of an experimental intervention (Emergency Informed Consent Exception, 21 CFR 50.24). The exception would apply to a limited class of research activities involving human subjects who are in need of emergency medical intervention but who cannot give informed consent because of their life-threatening medical condition, and who do not have a legally authorized person to represent them. The FDA undertook this action in response to growing concerns that acute care research can become difficult or impossible under a strict interpretation of the law, and that there is an urgent need for this research.

The Medical Device Amendments of 1976 [515(f)] include a provision for creating a product development protocol (PDP) whereby the investigation of a device and the development of information necessary for its approval are merged into one regulatory mechanism. This procedure was intended to be of assistance to small manufacturers, who have been responsible for a host of innovative and important devices that are used in limited circumstances and, thus, are not financially attractive to larger manufacturers.

The requirements for assurance of safety and effectiveness in the PDP are no less stringent than the requirements for an application for premarket approval, but the PDP provides for early and frequent interaction between the FDA and the developer while the device design is taking place. This procedure has not been greatly used, but it recently received renewed interest under the CDRH reengineering effort.

Another provision that might have application in pediatric AED research is the Humanitarian Use Device provision. Congress recognized that for diseases and conditions affecting small populations, a device manufacturer's research and development costs could exceed the potential market returns, thereby creating an impediment to the development of such devices. In the SMDA, Congress enacted an amendment to create an incentive for the development of devices intended to benefit patients by treating or diagnosing a disease or condition that affects or is manifested in fewer than 4000 individuals in the United States per year. Under this provision, there is an exemption from the effectiveness requirements of the act. The applicant must present convincing explanation showing that the probable benefits to health from the use of the device outweigh the risk of injury or illness from its use, taking into account the probable risks and benefits of currently available devices or alternate treatments. To determine if this provision is applicable, the manufacturer can request a determination from FDA's Office of Orphan Products Development. The request should include an estimate of the number of patients that would be required to generate data needed to support a full premarket approval application. It should also include an explanation of why such a study is not feasible, or an explanation of why the cost of conducting such a study could not reasonably be expected to be recovered.

In summary, the CDRH hopes to work with the research, clinical, and manufacturing communities to optimize the study design and regulating requirements to collect the necessary data to allow eventual approval for safe and effective use of AEDs in children. The AHA is to be commended for raising the sensitivity of the research, clinical, manufacturing, and regulatory communities to this issue.

References

1. Auble TE, Menegazzi JJ, Paris PM. Effect of out-of-hospital defibrillation by basic life support providers on cardiac arrest mortality: A meta-analysis. *Ann Emerg Med* 1995;25:642–648.
2. Gallehr J, Vukov LF. Defining the benefits of rural emergency medical technician-defibrillation. *Ann Emerg Med* 1993;22:108–112.
3. Eisenberg MS, Moore J, Cummins R. Use of automatic external defibrillator in homes of survivor of out-of-hospital ventricular fibrillation. *Am J Cardiol* 1989;63:443–446.
4. Brison RJ, Davidson JR, Dreyer JF et al. Cardiac arrest in Ontario: Circumstances, community response, role of prehospital defibrillation and predictors of survival. *Can Med Assoc J* 1992;14:191–199.
5. U.S. Department of Health and Human Services. *Federal Food, Drug, and Cosmetic Act, as Amended, and Related Laws.* Maryland: HHS Publication No. (FDA) 89–1051.
6. Office of the Federal Register National Archives and Records Administration. *21 Code of Federal Regulations, Parts 800 to 1299.* Washington, DC: US Government Printing Office; 1998.
7. Diack A, Wellborn WS, Rullman RG, et al. An automatic cardiac resuscitator for emergency treatment of cardiac arrest. *Med Instrumen* 1979;13: 78–81.
8. Gutgesell HP, Tacker HA, Geddes LA, et al. Energy dose for ventricular defibrillation of children. *Pediatrics* 1976;58:898–901.
9. Emergency Cardiac Care Committee and Subcommittees AHA. Guidelines for cardiopulmonary resuscitation and emergency cardiac care. Pediatric advanced life support. *JAMA* 1992;268:2172–2183, 2262–2275.
10. ACLS Task Force on Early Defibrillation. Automated external defibrillation. In: *Textbook of Advanced Cardiac Life Support.* Dallas: American Heart Association; 1990:287–299.
11. Chameides L, Hazinski MF (eds): *Advanced Pediatric Life Support. 2nd ed.* Dallas: American Heart Association; 1994.
12. Emergency Cardiac Care Committee and Advanced Cardiac Life Support and Subcommittees. In Cummins RO (ed): *Textbook of Advanced Cardiac Life Support. 3rd ed. Pediatric Guidelines.* Dallas: American Heart Association; 1994.
13. Atkins DL, Hartly LL, York DK. Accurate recognition and effective treatment of ventricular fibrillation by automated external defibrillators in adolescents. *Pediatrics* 1998;101:393–397.

Section VII

Pharmacologic Treatment

Chapter 19

Developmental Changes in the Cardiac Response to Pharmacologic Agents

Michael R. Rosen, MD

Few of the drugs prescribed for administration to children have been formally tested and approved by the Food and Drug Administration (FDA) for use in the pediatric population. Although the FDA has encouraged industry to perform studies in children, this is rarely done; the dangers and potential litigation that might result have been cited as justification. Moreover, FDA attempts to enforce resolutions that would require drug testing in children have been effectively countered by industry. The net result is that children still tend to be considered as small adults for whom the same methods and standards set for drug administration in adults are assumed to hold. To optimize drug therapy in children we need not only clinical information but very fundamental information about developmental changes in drug action and drug metabolism. With respect to drugs administered for heart disease, we need to know the developmental electrophysiology of the heart, the interaction of drugs with their target sites on the heart, the modulators of cardiac function, and the developmental changes that occur in metabolic enzyme systems, drug absorption, and drug excretion.

Coverage of the vast area of cardioactive drugs would require a book unto itself. Therefore, this chapter focuses on the interaction of a subset of cardioactive drugs with receptor sites on (although not limited to) the ventricles. To prepare the groundwork for this presentation, an initial introduction regarding the developmental electrophysiology of the ventricles is provided.

From: Quan L, Franklin WH (eds). *Ventricular Fibrillation: A Pediatric Problem.* Armonk, NY: Futura Publishing Company, Inc.; ©2000.

These studies were supported by USPHS-NHLBI Grant HL-28958 and by the Partnership for Women's Health.

Developmental Electrophysiology of the Ventricles

This is not an exhaustive review but rather a summary of those aspects of developmental electrophysiology that are deemed important for the discussion of pharmacology. The primary model referred to here is the postnatal canine heart, which is used for convenience and for its applicability to the human heart.

As shown in Figure 1, the newborn canine ventricular myocardial and specialized conducting (Purkinje) fiber action potentials have high resting potentials and a rapid rate of rise of phase 0 of the action potential.[1] Repolarization has three phases: an initial rapid repolarization, a plateau of varying duration, and a rapid phase of terminal repolarization. In the newborn, there is great homogeneity of the voltage-time course of repolarization across fiber types, so that there is little if any difference in action potential duration throughout the conducting system and ventricle.

The developmental evolution of the action potential is accompanied by a marked increase in heterogeneity.[1-3] This can be seen by comparing the upper panels in Figure 1 (the adult) with the lower panels, in which are displayed the action potential durations of the

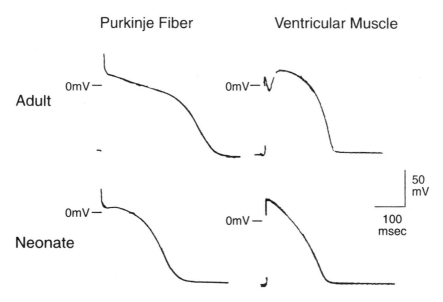

Figure 1. Adult and neonatal canine Purkinje fiber and left ventricular epicardial muscle action potentials. All experiments done at K+ = 4 mmol/L and at pacing cycle length of 1 second. Note the marked difference in duration of Purkinje and myocardial action potential durations in the adult, and the much greater homogeneity of repolarization in the neonate.

Purkinje system and myocardial fibers of the neonatal canine left ventricle. Note that in the Purkinje system, action potential duration increases markedly from neonate to adult. In the ventricle, action potential duration changes far less. It is to be stressed that the heterogeneity that has evolved in the conducting system and myocardium is magnified in the setting of isolated tissue studies[2-4]; that is, in the intact heart, where cell-cell interactions permit electrotonic flow of currents, the differences among cell types are minimized.[3,5-7] This is demonstrated in Figure 2, in which a transmural recording from the adult myocardial wall is shown. Here it is clear that despite the marked differences in action potential durations that are demonstrated in isolated tissues from the myocardium, there is a smooth and small gradient for repolarization across the normal adult myocardial wall in vivo. Under conditions that

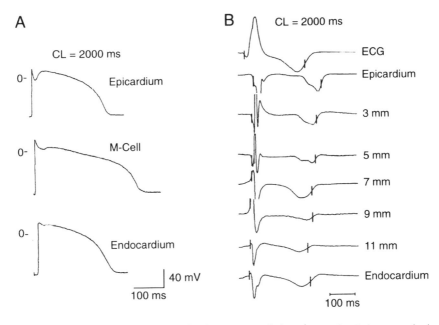

Figure 2. Adult canine left ventricular myocardial action potentials recorded from isolated tissues at K$^+$ = 4 mM (A) and activation-recovery intervals recorded simultaneously from left ventricle in situ via a multipolar needle electrode placed transmurally in the adult left ventricle (B). All records at pacing cycle length of 2000 ms. A. Note the large phase 1 notch of repolarization in the epicardial and midmyocardial (M cell) but not the endocardial recording, as well as the significantly greater duration of the M cell action potential. B. Note the minimal gradient across the myocardial wall in the heart in situ. Tick marks indicate points of measurement; mm scale is distance from epicardium that the individual activation-recovery intervals were recorded. Modified from Reference 3, by permission of the American Heart Association.

uncouple fibers (eg, myocardial fibrosis, ischemia, etc.) the expression of heterogeneity increases.[3]

The differences in action potential characteristics seen among cells in the neonate and the adult are the result of developmental evolution of the ion channels that control repolarization. Figure 3, modified from the Sicilian Gambit,[8] summarizes some of the currents responsible for the adult ventricular myocardial action potential. Phase 0 depolarization is the result of a rapid inward current carried by Na^+. The upstroke velocity of phase 0 (reflecting rapid Na^+ entry) is significantly lower in neonatal ($\approx$500 V/s) than adult myocytes (600 V/s), and the effect of tetrodotoxin (which blocks the Na^+ channel near its outer margin) to reduce upstroke velocity is greater on the neonatal fibers.[1] All this is consistent with a lesser inward Na^+ current in the neonate, which, in turn, would suggest the occurrence of a lower conduction velocity in neonatal fibers. This has been demonstrated to be the case (conduction velocity = 1.6 m/s in Purkinje fibers from 8-week-old dogs and 2.3 m/s in those from adults; $P<0.05$).[9]

In studies of single Na^+ channel currents of rat heart, a slower activation, time to peak and decay of ensemble, averaged currents is seen

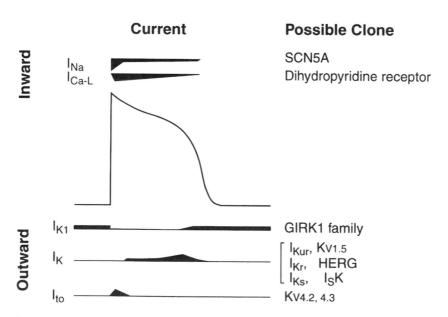

Figure 3. A schematized ventricular myocardial action potential with a subset of the inward and outward currents that contribute to it, as well as the possible clones. I_{Na} = fast inward sodium current; I_{Ca-L} = L-type calcium current; I_{K1} = inward rectifier; I_K = delayed rectifier, having three components, I_{Kur}, I_{Kr}, and I_{Ks}; I_{to} = transient outward current. Modified from Reference 8, by permission.

in the neonate[10]; this is consistent with the developmental changes described above in the canine Purkinje fiber action potential. Moreover, this evolution of Na^+ channel behavior is attributable to the development of the sympathetic nervous system,[10] with a particularly important role played by cyclic adenosine monophosphate.[11]

Repolarization is determined by a balance of inward currents carried by calcium and by sodium, and outward currents carried by potassium. The inward, L-type calcium current has been studied in neonatal and adult rabbit ventricular myocytes,[12] and when this is normalized to cell capacitance (to correct for differences in cell size), it shows a peak density in adults that is approximately twice that in the newborn. Hence, there is a developmental increase in the magnitude of inward Ca^{2+} current.

With respect to outward current components, the following changes are seen: the initial current responsible for the phase 1 notch of the action potential is a transient outward potassium current, referred to as I_{to}. I_{to} is not demonstrable in newborn dogs[13] or in rats,[14] and it is elicited after approximately 2 months of age in the dog.[13] Its evolution appears to be dependent on sympathetic innervation, as has been demonstrated in the rat.[14] The neonatal canine ventricle also manifests another outward K current, the identity of which is uncertain but which is not present in the adult.[13] With respect to the delayed rectifier, I_K, there is a postnatal increase in this current in the rat that is modulated by sympathetic innervation.[14] I_K, in turn, consists of three different components, one ultra rapidly activating, I_{Kur}, a second rapidly activating, I_{Kr}, and a third, slowly activating, I_{Ks}. Although major postnatal changes in these have not been described, there is a reported increase in I_{Ks} relative to I_{Kr} in late fetal murine myocytes.[15] Finally, whether the inward rectifier current, I_{K1}, changes importantly from neonate to adult is uncertain.

In summary, with growth and development, there are important changes in the depolarizing and repolarizing currents that contribute to the action potential. Because most antiarrhythmic drugs act by binding to the ion channels that carry these currents, the developmental evolution of these channels may be associated with changes in receptor sites for drugs, such that the expression of drug action will change developmentally. This is the subject of the following sections of this chapter.

Antiarrhythmic Drug Effects in the Neonatal and Adult Heart

To comprehend the changes that occur developmentally in drug effects, it is necessary first to understand the mechanisms whereby antiarrhythmic drugs achieve their actions on the heart. First discussed are those antiarrhythmics that are blockers of the fast inward Na$^+$ current. The Na$^+$ channel is presented schematically in Figure 4. Note that there is a narrowing, or selectivity filter, near the external mouth of the channel. Based on the diameter, configuration, and charge on the selectivity filter, entry of certain ions and their waters of hydration is favored.[16] Hence, the Na$^+$ channel is highly selective for Na$^+$, far less so for K.

Modulating the function of the inner mouth of the channel are two "gates." These were originally modeled mathematically by Hodgkin and Huxley[17,18] in experiments on squid axon, and, subsequently, have been the subject of a great deal of biophysical and molecular biological research that attempts to match the function of the gating proteins with their structure. In brief, in the resting state, the so-called m gate (or activation gate) is closed and the h gate (or inactivation gate) is open. When the cell is moved to its threshold potential, the m gate opens and

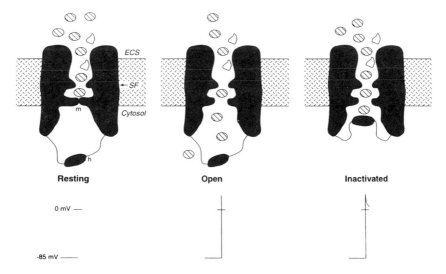

Figure 4. Schematic of a sodium channel (top panels) and the relationship of channel state to the action potential (bottom panels). In the resting state (left) the m gate is closed and the h gate is open. Na$^+$ (crosshatched symbols) is capable of crossing the selectivity filter (SF), while K$^+$ (unfilled symbols) is not. Because the m gate is closed, Na$^+$ cannot pass through the channel into the cytosol. In this setting, the cell is in the resting state, and only a highly negative resting membrane potential is recorded. In the open or activated state (center), the m gate has opened and the h gate remains open. Na$^+$ is now capable of passing through the channel pore into the cytosol, and as positive charge moves across the membrane, phase 0 of the action potential (bottom panel) is inscribed. In the inactivated state (right) the m gate remains open but the h gate has closed. Na$^+$ can no longer pass through the channel, and the action potential begins to repolarize.

Na$^+$ enters the cell, traveling down both concentration- and voltage-determined gradients (the interior of the cell has a low Na$^+$, the exterior, a high Na$^+$; the interior of the cell carries a negative charge and Na$^+$ is positively charged). As the membrane depolarizes during phase 0 and its potential moves into the positive range, the h gate, which was in the open state, closes. The channel is then said to be inactivated and will tend not to reopen until the membrane potential has decayed to a voltage negative to approximately −60 mV. With a return to the resting state, the m gate has closed and the h gate has opened. Hence, the transition from resting to open to inactivated states results in the onset and termination of phase 0 depolarization of the action potential.

The binding site for Na$^+$-channel-blocking antiarrhythmic drugs lies between the gates and the selectivity filter.[16] Hence, effectiveness of a drug to block a channel depends in large part on its ability to access the binding site and to prevent the channel from carrying inward Na$^+$ current. By blocking the Na$^+$ current, the drug slows conduction.

To exert its effects, a drug must equilibrate with the extracellular space, the cell membrane, and the cytosolic compartment. One major determinant of a drug's ease of access to a binding site on a channel is the extent to which it is ionized. Un-ionized molecules are highly lipid soluble and are able to approach the channel binding site via passage through the lipid membrane. Ionized molecules, which are water soluble rather than lipid soluble, most readily reach the binding site via the cytosol, traveling through the channel gates, passing from the bulk phase of the cytoplasm to the interior of the channel itself.

At physiological pH, local anesthetic antiarrhythmic drugs, such as lidocaine, that have a tertiary amino group exist as a charged, water-soluble form and an uncharged, lipid-soluble form. The former can best access the channel binding site when the channel is opening and closing frequently (ie, the more openings and closings per unit time, the more drug that can equilibrate across the channel gates). This type of channel block is referred to as frequency- or use-dependent.[19] The lipid-soluble form does not require the channel openings to occur for its equilibration; this type of block is referred to as tonic.[19]

To understand the extent to which there are developmental changes in drug access to the channels, it is instructive to use molecules that are permanently ionized, such as QX-314 (the quaternary derivative of lidocaine) and the uncharged, lipophilic local anesthetic, benzocaine. The effects of both drugs have been studied on neonatal and adult canine Purkinje fibers.[20] Benzocaine reduced $\dot{V}_{max}$ of phase 0 of the action potential comparably in neonates and adults; ie, there was no difference in tonic block. In contrast, QX-314 decreased $\dot{V}_{max}$ of the action potential upstroke more in adults than neonates, an effect that was attributable entirely to use-dependent blockade (Figure 5).

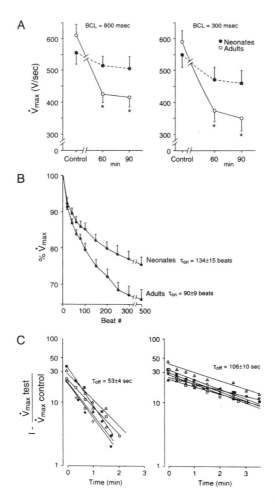

Figure 5. Effects of the permanently ionized local anesthetic, QX-314, on the neonatal and adult canine Purkinje fiber action potential. A. At constant drive cycle lengths of 800 (left) and 300 (right) ms, QX-314, 10 µmol/L, significantly reduces the $\dot{V}_{max}$ of six adult but not of seven neonatal action potentials at 60 and 90 minutes of superfusion. Moreover, the reduction of $\dot{V}_{max}$ is greater at the shorter cycle length, reflecting the use-dependent action of the drug. *$P<0.05$ cf control. B. Rate of development of use-dependent block with QX-314 (30 µmol/L). After a period of infrequent stimulation, the fibers were driven at a basic cycle length (BCL) of 500 milliseconds. The abscissa shows the number of beats, and the ordinate the percent block of $\dot{V}_{max}$ from the value during infrequent stimulation (100%). Symbols represent 5 adult and 5 neonatal fibers. C. Rate of recovery from use-dependent block with QX-314 (30 µmol/L). After a period of frequent stimulation (BCL = 500 ms), the fibers were stimulated at progressively longer intervals. The recovery is plotted as 1 minus the test $\dot{V}_{max}$/control $\dot{V}_{max}$ ratio (BCL = 500 ms) versus the recovery time. Different symbols represent different fibers (n=6 adults and 5 neonates). Reprinted from Reference 20, by permission.

Moreover, the neonatal fibers required more beats and therefore more time to develop blockade (134 beats in neonates versus 90 beats in adults at a cycle length of 0.5 s), and had a shorter time constant for recovery from blockade (53 versus 106 s). These results suggest that developmental changes in the actions of the local anesthetics not only occur, but can be attributed largely if not entirely to changes in the use-dependent actions of the charged molecule.[20] In other words, the effect of the drug is associated with developmental changes in the channel gating processes and in the interaction of the ionized drug and the receptor.

This result with permanently charged and uncharged molecules is directly applicable to experimental observations regarding lidocaine effects on canine Purkinje fibers. Despite the fact that at physiological pH, lidocaine exists in both charged and uncharged forms, the only developmental change in its effect on $\dot{V}_{max}$ is entirely consonant with the actions of QX-314 described above; that is, a longer time for development of block and a faster recovery from block are seen in the newborn.[21] Moreover, the threshold concentration for lidocaine to exert an effect on $\dot{V}_{max}$ is 5 µg/mL in neonatal Purkinje fibers as compared with 2 µg/mL in adults, and there is greater depression of $\dot{V}_{max}$ at any lidocaine concentration in the adult fibers.[22]

Results consistent with those described above are demonstrable in studies of the intact heart as well. At comparable plasma lidocaine concentrations from 3 to 9 µg/mL, there is interventricular conduction block that manifests use dependence in the adult and is not seen at all in the neonatal dog.[23] Also of interest are clinical pharmacologic differences in drug metabolism: for any dose, there is a lower total lidocaine concentration and lower free lidocaine concentration in the neonate than in the adult. In other words, to obtain comparable effects of lidocaine on the upstroke of the action potential and on conduction, a higher concentration of lidocaine is required in the neonate. Given that for any dose of lidocaine the neonate achieves lower free and total plasma concentrations, to achieve comparability of plasma levels, higher dosages are required in the neonate.[23]

Another antiarrhythmic drug with considerable clinical use is quinidine. In contrast to lidocaine, with quinidine there is no age-dependent difference in effect on the rate of onset and of offset of use-dependent block of $\dot{V}_{max}$ of phase 0 of neonatal and adult canine Purkinje fiber action potentials. The on rates are 1.6 and 1.8 seconds in neonates and adults, respectively, and the off rates are 4.5 and 4.0 seconds.[24] Similarly, in the intact heart, the effects of quinidine on induction of interventricular conduction block at plasma concentrations of 3.3 to 3.5 µg/mL and 5.6 to 6.2 µg/mL are equivalent.[23] Nor are there age-related differences in the dose of quinidine needed to achieve comparable total and free plasma concentration levels. The finding of no age-associated difference in drug action on $\dot{V}_{max}$ seen with quinidine characterizes still another antiarrhythmic drug, phenytoin,[25] while the occurrence of age-associated changes similar to those with lidocaine has also been described for procainamide.[26] These differing results highlight the importance of studying each drug in its own right.

The picture becomes even more complex when we consider the effects of drugs on repolarization. For example, with lidocaine, which markedly shortens the duration of repolarization, there is a greater effect on the adult than on the neonatal Purkinje fiber action potential.[22] This same effect is seen in the intact heart: comparable plasma concentrations of lidocaine shorten the electrocardiographic QT interval of adult canine hearts more than neonatal canine hearts.[23] Moreover, in isolated tissues, this effect to accelerate repolarization is most marked in the setting of initially long action potential durations and at long as opposed to short drive cycle lengths. In contrast, quinidine, which prolongs action potential duration, has a greater effect on neonatal canine Purkinje fibers than adult canine Purkinje fibers.[24] Similarly, in the intact heart, the prolongation of QT interval by quinidine is greater in the neonate than in the adult.

In summary, in considering the effects of different drugs on the action potential upstroke, on conduction, and on repolarization, it is clear that whether studied in isolated tissue or in intact heart, there are important age-associated differences for some drugs and no differences for others. Hence, no one drug can truly be considered a template.

Additional Complicating Factors with Respect to Drug Action

Thus far, this chapter has demonstrated that for drugs used as antiarrhythmics there are developmental changes that are manifested as lesser effects (lidocaine and procainamide) or greater effects (quinidine) on the neonate. For other drugs (eg, phenytoin), no developmental difference is seen. The complex events that determine the developmental evolution of normal electrophysiological properties and the actions of specific drugs are summarized above. Another complex factor comes into play as a child enters adolescence; this is the increase in gonadal steroids and their effects on the heart. Over a wide range of ages, females have faster heart rates and longer rate-corrected QT intervals (QTc) than males.[27–30] There are also gender-related differences in the incidence of some arrhythmias. For example, female gender is a

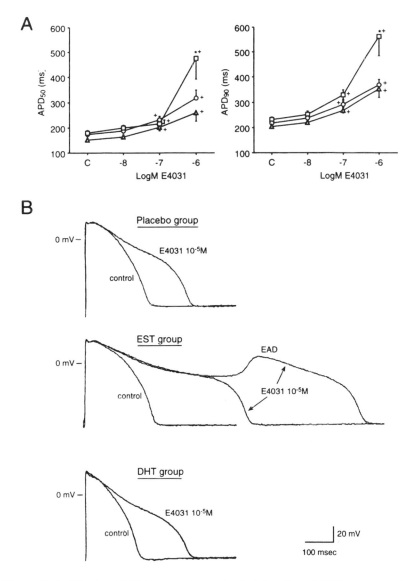

Figure 6. A. Effects of E4031 on action potential duration at 50% repolarization (APD$_{50}$) (left) and APD$_{90}$ (right) of papillary muscles from oophorectomized rabbits treated with placebo (O), estradiol (□), or dihydrotestosterone (DHT; △). Prolongation of APD$_{50}$ and APD$_{90}$ was greater in the estradiol group than the others ([+]$P<0.05$ cf control; [*]$P<0.05$ cf placebo and DHT). Basic cycle length (BCL) = 1 second. B. Representative experiments of the effects of E4031 on papillary muscles from rabbits treated with placebo, estradiol, or DHT. The prolongation of the action potential duration of the estradiol group was greater than the others, and early afterdepolarizations (EAD) were induced. BCL = 2 seconds. Modified after Reference 36, by permission.

risk factor for the occurrence of syncope and sudden death in the congenital long QT syndrome.[31] Moreover, female gender is also a risk factor for torsades de pointes associated with cardiovascular drugs that prolong repolarization.[32]

In a recent study of the effects of chronic administration of gonadal steroids (17-B estradiol or dihydrotestosterone) to rabbits that had been oophorectomized just before menarche, a dihydrotestosterone (DHT)-treated group had significantly shorter action potential durations than an estradiol-treated group, and a placebo-administered group was intermediate. Drici et al[33] showed that message levels for two potassium channels, HK2 and Isk, were downregulated in cardiac ventricular tissue from oophorectomized rabbits treated with estradiol or DHT. They also reported that in normal adult rabbits, the I_{K1} and I_{to} current densities were lower in females.[34] Differences in these repolarizing currents could contribute to the longer action potential durations seen in estradiol-treated rabbits as compared with DHT-treated rabbits, and also may provide a basis for the QT prolongation and proarrhythmia seen with some repolarization-prolonging antiarrhythmic drugs in female patients.[32,35]

The effects of E4031 (an antiarrhythmic drug and blocker of the I_{Kr} channel that expresses its effect by prolonging repolarization) in DHT- and estradiol-treated rabbits also has been studied.[36] E4031 prolonged the action potential duration of the estradiol-treated group to a significantly greater extent than the placebo or DHT-treated groups (Figure 6). Moreover, E-4031 induced early afterdepolarizations (the mechanism thought by many to be responsible for the drug-induced arrhythmia, torsades de pointes) to a significantly greater extent in the estradiol-treated group as well. These observations, considered in light of the work of Drici et al,[33,34] demonstrate not only the influence of estrogen and DHT on channel structure and function but also the interaction of channels with antiarrhythmic drugs. Clearly, the role of gender must be further incorporated in evolving strategies for drug evaluation and therapy, both in adults and developmentally.

Conclusions

This chapter has summarized some of the developmental changes that occur in the effects on the heart of antiarrhythmic drugs that are currently in use to treat patients in the pediatric age range. It has attempted to demonstrate that the root causes of the changes in drug effect are in part the result of developmental changes in the ion channels themselves, but that they also reflect differences among the drug-channel interactions and in drug metabolism. Finally, it has shown that, with adolescence, the presence of increased gonadal steroid levels adds further complexity to drug interactions with human subjects and animal models.

Some additional variables are important, especially in light of the consideration of ventricular fibrillation, for which there is not the space in this chapter. Nonetheless, the reader should be aware that pathologic conditions such as hypoxia and acidosis, which may be seen in heart disease and may facilitate ventricular fibrillation, have different effects on neonatal and adult fibers, with the neonate showing less deterioration in the setting of hypoxia.[37] With respect to acidosis, whereas adult Purkinje fibers tend to develop automatic and triggered arrhythmias at low pH, the neonatal fibers tend to become quiescent. The mechanisms responsible for these differences have yet to be identified. It is clear, however, that these require identification, as they too will contribute importantly to the milieu in which pharmacologic agents act after administration to the pediatric patient.

Acknowledgment   The author expresses his gratitude to Ms. Eileen Franey for her careful attention to the preparation of the manuscript.

References

1. Reder R, Miura D, Danilo P, et al. The electrophysiological properties of normal neonatal and adult canine cardiac Purkinje fibers. *Circ Res* 1981;48:658–668.
2. Antzelevitch C, Sicouri S, Litovsky SH, et al. Heterogeneity within the ventricular wall: Electrophysiology and pharmacology of epicardial, endocardial, and M cells. *Circ Res* 1991;69:1427–1449.
3. Anyukhovsky EP, Sosunov EA, Rosen MR. Regional differences in electrophysiological properties of epicardium, midmyocardium, and endocardium: In vitro and in vivo correlations. *Circulation* 1996;94:1981–1988.
4. Liu DW, Gintant GA, Antzelevitch C. Ionic bases for electrophysiological distinctions among epicardial, midmyocardial, and endocardial myocytes from the free wall of the canine left ventricle. *Circ Res* 1993;72:671–687.
5. Anyukhovsky EP, Sosunov EA, Feinmark SJ, et al. Effects of quinidine on repolarization in canine epicardium midmyocardium, and endocardium: II. In vivo study. *Circulation* 1997;96:4019–4026.
6. El-Sherif N, Caref E, Yin H, et al. The electrophysiological mechanism of ventricular arrhythmias in the long QT syndrome: Tridimensional mapping of activation and recovery patterns. *Circ Res* 1996;79:474–492.
7. Weissenburger J, Nesterenko VV, Antzelevitch C. Intramural monophasic action potentials (MAP) display steeper APD-rate relations and higher sensitivity to class III agents than epicardial and endocardial MAPs: Characteristics of M cells in vivo. *Circulation* 1995;92(suppl I):I300. Abstract.
8. Members of the Sicilian Gambit. *Antiarrhythmic Therapy: A Pathophysiologic Approach.* Armonk, NY: Futura Publishing Co., Inc.; 1994.
9. Rosen MR, Legato M, Weiss RM. Developmental changes in impulse conduction in the canine heart. *Am J Physiol* 1981;240:H546–H554.
10. Zhang J-F, Robinson RB, Siegelbaum SA. Sympathetic neurons mediate

developmental change in cardiac sodium channel gating through long-term neurotransmitter action. *Neuron* 1992;9:97–103.

11. Lipka LJ, Siegelbaum SA, Robinson RB, et al. An analogue of cAMP mimics developmental change in neonatal rat ventricular myocyte sodium current kinetics. *Am J Physiol (Heart Circ Physiol 39)* 1996;270: H194-H199.

12. Osaka T, Joyner RW. Developmental changes in the β-adrenergic modulation of calcium currents in rabbit ventricular cells. *Circ Res* 1992;70: 104–115.

13. Jeck CD, Boyden PA. Age-related appearance of outward currents may contribute to developmental differences in ventricular repolarization. *Circ Res* 1992;71:1390–1403.

14. Liu Q-Y, Rosen MR, McKinnon D, et al. Sympathetic innervation modulates repolarizing K$^+$ currents in rat epicardial myocytes. *Am J Physiol (Heart Circ Physiol 43)* 1998;274:H915-H922.

15. Davies MP, An RH, Doevendans P, et al. Developmental changes in ionic channel activity in the embryonic murine heart. *Circ Res* 1996;78:15–25.

16. Hille B. *Ionic Channels of Excitable Membranes.* 2nd ed. Suderland, MA: Sinauer Associates, Inc.; 1992.

17. Hodgkin AL, Huxley AF. The components of membrane conductance in the giant axon of Loligo. *J Physiol (Lond)* 1952;116:473–496.

18. Hodgkin AL, Huxley AF. The dual effect of membrane potential on sodium conductance in the giant axon of Loligo. *J Physiol (Lond)* 1952;116: 497–506.

19. Hondeghem LM, Katzung BG. Time- and voltage-dependent interactions of antiarrhythmic drugs with cardiac sodium channels. *Biochim Biophys Acta* 1977;472:377–398.

20. Spinelli W, Danilo P, Rosen MR. Reduction of $\dot{V}_{max}$ by QX-214 and benzocaine in neonatal and adult canine cardiac Purkinje fibers. *J Pharmacol Exp Ther* 1988;245:381–387.

21. Morikawa Y, Rosen MR. Developmental changes in the effects of lidocaine on the electrophysiological properties of canine Purkinje fibers. *Circ Res* 1984;55:633–641.

22. Mary-Rabine L, Rosen MR. Lidocaine effects on action potentials of Purkinje fibers from neonatal and adult dog. *J Pharmacol Exp Ther* 1978;205: 204–211.

23. Morikawa Y, Rosen TS, Hordof AJ, et al. Developmental changes in the effects of lidocaine and quinidine on the canine heart. *J Cardiovasc Pharmacol* 1987;10:450–455.

24. Morikawa Y, Rosen MR. Effects of quinidine on the transmembrane potentials of young and adult canine cardiac Purkinje fibers. *J Pharmacol Exp Ther* 1986;236:832–837.

25. Spinelli W, Rosen M. Frequency dependent actions of phenytoin in adult and young canine Purkinje fibers. *J Pharmacol Exp Ther* 1986;238:794–801.

26. Ezrin AM, Epstein K, Bassett AL, et al. Effects of procaine amide on cellular electrophysiology of neonatal and adult dog myocardium. *Dev Pharmacol Ther* 1980;1:352–363.

27. Ashman R. The normal duration of the Q-T interval. *Am Heart J* 1942; 23:522–534.

28. Adams W. The normal duration of the electrocardiologic ventricular complex. *J Clin Invest* 1936;15:333–342.

29. Merri M, Benhorin J, Alberti M, et al. Electrocardiographic quantitation of ventricular repolarization. *Circulation* 1989;80:1301–1308.
30. Rautaharju PM, Zhou SH, Wong S, et al. Sex differences in the evolution of the electrocardiographic QT interval with age. *Can J Cardiol* 1992;8:690–695.
31. Moss A, Schwartz PJ, Crampton RS, et al. The long QT syndrome: A prospective international study. *Circulation* 1985;71:17–21.
32. Waldo AL, Camm AJ, deRuyter H, et al, for the SWORD Investigators. Effect of d-sotalol on mortality in patients with left ventricular dysfunction after recent and remote myocardial infarction. *Lancet* 1996;348:7–12.
33. Drici MD, Burklow TR, Haridasse V, et al. Sex hormones prolong the QT interval and downregulate potassium channel expression in the rabbit heart. *Circulation* 1996;94:1471–1474.
34. Drici MD, Ducic I, Morad M, et al. Gender differences in cardiac repolarization depends on I_{K1} and I_{to} K^+ channel currents in rabbit. *Circulation* 1996;94:I473. Abstract.
35. Lehmann MH, Hardy S, Archibald D, et al. Sex difference in risk of torsade de pointes with d,l-sotalol. *Circulation* 1996;94:2535–2541.
36. Hara M, Danilo P Jr, Rosen MR. Effects of gonadal steroids on ventricular repolarization and on the response to E4031. *J Pharmacol Exp Ther* 1998;285:1068–1072.
37. Chevalier P, Geller JC, Rosen MR. The basis for normal cardiac electrical activity and the effects thereon of hypoxia and acidosis. In Haddad GG, Lister G (eds): *Tissue Oxygen Deprivation. From Molecular to Integrated Function.* New York: Marcel Dekker, Inc.; 1996:479–496.

Chapter 20

Pharmacologic Therapy of Ventricular Fibrillation

James C. Perry, MD

It is fairly easy to say that very little is known regarding appropriate drug therapy for pediatric ventricular fibrillation (VF). Given the relatively low incidence of the disease in young patients compared with the adult population, prospective studies of drug effectiveness for the acute termination and subsequent prevention of recurrences of VF are difficult to conceptualize, let alone perform. Such studies would require large multicenter, collaborative efforts due to the low volume of patients at any one center. Additionally, the etiologies and substrates underlying pediatric VF are varied to such an extent that meaningful conclusions from such studies may be tenuous due to confounding variables. In examining new approaches to pediatric VF therapy, one would surely encounter ethical difficulties in randomizing patients away from anecdotally "proven," older forms of therapy and in enrolling patients in any long-term study that did not include defibrillator therapy.

In this context, an examination of the pharmacologic therapy of VF must consider the following realities: 1) there is no current volume of literature on the subject from which to draw definitive conclusions; 2) determination of the "best" mode of acute and chronic VF therapy in children would require a massive, multicenter, collaborative effort and a commitment extending well beyond the primary investigators at each institution; 3) most advances in the acute therapy for pediatric VF will, of necessity, be derived from larger adult studies; 4) a study of the prevention of VF recurrence is far more likely to be achieved, due to advances in defibrillator therapy as back-up support; 5) the pace of continued advances in defibrillator technology may be a great deal faster

From: Quan L, Franklin WH (eds). *Ventricular Fibrillation: A Pediatric Problem.* Armonk, NY: Futura Publishing Company, Inc.; ©2000.

than the ability to conclude such a study in a timely fashion; and 6) drug therapy for VF prevention must be recognized as *adjunct* therapy with defibrillators.

Etiologies of Pediatric VF

Underlying factors that result in VF in children can be broken down into four separate groups (Table 1): 1) primary electrical abnormalities; 2) cardiomyopathies; 3) postoperative congenital heart disease; and 4) drugs.

Primary Electrical Abnormalities

Of the primary electrical abnormalities, the long QT syndrome (LQTS) is foremost and potentially the most under-recognized. The abnormalities of cardiac ion channel function responsible for producing LQTS are being elucidated and currently include both sodium and potassium channels.[1,2] As the molecular bases for the arrhythmias in LQTS are identified, ion channel-specific forms of long-term therapy are emerging. For the patient with known LQTS, this will prove helpful; however, for the initial presentation of torsades de pointes in such a patient, basic approaches to acute VF therapy are still operative.

Wolff-Parkinson-White syndrome (WPW) may account for a small fraction of pediatric VF cases. Rapid antegrade conduction down the accessory pathway during atrial fibrillation is a likely cause of induction of VF, but in a compromised patient, for example the patient with WPW and cardiomyopathy or congenital heart disease, poor myocardial perfusion during orthodromic supraventricular tachycardia may also lead to VF. In the acute setting, standard approaches to VF apply.

Table 1

Underlying Causes of Pediatric Ventricular Fibrillation

Electrical: long QT syndrome, Wolff-Parkinson-White syndrome, "primary electrical disease"

Cardiomyopathies: hypertrophic cardiomyopathy, dilated cardiomyopathy, arrhythmogenic right ventricular dysplasia, Brugada syndrome

Postoperative congenital heart disease: tetralogy of Fallot, left-sided lesions with thick ventricles, single ventricle physiology

Drugs: cocaine, crystal methamphetamine, antiarrhythmic agents (Class Ia, Ic, III, digoxin), imipramine, cisapride

---

Chronic therapy in this setting has become inappropriate, as the accessory pathway should be eliminated by radiofrequency catheter ablation techniques. So-called "primary electrical disease" is a diagnosis of exclusion.[3] This rare phenomenon may occur in young patients in whom other explanations are lacking. The electrocardiogram is normal at rest, without even the often subtle T wave abnormalities found in arrhythmogenic right ventricle. Most patients undergo cardiac catheterization, angiography (including the coronaries), and electrophysiological assessment, along with endomyocardial biopsy, with unremarkable findings.

Cardiomyopathies

Several forms of cardiomyopathy may result in VF. These include hypertrophic cardiomyopathy (obstructive or nonobstructive), dilated cardiomyopathy (multiple etiologies), arrhythmogenic right ventricular dysplasia,[4,5] and Brugada syndrome.[6]

Myocarditis can also result in ventricular tachycardia (VT) and VF, and can be very resistant to acute therapeutic measures.[7]

Postoperative Congenital Heart Disease

As surgery for complex congenital heart disease has advanced, patients live longer and reach a decade or more of postoperative life. In some settings, they may be at risk for "late" onset of VF. These patients include those with right heart obstruction who undergo resection of infundibular muscle and often closure of a ventricular septal defect, as in tetralogy of Fallot. Much has been published about the tetralogy patient, in attempts to identify those at risk for subsequent VF. Persistent right heart obstruction,[8] significant pulmonary insufficiency,[9] complex ventricular arrhythmia on ambulatory monitoring or electrophysiology study,[10] atrial flutter,[11] and very wide QRS complexes in sinus rhythm[12] may help identify patients at risk. The place of electrophysiological testing in this group is unclear. A large study by Chandar et al[13] from the Pediatric Electrophysiology Society failed to show any predictive value of electrophysiology study for patients who subsequently died suddenly. Deal et al[8] showed some help from electrophysiological assessment, but not for the patient with persistent hemodynamic abnormalities, in whom no drug was truly effective until the residual abnormality was repaired.

Other postoperative patients at risk of VF include those with thick ventricles and left-sided lesions. These include those following aortic valve operations, Konno-Rastan type procedures, and some Damus operations. Patients with single ventricle physiology can develop ventricular arrhythmias late after repair,[14] particularly if ventricular function is depressed.

Drugs

Several "street" drugs, including cocaine and crystal methamphetamine, can cause VF; the arrhythmia is a result of coronary vasoconstriction and/or direct cellular effects. Antiarrhythmic agents may have proarrhythmic effects, resulting in VF. Most notably, these include the Class IA drug quinidine,[15] the Class IC agents flecainide and encainide,[16,17] the intravenous agent ibutilide,[18] and, less frequently, amiodarone[19] and sotalol.[20] The drugs imipramine and cisapride may also cause VF.

Acute Therapy for Pediatric VF

On a practical level, the approach to the acute therapy of pediatric VF depends upon the Advanced Cardiac Life Support guidelines, whether the event is witnessed in the hospital, whether any potential initiating factors are recognizable, and personal past experience with successful techniques. Again, there are no organized studies of effective antifibrillatory medical therapy in young patients.

Lidocaine

One of the first drugs used to treat VF in nearly every center in the US is lidocaine. The reason for this fact rests more in the physician's comfort level using a "safe" antiarrhythmic agent than a proven efficacy. Questions have been raised about lidocaine's true place in the antiarrhythmic spectrum for sustained VT.[21] Lidocaine is probably best used in the setting of ischemic myocardium causing VF rather than reentrant VT, in which a case has been made that procainamide may be preferable.[22] Lidocaine is also useful for digoxin toxicity. Lidocaine blocks the fast sodium channel and shows use dependence. It has little or no effect on structures above the bundle of His. Lidocaine causes a shortening of repolarization, especially in cells with the long action potential duration, resulting in an overall homogeneity of repolarization.

Lidocaine is given as an intravenous bolus of 1 mg/kg and can be repeated after several minutes. Infusions of lidocaine are usually 20 to 50 μg/kg/min.

The predominant adverse drug reactions to lidocaine are in the central nervous system, and include seizures, apnea, and changes in mental status. Plasma levels often exceed 7 µg/mL in this setting.[23]

Bretylium

Bretylium is used in resuscitative settings as therapy for polymorphic VT, VF, or monomorphic VT that is resistant to standard forms of therapy. The drug has reported use in the setting of ventricular arrhythmias due to digitalis intoxication.[24] Bretylium causes an initial release of norepinephrine stores from sympathetic ganglia, but then prevents norepinephrine release and reuptake. It has relatively equal effects on prolongation of action potential duration and repolarization, much like amiodarone.

The intravenous dose of bretylium is 5 mg/kg as a rapid push during VF. There are hypotensive effects such that in cases of hemodynamically stable VT, it should be diluted in 5% dextrose and given more slowly. The total dose should not exceed 30 mg/kg. A continuous infusion can be used at 15 to 30 µg/kg/min. The specific dosing for children has not been established. Although bretylium is used to treat digoxin-induced arrhythmias, the drug may worsen these rhythms initially due to the early release of norepinephrine. Tricyclic antidepressants block bretylium's synaptic effects.

Intravenous Amiodarone

Amiodarone is a potent agent for control of a wide spectrum of cardiac tachyarrhythmias. It was recently released in the US for intravenous use, and a body of literature for its safety and effectiveness in resistant arrhythmias in children has been published.[25,26] In addition to prolonging refractory periods, the drug also is a sodium channel blocker, a noncompetitive α- and β-adrenergic receptor blocker, and an inhibitor of the release of presynaptic norepinephrine. Amiodarone affects potassium channels, with interference with the delayed outward current, causing most of amiodarone's prolongation of refractoriness. The drug is metabolized to an active agent, desethylamiodarone, in the liver.

Amiodarone shows a rapid onset of action, and the antiarrhythmic effect lasts 1 to 6 hours. In the largest study of intravenous amiodarone to date in young patients, a 5-mg/kg bolus was used and divided into five 1 mg/kg aliquots.[26] As no adverse effect was seen in the first 1- to 3-mg/kg bolus, the drug can probably be given in initial bolus at least as two 2.5-mg/kg boluses. The average successful load was 6 to 7 mg/kg. Infusions of amiodarone were used predominantly in those with ventricular tachyarrhythmias, at 10 to 15 mg/kg/day. Side effects of intravenous therapy are predominantly related to hypotension.

Magnesium Sulfate

Reports of the use of magnesium sulfate for ventricular arrhythmias relate to torsades de pointes.[27] Magnesium can suppress early afterdepolarizations. It may be effective by means of a membrane stabilizing effect or calcium channel blockade.

The dose of magnesium sulfate in adults is a single bolus of 1 to 2 g. An infusion of 2 to 10 mg/min is reported.[27] For children, this author and others have used a bolus of 10 to 20 mg/kg.

Chronic Therapy for VF

Summary of Adult Antiarrhythmic Drug Trials

Given the large number of adult-age patients with VT/VF, randomized studies are plentiful. Early studies investigated whether empiric antiarrhythmic therapy alone or that guided by invasive electrophysiology study was preferable. The study by Steinbeck et al[28] shows that the best results, with decreased mortality, occurred when an inducible ventricular tachyarrhythmia was suppressed at follow-up electrophysiology study. The Electrophysiology Study versus Electrocardiographic Monitoring (ESVEM) trial[29] examined the benefit of therapy guided by electrophysiology study versus ambulatory Holter monitoring for a wide variety of antiarrhythmic agents. The study concluded that there was no difference in the means of monitoring the effect of therapy, that sotalol was a better agent than the Class I agents, and that sotalol and a Class I agent combined with a β-blocker resulted in the same annual mortality, approximately 3% to 4%. The patients in the ESVEM trial were those with prior cardiac arrest and decreased ejection fraction. There were so many drugs included in the ESVEM trial that definitive statements about each drug are probably best taken lightly. The Cardiac Arrest Seattle: Conventional versus Amiodarone Drug Evaluation (CASCADE) trial compared the freedom from events in VF survivors for conventional therapy versus amiodarone.[30] Amiodarone was superior for the 2-, 4-, and 6-year follow-up period. Freedom from events were 82%, 66%, and 53% for amiodarone and 69%, 52%, and 40% for conventional drugs at these intervals.

Therapy in Patients with Implantable Cardioverter-Defibrillators

More recently, two specific studies have examined the role of defibrillator therapy for patients with VT/VF. One study was the Multicenter Automatic Defibrillator Implantation Trial (MADIT).[31] Patients enrolled in MADIT had a positive electrophysiology study and low ejection fraction; the study showed that an implantable cardioverter-defibrillator (ICD) decreased sudden death by 54%. The Antiarrhythmics versus Implantable Defibrillators (AVID) trial[32] also showed a decrease in sudden death in the defibrillator group by 31% at 3 years. The problems with both of these studies are that they do not shed light on the benefits of defibrillators plus anitarrhythmics and they examine only the highest known risk groups.

Young patients with defibrillators have improved survival, but the high-risk group, again, is the group of people who have poor ventricular function.[33] In a report by Silka et al,[33] no benefit to electrophysiology study was observed. Of the reported group of 125 patients (less than 20 years old), 84% were given an antiarrhythmic agent as well as an ICD; however, no breakdown of specific drugs was provided. Most patients received β-blockers, and amiodarone and sotalol were not readily available at the time.

Summary of Medical Therapy Principles

For acute therapy of pediatric VF (Table 2), there are no apparent contraindications to use of lidocaine, but its true efficacy is in question. The drug is helpful for digoxin toxicity. Bretylium is a useful agent for the patient with poor ventricular function, such as those with dilated cardiomyopathy, arrhythmogenic right ventricular dysplasia, and single ventricle. Amiodarone is useful for patients with thick ventricles, such as those with hypertrophic cardiomyopathy and postoperative congenital heart disease.

For chronic VF therapy, nearly all patients will have concomitant ICD therapy. β-Blockers are appropriate for nearly all patients, with the exception of those with poor ventricular function. The place of sotalol in these patients is uncertain at present, but it may be appropriate for primary electrical disease, postoperative congenital heart disease, and hypertrophic cardiomyopathy. The therapy for LQTS is evolving due to the dramatic advances made in identification of specific ion channel defects.

Table 2

Drug Therapy for Pediatric VF

	Acute Drug	Chronic Drug
Electrical		
"PED"	Lido, bretylim, amio	β-Blocker, sotalol?
LQTS	Lido, Mg, Na (bretylium?)	β-Blocker, Na blocker, K?
WPW	Lido, amio	–
Cardiomyopathies		
Hypertrophic	Lido, amio, β-blocker	β-Blocker, amio, sotalol?
Dilated	Lido, bretylium	Amio
ARVD	Lido, bretylium, amio	β-Blocker, amio, mexiteline
Brugada	Lido, bretylium, amio	β-Blocker, amio, mexiteline
Postoperative CHD		
Tetralogy	Lido, amio	Amio, mexiteline, sotalol?
Left-sided	Lido, amio	β-Blocker, amio
Single ventricle	Lido, bretylium	Amio
Drugs		
"Street"	Lido, β-blocker	–
Ia, Ic	Bretylium, Na, Mg, lido	–
Imipramine	Sodium	
Cisapride		

ARVD = arrhythmogenic right ventricular dysplasia; CHD = congenital heart disease; LQTS = long QT syndrome; PED = primary electrical disease; VF = ventricular fibrillation; WPW = Wolff-Parkinson-White.

What is Needed?

Without suggesting a catchy name, a "Cardiac Arrest Study" is needed to address the issue of acute therapy for VF in children. One suggested means of gathering enough data would be an agreement by many investigators to select one antiarrhythmic agent (eg, bretylium) as their firstline agent for any VF case they encounter for the next 1 to 2 years. The data could be tabulated and compared with results with another agent (eg, amiodarone) over the following 1 to 2 years.

Since it is generally accepted that defibrillators are now an integral part of VF therapy in children, future studies must examine which chronic antiarrhythmic drugs are best and for which patients. Two studies to be considered are a study of ICD plus β-blocker versus ICD alone, followed by ICD plus β-blocker versus ICD plus amiodarone. For young patients with cardiomyopathies, the risk of recurrent VF that prompts placement of an ICD probably dictates serious consideration of cardiac transplantation. In the population with postoperative congestive heart disease, the risk group is unclear, and therefore only VF survivors could be included. For the majority of LQTS patients, there are other effective, non-ICD therapies available, and gene-specific therapeutic trials are under way.

References

1. Wang Q, Shen J, Splawski I, et al. SCN5A mutations associated with an inherited cardiac arrhythmia, long QT syndrome. *Cell* 1995;80:805–811.
2. Curran ME, Splawski I, Timothy KW, et al. A molecular basis for cardiac arrhythmia: HERG mutations cause long QT syndrome. *Cell* 1995;80: 795–803.
3. Wever EFD, Hauer RNW, Oomen A, et al. Unfavorable outcome in patients with primary electrical disease who survived an episode of ventricular fibrillation. *Circulation* 1993;88:1021–1029.
4. Wichter T, Borggrefe M, Haverkamp W, et al. Efficacy of antiarrhythmic drugs in patients with arrhythmogenic right ventricular disease. Results in patients with inducible and noninducible ventricular tachycardia. *Circulation* 1992;86:29–37.
5. Corrado D, Basso C, Thiene G, et al. Spectrum of clinicopathologic manifestations of arrhythmogenic right ventricular cardiomyopathy/dysplasia. A multicenter study. *J Am Coll Cardiol* 1997;30:1512–1520.
6. Brugada P, Brugada J. Right bundle branch block persistent ST segment elevation and sudden cardiac death: A distinct clinical and electrocardiographic syndrome. *J Am Coll Cardiol* 1992;20:1391–1396.
7. Friedman RA, Moak JP, Fenrich AR, Perry JP. Persistence of ventricular arrhythmias beyond resolution of occult myocarditis in children. *Am J Cardiol* 1993;72:501.
8. Deal BJ, Scagliotto D, Miller SM, et al. Electrophysiologic drug testing in symptomatic ventricular arrhythmias after repair of tetralogy of Fallot. *Am J Cardiol* 1987;59:1380–1385.
9. Harrison DA, Harris L, Sui SC, et al. Sustained ventricular tachycardia in adult patients late after repair of tetralogy of Fallot. *J Am Coll Cardiol* 1997;30:1368–1373.
10. Deanfield JE, McKenna WJ, Hallidie-Smith KA. Detection of late arrhythmia and conduction disturbance after correction of tetralogy of Fallot. *Br Heart J* 1980;44:248–253.
11. Roos-Hesselink J, Perlroth MG, McGhie J, Spitaels S. Atrial arrhythmias in adults after repair of tetralogy of Fallot. Correlation with clinical, exercise and echocardiographic findings. *Circulation* 1995;91:2214–2219.
12. Gatzoulis MA, Till JA, Redington AN. Depolarization-repolarization inhomogeneity after repair of tetralogy of Fallot: The substrate for malignant ventricular tachycardia? *Circulation* 1997;95:401–404.
13. Chandar JS, Wolff GS, Garson A Jr, et al. Ventricular arrhythmias in postoperative tetralogy of Fallot. *Am J Cardiol* 1990;65:655–661.
14. Stelling JA, Danford DA, Kugler JD, et al. Late potentials and inducible ventricular tachycardia in surgically repaired congenital heart disease. *Circulation* 1990;82:1690–1696.
15. Webb CL, Dick M III, Rocchini AP, et al. Quinidine syncope in children. *J Am Coll Cardiol* 1987;9:1031.
16. Fish FA, Gillette PC, Benson DW Jr, et al. Proarrhythmia, cardiac arrest

and sudden death in young patients receiving encainide and flecainide. *J Am Coll Cardiol* 1991;18:356–365.

17. Perry JC, Garson A Jr. Flecainide acetate for treatment of tachyarrhythmias in children: Review of world literature on efficacy, safety and dosing. *Am Heart J* 1992;124:1614–1621.
18. Murray KT. Ibutilide. *Circulation* 1998;97:493–497.
19. Fananapazir L, Leon MB, Bonow RO, et al. Sudden death during empiric amiodarone therapy in symptomatic hypertrophic cardiomyopathy. *Am J Cardiol* 1991;67:169–174.
20. Pfammater JP, Paul T, Lehmann C, Kallfelz HC. Efficacy and proarrhythmia of oral sotalol in pediatric patients. *J Am Coll Cardiol* 1995;26:1002–1007.
21. Josephson ME. Lidocaine and sustained monomorphic ventricular tachycardia: Fact or fiction. *Am J Cardiol* 1996;78:82–83.
22. Gorgels APM, van den Dool A, Hofs A, et al. Comparison of procainamide and lidocaine in terminating sustained monomorphic ventricular tachycardia. *Am J Cardiol* 1996;78:43–46.
23. Denaro CP, Benowicz NL. Poisoning due to Class IB antiarrhythmic drugs. Lignocaine, mexiletine, and tocainide. *Med Tox Adv Drug Exp* 1989;4:412.
24. Vincent JL, Dufaye P, Berre J, et al. Bretylium in severe ventricular arrhythmias associated with digitalis intoxication. *Am J Emerg Med* 1984;2:504–506.
25. Perry JC, Knilans TK, Marlow D, et al. Intravenous amiodarone for life-threatening tachycardias in children and young adults. *J Am Coll Cardiol* 1993;16:2007–2011.
26. Perry JC, Fenrich AL, Hulse JE, et al. Pediatric use of intravenous amiodarone: Efficacy and safety in critically ill patients from a multicenter protocol. *J Am Coll Cardiol* 1996;27:1246–1250.
27. Tzivoni D, Banai S, Schuger C, et al. Treatment of torsade de pointes with magnesium sulfate. *Circulation* 1988;77:392.
28. Steinbeck G, Andersen D, Bach P, et al. A comparison of electrophysiologically guided antiarrhythmic drug therapy with beta-blocker therapy in patients with symptomatic, sustained ventricular tachyarrhythmias. *N Engl J Med* 1992;327:987–392.
29. Mason JW, for the ESVEM Investigators. A comparison of electrophysiologic testing with Holter monitoring to predict antiarrhythmic efficacy for ventricular tachyarrhythmias. *N Engl J Med* 1993;329:445–451.
30. CASCADE Investigators. Randomized antiarrhythmic drug therapy in survivors of cardiac arrest (the CASCADE study). *Am J Cardiol* 1993;72:280–287.
31. Moss AJ, Hall WJ, Cannom DS, et al, and the MADIT Investigators. Improved survival with an implanted defibrillator in patients with coronary artery disease at high risk for ventricular arrhythmia. *N Engl J Med* 1996;335:1333–1340.
32. The Antiarrhythmics versus Implantable Defibrillators (AVID) Investigators. A comparison of antiarrhythmic drug therapy with implantable defibrillators in patients resuscitated from near-fatal ventricular arrhythmias. *N Engl J Med* 1997;337:1576.
33. Silka MJ, Kron J, Dunnigan A, et al. Sudden cardiac death and the use of implantable cardioverter-defibrillators in pediatric patients. *Circulation* 1993;87:800–807.

Section VIII

Outcomes

Chapter 21

Survival Following
Ventricular Fibrillation

Michael J. Silka, MD and John H. McAnulty, MD

The very low overall salvage rate for pediatric patients who undergo attempted cardiopulmonary resuscitation (CPR) would suggest that a discussion of survival of these patients would be based primarily, if not exclusively, on speculative data. However, as public awareness as well as resuscitation times and methods have improved, some data have become available to allow for discussion of this topic.[1,2] This issue becomes increasingly salient as treatment methods such as implantable cardioverter-defibrillators (ICDs) become an option for patients resuscitated from ventricular fibrillation (VF). In this chapter, three questions are considered: 1) What are the characteristics of pediatric patients who are resuscitated from an episode of VF? 2) What are the risks of a recurrent tachyarrhythmic event following resuscitation? 3) Is therapy helpful in altering the long-term prognosis?

Pediatric Survivors of VF: General Considerations

The factors that are predictive of survival and functional neurologic status following cardiopulmonary arrest in young patients have been the subject of multiple studies (Table 1). The factors that appear to be associated with a potentially favorable outcome include: 1) an in-hospital versus out-of-hospital arrest; 2) the presence of an active cardiac rhythm (pulseless ventricular tachycardia [VT] or VF) rather than asystole as the initial cardiac rhythm at attempted resuscitation; and 3) a primary respiratory cause rather than cardiac etiology of arrest.

From: Quan L, Franklin WH (eds). *Ventricular Fibrillation: A Pediatric Problem.* Armonk, NY: Futura Publishing Company, Inc.; ©2000.

Table 1

Prognostic Factors Following Attempted Resuscitation in Pediatric Patients

	Favorable	Unfavorable
Site	In-hospital	Out of Hospital
Cardiac rhythm	Ventricular tachycardia/fibrillation	Asystole
Primary etiology	Respiratory	Cardiac

The prevalence of VF as the cause of cardiopulmonary arrest in pediatric patients has ranged between 4% and 22% in different series.[3–7] This variance is based on in-hospital or out-of-hospital studies, case selection, which includes or excludes sudden infant death syndrome or trauma victims, and the proportion of patients with underlying cardiovascular disease (Table 2). The following trends appear to be consistent in the medical literature: 1) the probability that the initial cardiac rhythm will be VF at initial attempted resuscitation increases with an earlier response time[6]; 2) the probability that VF will be the initial cardiac rhythm at attempted resuscitation is higher in patients with heart disease[7]; and 3) the proportion of patients whose initial cardiac rhythm is VF at attempted resuscitation increases with age.[8]

The study by Walsh and Krongrad[7] provides some perspective regarding the limitations that exist in the determination of whether a pediatric patient expires due to asystole or pulseless VT/VF. This was an in-hospital study of the terminal cardiac rhythm in 100 consecutive infants and children, in which VF was considered to be the terminal cardiac rhythm in only 6 cases (6%). However, in another 16 patients, the terminal rhythm was pulseless VT or VF preceding asystole. Furthermore, 32 of the 100 patients were infants who weighed less than 2.23 kg,

Table 2

Prevalence of Ventricular Fibrillation Among Pediatric Patients at Attempted Resuscitation

Author[ref]	# Ventricular # Patients	% Ventricular Fibrillation	In or Out of Fibrillation	Hospital
Hickey et al[3]	95	14	15	out
Innes et al[4]	33	4	11	in
Schindler et al[5]	101	8	8	out
Mogayezi et al[6]	157	29	19	out
Walsh et al[7]	100	6	6	in

a group in whom VT/VF was not observed. Therefore, of the remaining 68 patients, 22 (31%) could have been classified as having VT/VF as the terminal cardiac rhythm, based on the recognition that pulseless VT/VF is a transient rhythm, rarely lasting longer than 3 minutes in young patients.[9]

Thus, given the increased probability that VF will be the initial cardiac rhythm in patients in whom earlier resuscitative efforts are instituted, and that VF will terminate as asystole or pulseless electrical activity after approximately 3 minutes (the time generally cited for irreversible neurologic injury), it should be anticipated that some pediatric patients who are resuscitated from VF may survive with normal or near-normal neurologic status. This proposal has been validated by studies that have compared the initial rhythm and outcome of pediatric patients following out-of-hospital resuscitation.[4,6] In adults, the estimated proportion of patients who survive VF with an intact neurologic status is 20% to 25%.[10] Thus, a major question for the survivor of VF with an intact neurologic status becomes the risk of a recurrent cardiac event.

Patient Characteristics and the Risk of a Recurrent Event

Most studies of pediatric survivors of VF have been isolated case reports, at times summarized as literature reviews. As early as 1949, Moe[11] reported survival following VF in the case of a young man with recurrent syncope and electrocardiogram-documented VF without identifiable heart disease. This same patient was again reported on in 1990, as a long-term survivor of VF without apparent cause who had been asymptomatic on oral antiarrhythmic therapy with quinidine.[12] However, although such cases are interesting, they are exceptional and do not fit the general profile of young patients who are survivors of VF.

There appear to be two major groups of young patients who survive an episode of VF with minimal neurologic sequelae. The first are patients without intrinsic cardiovascular disease who experience VF either as a consequence of an "electrical accident" or who develop pathologic prolongation of cardiac repolarization due to idiosyncratic responses to prescribed medications or illicit street drugs. The second group consists of patients with intrinsic cardiovascular diseases such as cardiomyopathies, primary electrical diseases, or congenital heart disease, who may be predisposed to VF due to myocardial ischemia or to inherent electrical instability. As these two groups appear to have a different risk of a recurrent event, they are discussed separately in this chapter.

VF in Pediatric Patients with an Ostensibly Normal Heart

VF may occur in the absence of defined heart disease on the basis of normal cardiac electrophysiology—that is, the capability to fibrillate is inherent to the human myocardium.[13] This is due to the fact that the process of cardiac repolarization is nonuniform, which may render segments of the ventricle susceptible to fibrillation if a stimulus occurs during a vulnerable period. One probable example of VF in the normal heart as the result of stimulus during the ventricular vulnerable period is described in two recent reports, by Maron et al,[14,15] of minor blunt chest trauma during sports activities. In these studies of 28 patients aged 3 to 19 years (mean 11), cardiac arrest occurred immediately after an unexpected blow to the chest that was insufficient to produce structural injury. Although the cardiac rhythm was infrequently recorded due to delayed onset of CPR and call for advanced support, VF was documented in the few survivors who did receive prompt and effective bystander resuscitation and early defibrillation.

Another transient and potentially reversible substrate for VF in pediatric patients who do not have heart disease may be idiosyncratic responses to the use of conventional medical therapies. Several unexplained sudden deaths have occurred in young patients that are associated with the use of tricyclic antidepressants, as well as with terfenadine, erythromycin, and pentamidine.[16,17] The proposed mechanism of VF is prolongation of the QT interval due to potassium channel blockade that results in increased dispersion of ventricular refractoriness.[17] A secondary mechanism may be elevation of serum catecholamine levels due to either reduced synaptic uptake or impaired metabolism.[16] Although these associations are presumptive, they have been supported by basic science investigations and provide a rationale for otherwise unexplained VF in these patients.

Finally, there is increasing recognition of the occurrence of unexplained cardiac arrest due to VF in young patients in the absence of any clearly defined etiology or precipitating event. The estimated incidence of idiopathic VF is 3% to 9% in cases unrelated to myocardial infarction, and in 10% to 15% of all VF resuscitations for patients under the age of 40 years.[18] A number of unique clinical syndromes have been proposed to account for idiopathic VF, including the Brugada syndrome of right bundle branch block, ST elevation, and sudden death,[19] or Leenhardt's[20] report of torsades de pointes in patients without QT interval prolongation.

Recently, diagnostic criteria for the diagnosis of idiopathic VF have been proposed along with establishment of an international registry to evaluate the outcome of these patients.[21] This issue is critical, as the literature is inconsistent with regard to the risk of a recurrent event; The Unexplained Cardiac Arrest Registry (UCARE) reports a 30% recurrence rate within 3 years of follow-up, and inadequate response to antiarrhythmic agents. Conversely, Viskin and Belhassen[22] report a low recurrence rate in patients with idiopathic VF who are treated with Class IA agents.

The following case reflects some of the difficulties in the evaluation of such a patient. In 1990, a teenage boy was referred to us for evaluation following resuscitation from VF. An extensive hemodynamic and electrophysiological investigation failed to identify the cause of aborted sudden death. Although the association was not recognized at that time, the patient had been placed on terfenadine 10 days prior to his arrest. In the absence of a plausible explanation for VF, a decision was made to proceed with implantation of an ICD. Since then, the device has never been used, and the device is now at elective replacement. The question is, was VF in this patient due to drug effect or was the patient a victim of idiopathic VF, and, based on the UCARE data, should he undergo ICD generator replacement due to the risk of recurrent VF?

In conclusion, cardiac arrest due to VF in the pediatric patient in the absence of defined cardiovascular disease requires a careful and in-depth investigation. The optimal evaluation and definition of treatment strategies must be based on the premise that the episode of VF may have been related to a potentially transient or reversible electrophysiological disturbance rather than to intrinsic structural or functional cardiovascular disease. In the presence of a clearly defined and transient or reversible etiology, a low risk of recurrent VF would be anticipated. However, in the absence of a defined etiology, the risk of recurrence remain uncertain.

VF in Pediatric Patients with Cardiovascular Disease

A larger and somewhat better defined group of pediatric patients who are VF survivors is the group of pediatric patients with cardiovascular disease. Even within this group there is significant heterogencity, as related to causes of VF as well as to the risk of recurrent event.

In 1983, Benson et al[23] reported a series of 11 young patients (mean age 18 years) in whom cardiac arrest was the initial manifestation of cardiovascular disease. A number of diverse forms of subtle cardiovascular disease was identified in these patients, and included viral myocarditis, dilated cardiomyopathy, previously asymptomatic Wolff-

Parkinson-White syndrome, and connective tissue disease. In this study, there were four patients with inducible ventricular arrhythmias who were treated with empiric regimens of antiarrhythmic drugs: 2 of these patients had recurrent cardiac arrest and resuscitation and the other 2 died suddenly.

In 1990, Silka et al[24] reported the assessment of 15 pediatric survivors of tachyarrhythmic sudden death (VT/VF), evaluating both hemodynamic and electrophysiological factors. Of these 15 patients, 5 had undergone prior surgical treatment of congenital heart disease, 4 had cardiomyopathies (3 dilated, 1 hypertrophic), and 6 had primary electrical abnormalities. Sustained tachyarrhythmias were inducible in 13 of 15 patients: VT (n=8), orthodromic reciprocating tachycardia in association with the Wolff-Parkinson-White syndrome (n=3), and atrial flutter (n=2). Surgical or catheter ablation of the accessory pathway was performed in the patients with Wolff-Parkinson-White syndrome, while VT was rendered noninducible with treatment (antiarrhythmic drug, pacemaker, and/or surgery) in 6 of 8 patients with ventricular arrhythmias inducible during programmed stimulation. There were no recurrent events in these nine patients during more than 3 years of follow-up. However, similar to the study by Benson et al,[23] of the remaining 6 patients with persistent inducibility or empiric drug therapy, 2 died suddenly and 3 required a second resuscitation from pulseless VT or VF. The findings of these studies suggest there is significant risk of recurrent VT/VF in young patients when the cause of cardiac arrest is undefined or therapy is empiric. Conversely, the data could also be interpreted to suggest that certain patients were "healthy responders"; that is, some patients had an inherently better prognosis, suggested by the fact that VT could be rendered noninducible by conventional methods.

During the 1990s there were exponential increases in the use of ICDs in patients who had been resuscitated from tachyarrhythmic sudden death, along with increased concerns regarding the proarrhythmic potential of cardiac antiarrhythmic drugs in children as well as adults.[25,26] A multicenter study of pediatric patients who had received ICDs was initially reported in 1990[27] and was expanded in 1993.[28] These studies provide the bases for many of our current recommendations regarding the use of these devices in young patients. In this registry, 125 pediatric patients were identified who had been resuscitated from pulseless VT or VF. Three forms of cardiovascular disease were identified: 1) hypertrophic or dilated cardiomyopathies; 2) primary electrical diseases (long QT syndromes or idiopathic VF); and 3) congenital heart disease. Although this study was limited by constraints and inaccuracies inherent to any voluntary registry, it did provide a large database of pediatric patients who were survivors of sudden death. Several trends related to both the risk of a recurrent event and long-term survival were identified and are listed below.

Risk of Recurrent VT/VF

During a mean follow-up of 31 ± 23 months, 59% of patients received at least one ICD shock for what was interpreted to be a sustained ventricular arrhythmia. Appropriate ICD shocks were correlated with longer length of follow-up and induction of a sustained ventricular arrhythmia during programmed stimulation. ICD discharges were not related to type of heart disease or ventricular function.

Survival Following ICD Implantation

There were nine deaths among the 125 patients during the follow-up period. The primary risk factor for death due to cardiovascular disease was impaired ventricular function. Survival was not related to type of cardiovascular disease or inducibility of arrhythmias at electrophysiological testing.

Thus, the primary conclusions of these studies were that: 1) The risk of a recurrent sustained ventricular arrhythmia in young patients following resuscitation during the first 2 to 3 years following resuscitation is approximately 50%, and 2) the primary risk of death following ICD implant is related to impaired ventricular function rather than recurrence of the arrhythmia itself. Therefore, survival should be anticipated in patients with relatively normal ventricular function. Conversely, heart transplantation may be a reasonable option for the patient with impaired ventricular function who is resuscitated from VF. The primary role of the ICD in such patients may be to provide a "bridge to transplant" until an acceptable donor is procured.[29]

Is Therapy Necessary for All Patients and Does it Alter the Prognosis?

In the preceding discussion, some of our uncertainties regarding evaluation of the causes of VF and risks of empiric therapy post resuscitation have been presented. Similar limitations and concerns persist for adult survivors of VF; the ICD has become the preferred option for patients both resuscitated from and perceived to be at high-risk for VF.[30,31]

However, there are certain instances in which an ICD is not necessary following resuscitation. Perhaps the most convincing example is the patient with Wolff-Parkinson-White syndrome and a short antegrade refractory period who undergoes ablation of the accessory pathway. A similar case could be made for the patient with drug-induced QT prolongation who experiences documented VF, in whom there is no evidence of other cardiovascular disease and no inducible arrhythmia, and where the QT interval returns to normal with drug discontinuation.

A third and unusual group of pediatric patients are those experience VT or VF in the setting of an acute myocardial infarction. The causes of such an event in young patients include Kawasaki disease or anomalous origin of left coronary artery, either from the left pulmonary artery or the right sinus of Valsalva. Johnsrude et al,[32] in a series of 96 children with myocardial infarction, report a 28% incidence of peri-infarction VT/VF. Although the combination of acute infarction and VT/VF was associated with an 80% mortality, survival for nearly 5 years in the remaining 61 patients was notable for the absence of either recurrent ventricular arrhythmias or late sudden death. Thus, it would appear that survival beyond the acute ischemic event may imply a better long-term prognosis than generally cited for adult patients. This may be due to the fact that most cases of infarction in pediatric patients are due to coronary hypoperfusion due to "steal" syndromes or major arterial obstruction rather than diffuse atherosclerotic disease.

Finally, a group of patients that is very difficult to treat is the group with long QT syndromes, particularly when VF is the initial presentation of their disease. Considerable controversy exists as to whether these patients should be treated with β-blockade and perhaps cardiac pacing or whether they have declared themselves as "high-risk" and thus should undergo ICD implantation.[33,34]

Conclusions and Suggestion for Research

In this era of increased public awareness, improved response times and resuscitation techniques, and automated external defibrillators, it is reasonable to anticipate that there may be an increased number of neurologically intact survivors of VF, both children and adults.[35] Following resuscitation, the major issue is to define the cause of the cardiac arrest and the risk of a recurrent event (Table 3). A reversible etiology of VF may be established in some patients without identifiable cardiovascular disease, such as those who have experienced trauma or idiosyncratic drug response. In others, there may be a remediable cause, such as atrial fibrillation in association with the Wolff-Parkinson-White syndrome or severe bradycardia in the setting of advanced atrioventricular block. In other patients, the risk of recurrence may be reduced by therapy, such as revascularization in the setting of myocar-

Table 3

Proposed Risk Stratification for Recurrent Ventricular Fibrillation in Pediatric Patients

Low risk

Transient etiology:	Drug-induced QT prolongation
	Commitio cordis
Reversible etiology:	Wolff-Parkinson-White (post ablation)
	Third-degree AV block (post pacemaker)

Moderate risk

Unknown etiology:	Idiopathic VF
Ischemia:	Remote myocardial infarction

High Risk

Cardiovascular disease:	Impaired ventricular function
	Family history of sudden death (long QT, HCM)
	Persistent ventricular arrhythmias ($\pm$ drug Rx)

AV = atrioventricular; HCM = hyopertrophic cardiomyopathy; VF = ventricular fibrillation.

dial ischemia or β-blockade with or without concomitant pacemaker therapy in patients with prolonged QT syndromes. Prospective and unbiased long-term evaluation will be necessary to determine the efficacy of these therapies.

For patients with known cardiovascular disease and relatively normal ventricular function, the risk of recurrent VF may exceed 50% during the subsequent 2 to 3 years of follow-up. In these patients, the ICD would appear to offer a significant benefit, particularly as compared with conventional antiarrhythmic therapy. The smaller numbers of patients would suggest a that similar approach may be indicated in patients with idiopathic VF. Finally, patients with impaired ventricular function appear to be at the greatest risk of recurrent VF. The ICD may improve short-term survival in this subgroup; however long-term survival may not be improved in these patients, as has been suggested in adults.[36]

Many of these suggestions are based on clinical experience combined with extrapolation of data derived from adult survivors of VF. As the substrate of VF is different in pediatric patients than in adults, novel or unique approaches need to be developed once a patient has been identified as "high-risk." Prospective evaluation of all pediatric survivors of VF is needed to determine the need for therapy (ICD) and whether such therapy truly improves the long-term prognosis. Conversely, the question of whether certain patients can be defined who are at a very low risk of a recurrent event is equally relevant.

References

1. Nadkarni V, Hazinski MF, Zideman D, et al. Pediatrics resuscitation: An advisory statement from the pediatric working group of the International Liaison Committee on Resuscitation. *Circulation* 1997;95:2185–2195.
2. Eisenberg M, Bergner L, Hallstrom A, et al. Epidemiology of cardiac arrest and resuscitation in children. *Ann Emerg Med* 1983;12:672–674.
3. Hickey RW, Cohen DM, Strausbaugh S, et al. Pediatric patients requiring CPR in the prehospital setting. *Ann Emerg Med* 1995;25:495–501.
4. Innes PA, Summers CA, Boyd IM, et al. Audit of paediatric cardiopulmonary resuscitation. *Arch Dis Child* 1993;68:487–491.
5. Schindler MB, Bohn D, Cox PN, et al. Outcome of out of hospital cardiac or respiratory arrest in children. *N Engl J Med* 1996;335:1473–1479.
6. Mogayzel C, Quan L, Graves JR, et al. Out of hospital ventricular fibrillation in children and adolescents: Causes and outcomes. *Ann Emerg Med* 1995;25:484–491.
7. Walsh CK, Krongrad E. Terminal cardiac electrical activity in pediatric patients. *Am J Cardiol* 1983;51:557–561.
8. Safranek DJ, Eisenberg MS, Larsen MP. The epidemiology of cardiac arrest in young adults. *Ann Emerg Med* 1992;21:1102–1106.
9. Nikolic G, Bishop RL, Singh JB. Sudden death recorded during Holter monitoring. *Circulation* 1982;66:218–225.
10. Cobb LA, Weaver WD, Fahrenbruch CE, et al. Community-based interventions for sudden cardiac death: Impact, limitations and changes. *Circulation* 1992; 85(suppl I):98–102.
11. Moe T. Morgagni-Adams-Stokes attacks caused by transient recurrent ventricular fibrillation in a patient without apparent organic heart disease. *Am Heart J* 1949;37:811–818.
12. Kontny F, Dale J. Self-terminating idiopathic ventricular fibrillation presenting as syncope: A 40-year follow-up report. *J Intern Med* 1990;227: 211–213.
13. Zipes D. Electrophysiological mechanisms involved in ventricular fibrillation. *Circulation* 1975;52(6 suppl)III120–III130.
14. Maron BJ, Poliac LC, Kaplan JA, et al. Blunt impact to the chest leading to sudden death from cardiac arrest during sports activities. *N Engl J Med* 1995;333:337–342.
15. Maron BJ, Strasburger JF, Kugler JD, et al. Survival following blunt chest impact-induced cardiac arrest during sports activities in young athletes. *Am J Cardiol* 1997;79:840–841.
16. Martyn R, Somberg JC, Kerin NK. Proarrhythmia of nonantiarrhythmic drugs. *Am Heart J* 1993;126:201–205.
17. Berul CI, Morad M. Regulation of potassium channels by nonsedating antihistamines. *Circulation* 1995;91:2220–2225.
18. Kasanuki H, Ohnishi S, Ohtuka M, et al. Idiopathic ventricular fibrillation induced with vagal activity in patients without obvious heart disease. *Circulation* 1997;95:2277–2285.
19. Brugada J, Brugada R, Brugada P. Right bundle-branch block and ST-segment elevation in leads V1 through V3: A marker for sudden death in patients without demonstrable structural heart disease. *Circulation* 1998;97: 457–460.
20. Leenhardt A, Lucet V, Denjoy I, et al. Catecholaminergic polymorphic ventricular tachycardia in children. A 7-year follow-up of 21 patients. *Circulation* 1995;91:1512–1519.

21. Priori SG. Survivors of out of hospital cardiac arrest with apparently normal heart. *Circulation* 1997;95:265–272.
22. Viskin S, Belhassen B. Idiopathic ventricular fibrillation. *Am Heart J* 1990;120:661–671.
23. Benson DW, Benditt DG, Anderson RW. Cardiac arrest in young, ostensibly healthy patients: Clinical, hemodynamic, and electrophysiologic findings. *Am J Cardiol* 1983;52:65–69.
24. Silka MJ, Kron J, Walance CG, et al. Assessment and follow-up of pediatric survivors of sudden cardiac death. *Circulation* 1990;82:341–349.
25. Echt DS, Liebson PR, Mitchell LB, et al. Mortality and morbidity in patients receiving encainide, flecainide, or placebo. *N Engl J Med* 1991;324:781–788.
26. Fish FA, Gillette PC, Benson DW Jr. Proarrhythmia, cardiac arrest and death in young patients receiving encainide and flecainide. *J Am Coll Cardiol* 1991;18:356–365.
27. Kron J, Oliver RP, Norsted S, et al. The automatic implantable cardioverter-defibrillator in young patients. *J Am Coll Cardiol* 1990;16:896–902.
28. Silka MJ, Kron J, Dunnigan A, et al. Sudden cardiac death and the use of implantable cardioverter-defibrillators in pediatric patients. *Circulation* 1993;87:800–807.
29. Jeevanandam V, Bielefeld MR, Auteri JS, et al. The implantable defibrillator: An electric bridge to cardiac transplantation. *Circulation* 1992;86 (suppl):II276–II279.
30. The AVID Investigators. A comparison of antiarrhythmic-drug therapy with implantable defibrillators in patients resuscitated from near-fatal ventricular arrhythmias. *N Engl J Med* 1997;337:1576–1583.
31. Moss AJ, Hall WJ, Cannom DS, et al. Improved survival with an implanted defibrillator in patients with coronary disease at high risk for ventricular arrhythmia. *N Engl J Med* 1996;335:1933–1940.
32. Johnsrude CL, Towbin JA, Cecchin F, et al. Postinfarction ventricular arrhythmias in children. *Am Heart J* 1995;129:1171–1177.
33. Eldar M, Griffin JC, Van Hare GF, et al. Combined use of beta-adrenergic blocking agents and long-term cardiac pacing for patients with the long QT syndrome. *J Am Coll Cardiol* 1992;20:830–837.
34. Groh WJ, Silka MJ, Oliver RP, et al. Use of implantable cardioverter-defibrillators in congenital long QT syndrome. *Am J Cardiol* 1996;78:703–705.
35. Morris RD, Krawiecki NS, Wright JA, Walter LW. Neuropsychological, academic and adaptive functioning in children who survive in-hospital cardiac arrest and resuscitation. *J Learn Disabil* 1993;26:46–51.
36. Kim SG, Fisher JD, Furman S, et al. Benefits of implantable defibrillators are overestimated by sudden death rates and better represented by the total arrhythmic death rate. *J Am Coll Cardiol* 1991;17:1587–1592.

Chapter 22

Cost-Effectiveness of the Implantable Cardioverter-Defibrillator in the Young

Richard A. Friedman, MD
and Arthur Garson, Jr., MD, MPH

The incidence of sudden cardiac death in pediatric-aged patients is uncommon compared with that seen in adults. It is estimated that approximately 300,000 adults will suffer a sudden cardiac death in the United States each year, an overall incidence of 0.1% to 0.2% per year in the total adult population.[1] Compare this with the last published estimate of one to eight sudden cardiac death events per 100,000 patient years,[2] and the overall impact on the US healthcare system is underwhelming. Studies of the cost-effectiveness of the use of implantable cardioverter-defibrillators (ICDs) in adults have demonstrated that this therapy is appropriate for selected patients.[3,4] However, to date there have been no randomized clinical trials in pediatric patients or in young adults with congenital heart disease to address whether the therapy is warranted or cost-effective.

The aim of this chapter is to briefly review some of the methods of calculating measures of cost-effectiveness and to relate them to the potential for developing a strategy to study whether the use of ICDs in a population of young patients without coronary artery disease is cost-effective. The interested reader is referred to several references for a more complete understanding.[5,6]

Measures of Cost

The term "cost" is frequently misused, and incompletely understood. Specifically, it is not another term for "charges," whether they be

From: Quan L, Franklin WH (eds). *Ventricular Fibrillation: A Pediatric Problem*. Armonk, NY: Futura Publishing Company, Inc.; ©2000.

hospital- and/or physician-based. To be certain, these two components are a significant percentage of the cost, but there are a number of other considerations that must be accounted for in the calculation.

Direct medical costs include physicians' work, hospital charges, and laboratory work. *Direct nonmedical costs* include costs borne by the patient for transportation, special diets, tutors, and any home improvements needed for his or her support. *Indirect costs* involve lost wages (lost productivity) by the parent(s) or patient and loss of potential advancement that would not have been incurred in the absence of the intervention. *Induced costs* include the cost of treating side effects of a medication and ongoing treatment of the patient who lives longer because of the intervention.[5] *Intangible costs*, which are difficult to measure, involve pain, suffering, and anxiety. Some authors consider this last category within the realm of an indirect cost.[5]

It is also important to note from whose perspective the costs are evaluated. Potential parties include the insurance company, the patient, the hospital, and society. The insurance company would not be associated with the cost of lost productivity of the patient, as that is not its concern. On the other hand, society would evaluate the total costs for all patients for a given intervention and then attempt to include in the analysis the potential gain to society from that intervention if it results in enhanced longevity for the patient. In the case of a health maintenance organization (HMO), evaluation of an intervention for a given patient may have to take into account the projected length of time that patient may be covered. For example, rather than pay a large one-time cost for a radiofrequency ablation procedure, an HMO may decide that it is more cost-effective to pay for medication for control of supraventricular tachycardia if it is determined that the patient may only be covered for 5 years within its plan. From a societal perspective, the radiofrequency ablation has shown to be more cost-effective.[7]

Cost should be reported with respect to a *discount of future costs*, which takes into account costs and health outcomes that occur during different periods. Discounting adjusts future costs and expresses all cost and monetary benefits in terms of their present value.[5] For the purpose of most studies, the recommendation is to use a 3% discount rate and then apply a sensitivity analysis using a range of 0% to 7%.[8] A *sensitivity analysis* is a statistical tool to check the effect of assumptions made during the analysis of data. In this example, one would do a cost-effectiveness analysis using several discount rates, and report the results of the analysis in a table showing the differences using each discount rate.

Estimates of costs may be difficult to obtain, as they vary significantly from locale to locale. Aside from the scrupulous gathering of all billing records for a patient for a given intervention and follow-up care, estimates may have to be obtained from Medicare or Medicaid payments based on diagnosis-related groups. Problems with this approach include multiple diagnostic-related groups for a given diagnosis; location of the provider will also affect payment. For a study of defibrillators, the cost of the device should be available to a registry. However, differences in price may still exist because of large buying programs of which the hospital is a member. In lieu of "hard numbers," average charges for goods and services may have to be applied.

Measures of Effectiveness

At first glance, most people would rate a potentially life-saving treatment as effective if it accomplished that goal. In fact, the two studies discussed below which involved randomized clinical trials of defibrillators versus drug therapy in adult patients with coronary artery disease and ventricular tachycardia (VT) did just that; ie, calculation of life years saved by the intervention. However, the value of *effectiveness* is a much more complicated issue and deserves more attention here. Quality-adjusted life years (QALYs) are the commonly accepted unit of measurement of the effect of an intervention. It measures the number of life years added and modifies it by a factor estimating the quality of life those additional years provide. The scale is from 0 to 1 with death = 0 and perfect health = 1 (Figure 1). The question that arises is, who determines what the quality of life is during those years—the patient, family members (in the case of a child), physicians, or the general community? For the most part, investigators prefer to use patient assessment of quality of life.[9] Dollars expended per QALY are then calculated and used to determine whether a particular intervention is "cost-

QALYs

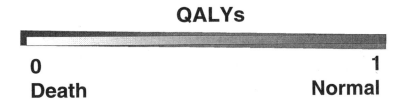

0   **1**
Death   **Normal**

Added years of life X Quality of those years

Repair of ToF adds 50 years X 0.75 = 37.5 QALYs
Norwood for HLHS adds 15 y X 0.5 = 7.5 QALYs

Figure 1. ToF = tetralogy of Fallot; HLHS = hypoplastic left heart syndrome; QALY = quality-adjusted life year. See text for details.

effective." Societal pressures sometimes create situations in which the cost/QALY, though excessive, are still favored. This would be the case in the testing of female blood donors in the general population—$1.5 million/QALY compared with heart transplantation ($20,000/QALY). Generally, a $30,000/QALY is in the range of reasonable whereas when the cost starts to exceed $50,000/QALY, cost-effectiveness is considered low. This clearly becomes an emotional issue, especially in the pediatric patient, and deserves further study.

Many other complex ethical issues arise in the use of QALYs in cost-effectiveness; these are discussed in detail elsewhere.[5,9–11] In the case of defibrillators in pediatric patients with congenital heart disease, the issue is further complicated by the fact that there is no baseline from which to compare quality of life issues. That is, before assessing quality of life in a congenital heart disease patient with an ICD, one would need to use a base of patients with congenital heart disease or other chronic diseases for comparison, rather than the general population, whose health, on a scale of 0 to 1, is closer to 1. Unfortunately, at present, no database exists to refer to in forming this analysis.

Although the QALY is surrounded by many problematic issues, as Danford[10] points out, without it *"those who implement health care policy could not be held to quantitative justification of resource allocation. . . ."* Thus, whether it is the QALY that is to be used, or some other iteration, a useful measure of benefit to patient and society must be applied in the denominator of the cost-effectiveness ratio to help formulate a basis for rational decision making.

Cost-Effectiveness

In order to determine whether a particular intervention is cost-effective, more than one therapy should be evaluated so that one alternative may be considered against another. This would be best served by a randomized clinical trial of two or more therapies for the same condition. In the absence of a prospective study, meta-analysis can be used. Unfortunately, the term "cost-effective" is often misused to imply "cheap." As Petitti[5] nicely summarized from the work of Doubilet et al,[12] misuse includes applying the term 1) in the absence of data on both cost and effectiveness; 2) when effectiveness is demonstrated in the absence of data on cost; and 3) as restricted to a situation where it is merely cost saving relative to its alternatives and does not apply to a medical situation. Proper application of the term occurs when an intervention is 1) less costly and at least as effective; 2) more effective and more costly where the added benefit is felt to be "worth the cost"; 3) less effective and less costly where the alternative is felt to be not "worth the added cost"; and 4) cost saving with an equal or better outcome.

A useful way to visualize the complexity of the issue of cost-effectiveness is shown in Figure 2. This four-quadrant grid comprises two "easy" quadrants and two difficult ones. The two easy quadrants are the ones with high cost and low effectiveness (lower right), and low cost, high effectiveness (upper left). In the former is the example of the CAST trial, in which use of Class IC agents for the treatment of asymptomatic premature ventricular contractions in patients with coronary heart disease was associated with an increased expense and mortality as compared with placebo. In the latter is the use of radiofrequency catheter ablation for Wolff-Parkinson-White supraventricular tachycardia in children,[7] shorter hospital stays achieved through improved scheduling, and flexible shifts for certain hospital departments.

The two "difficult" quadrants—upper right (high cost, increased effectiveness) and lower left (decreased cost, decreased effectiveness)—call for a complex interaction between patient, physician, payor for services, and, ultimately, the community at large. Trade-offs between cost and effectiveness are not simple and involve complex inputs and judg-

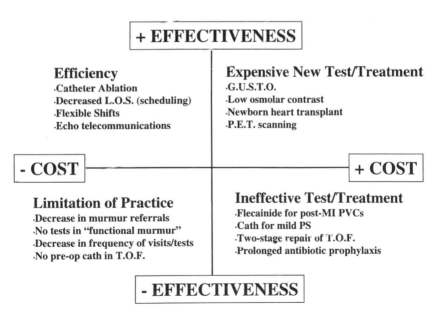

+ EFFECTIVENESS

Efficiency
·Catheter Ablation
·Decreased L.O.S. (scheduling)
·Flexible Shifts
·Echo telecommunications

Expensive New Test/Treatment
·G.U.S.T.O.
·Low osmolar contrast
·Newborn heart transplant
·P.E.T. scanning

- COST   **+ COST**

Limitation of Practice
·Decrease in murmur referrals
·No tests in "functional murmur"
·Decrease in frequency of visits/tests
·No pre-op cath in T.O.F.

Ineffective Test/Treatment
·Flecainide for post-MI PVCs
·Cath for mild PS
·Two-stage repair of T.O.F.
·Prolonged antibiotic prophylaxis

- EFFECTIVENESS

Figure 2. The cost-effectiveness grid. G.U.S.T.O. = Global Utilization of Streptokinase and Tissue Plasminogen Activator for Occluded Coronary Arteries; L.O.S. = length of stay; MI = myocardial infarction; P.E.T. = positron emission tomography; PS = pulmonary stenosis; PVCs = premature ventricular contractions; T.O.F. = tetralogy of Fallot.

ments from the physician, the payor, whether it be "third party" or government, and the patient/family.

Previous Studies

Two recent studies are worth mentioning prior to addressing the issue in a pediatric population. Wever et al[4] performed a randomized clinical trial in adults with coronary artery disease and compared the effectiveness, as measured by total mortality, of tiered therapy with antiarrhythmic drugs guided by electrophysiological testing versus implantation of an ICD. Costs were calculated using the lowest class scale rates of Dutch private healthcare insurance. Cost-effectiveness was gauged by using the median total costs per patient day alive divided by the number of days the patient was alive. The electrophysiology-testing-guided group included patients who were treated with predominantly Class III agents, VT surgery, or late ICD implantation if all previous therapies failed. Overall, the electrophysiology study group suffered a very high mortality, 7 of 11 patients with antiarrhythmics as sole therapy, compared with the ICD group (4 of 29 patients); the drug only group had a lower cost-effectiveness ratio. Except for the first 3 months of therapy when costs of device implantation and follow-up were included, the ICD was significantly more cost-effective: $63 per patient versus $94 per patient day alive. If calculated on a net cost-effectiveness ratio, the result was $11,300 per patient per life year saved. Quality of life aspects were also used to determine that the ICD group had a significantly improved exercise tolerance, shorter hospitalizations, fewer invasive procedures, and no recurrent cardiac arrests or referrals for heart transplantation.

The results of the Multicenter Automatic Defibrillator Implantation Trial (MADIT) were recently reported by Mushlin et al.[3] Costs were determined based on services rendered including patient bills, emergency department visits, physician office visits, outpatient tests/procedures, medication, and other disease-/treatment-related service. Community services, including nursing home care and occupational or physical therapy were also included. The actual amount estimated for each service was based on a national study of Medicare claims that calculated the ratio of physician to hospital costs for each diagnostic-related group. Outpatient tests and community services were similarly calculated while emergency room visits were based on the Medicare Resource-Based Relative Value Scale with geographic adjusters. Drug costs were estimated by use of a published source of wholesale prices for each medication prescribed. The MADIT study previously showed improved survival in the ICD group versus conventional therapy.[13] With use of these data and the increased longevity of the ICD survivors of 3.66 years versus 2.80 years for the conventional therapy group, an incremental cost-effectiveness ratio of $27,000 per life year saved was calculated. A sensitivity analysis showed an even better result of $23, 000 per life year saved if the cost of the defibrillators was based on transvenous devices only. Of note is that no attempt was made in this study to qualify the results based on a value system of the quality of the life years saved, ie, no QALY analysis was performed. The authors also cautioned that this was a randomized clinical trial of a specific group of patients and that application of this therapy to other groups of patients might not yield the same cost-effectiveness.

Cost-Effectiveness in the Pediatric Population

There is a paucity of data on the use of ICDs in the young. Kron et al[14] reported on a database of 40 patients less than 20 years of age who had undergone implantation of an ICD for a variety of diseases including long QT syndrome, dilated cardiomyopathy, hypertrophic cardiomyopathy, and primary ventricular fibrillation. They concluded that the ICD was an effective form of therapy in terms of prolonging survival in this nonselected population. In another report that included 177 patients,[15] some of which were from the previous study, the investigators found that pediatric survivors of sudden cardiac death remained at risk for recurrence and that this therapy was useful for those patients. They estimated that 60% of the sudden cardiac death survivors who receive an ICD will receive an appropriate shock within 36 months. Given those numbers, it follows that if a defined population can be identified, there exists the potential for ICD implantation to have a significant effect on life years saved. The major issue then remains to determine whether such therapy is cost-effective.

It appears unlikely that a randomized clinical trial of a specific population of children and young adults comparing ICD implantation and conventional therapy will take place. Reasons include too small a subset of patients with similar disease, unwillingness of physicians to reserve ICD therapy for some patients because of a widespread bias toward implantation, and unwillingness of patients and/or families to be part of such a trial. In addition, no standard assessment of quality of life indicators exists for young patients, whether they have had palliated congenital heart disease or acquired heart disease. A detailed analysis of costs, especially future costs after an intervention, will be complex because of the need for long-term follow-up. Thus, there are several questions that should be addressed.

First, *is it necessary to do such a study?* From the perspective of the patient, it would be most beneficial to have a clearer concept of whom would really benefit from this therapy, as the untoward effects, both physical (infection, erosion, inappropriate shocks) and psychological, are considerable. However, compared with the adult population of potential patients who could benefit from an ICD, implants in the young would account for no more than 2% to 3% of the total implants in the population as a whole.

Second *how can this study be done?* If a study is to be done, then the first logical step would be to establish a registry of young patients with congenital and acquired heart disease who have already had a device implanted. Careful follow-up of these patients will go a long way toward answering who is most likely to benefit from the device. Figure 3

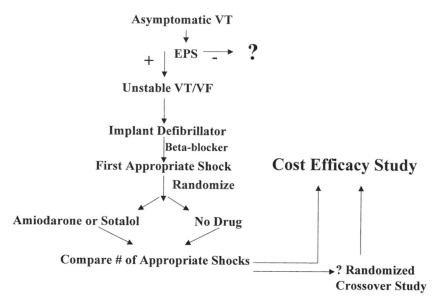

Figure 3. Proposed study of cost-effectiveness of implantable cardioverter-defibrillators (ICDs) in young patients with congenital heart disease. Patients with congenital heart disease and asymptomatic ventricular tachycardia (VT) undergo electrophysiology studies (EPS). Those with a "+" study, i.e., induction of unstable VT or ventricular fibrillation (VF), undergo implantation of an ICD. There is still a question as to those with a "−" study. All patients would receive a β-blocker but no other antiarrhythmic therapy. Following the first appropriate shock, patients would be randomized to a Class III drug or to no drug. A longitudinal assessment of the number of subsequent appropriate shocks would then take place. The assumption is that an appropriate shock represents a "sudden death" event. The data could then be assessed for cost-effectiveness, including quality of life issues. Alternatively, some or all of the patients could enter a randomized crossover study and then proceed to the cost-effectiveness study.

is an outline of a potential study for those patients with asymptomatic VT in whom a bias toward implantation has already resulted in the implantation of a device following induction of hemodynamically unstable VT. In this scenario, all patients get an ICD and then are "randomized" to additional therapy with either a Class III agent or other appropriate drug or to no drug. If the patients who receive a drug have a significantly lower number of shocks than the ICD, no-drug group, the effect of antiarrhythmic therapy alone can be surmised, and life years saved by the two therapies are compared.

Finally, *how do we assess effectiveness?* Mortality certainly would continue to be the most important determinant, but quality of life issues must also be addressed. Therefore, it seems equally as logical, as was the case in developing a registry of young ICD patients, to establish a registry of young patients with heart disease that pertains to their quality of life. Questionnaires and other instruments to measure the effects of interventions on quality of life of the patients and their families will need to be developed in order to attempt some sort of standardization. In the absence of this component, rational decision making will suffer and the implantation of ICDs will continue to be subject to a lower standard than our patients deserve.

References

1. Myerburg RJ, Interian A, Mitrani RM, et al. Frequency of sudden cardiac death and profiles of risk. *Am J Cardiol* 1997;80(5B):10F-19F.
2. Silka MJ, Kron J, Dunnigan A, et al. Sudden cardiac death and the use of implantable cardioverter-defibrillators in pediatric patients. *Circulation* 1993;87:800–807.
3. Mushlin AI, Hall J, Zwanziger J, et al. The cost-effectiveness of automatic implantable cardiac defibrillators. Results from MADIT. *Circulation* 1998; 97:2129–2135.
4. Wever EFD, Hauer RNW, Schrijvers G, et al. Cost-effectiveness of implantable defibrillator as a first-choice therapy versus electrophysiologically guided, tiered strategy in postinfarct sudden death survivors. *Circulation* 1996;93:489–496.
5. Petitti Diana B. *Meta-Analysis, Decision-Analysis, and Cost-Effectiveness. Methods for Quantitative Synthesis in Medicine.* New York: Oxford University Press; 1994:169–186.
6. Feldstein PJ. *Health Care Economics.* 4th ed. Albany, NY: Delmar Publishers, Inc.; 1993.
7. Weinstein MC, Siegel JE, Gold MR, et al. Recommendations of the Panel on Cost-Effectiveness in Health and Medicine. *JAMA* 1996;276:1253–1258.
8. Garson A. Children with Wolff Parkinson White and supraventricular tachycardia: A model cost-effectiveness analysis for pediatric chronic disease. *Am J Cardiol* 1993;72(suppl):302.
9. Russell LB, Gold MR, Siegel JE, et al. The role of cost-effectiveness analysis in health and medicine. Consensus statement. *JAMA* 1996;276: 1172–1177.

10. Danford DA. QALYs: Their ethical implications. *JAMA* 1990;264:2503.
11. LaPuma J, Lawlor EF. Quality adjusted life years: Ethical implications for physicians and policymakers. *JAMA* 1990;263:2917–2921.
12. Doubilet P, Weinstein MC, McNeil BJ. Use and misuse of the term "cost-effective" in medicine. *N Engl J Med* 1986;314:253–256.
13. Moss AJ, Hall WJ, Cannom DS, et al. Improved survival with an implanted defibrillator in patients with coronary artery disease at high risk for ventricular arrhythmia. *N Engl J Med* 1996;335:1933–1940.
14. Kron J, Liver RP, Norsted S, Silka MJ. The automatic implantable cardioverter-defibrillator in young patients. *J Am Coll Cardiol* 1990;16: 896–902.
15. Silka MJ, Kron J, Dunnigan A, Dick M 2d, et al. Sudden cardiac death and the use of implantable cardioverter-defibrillators in pediatric patients. *Circulation* 1993;87:800–807.

Section IX

Prevention

Chapter 23

The Genetics
of Brugada Syndrome

Jeffrey A. Towbin, MD

Sudden cardiac death is a significant problem in the United States, with an incidence reported to be greater than 300,000 persons per year.[1] Interest in identifying the underlying cause of the death has been focused on cases of unexpected arrhythmogenic death, which is estimated to represent 5% of all sudden deaths.[2] In cases in which no structural heart disease can be identified, the long QT syndrome and ventricular preexcitation are most commonly considered as likely causes. Recently, Brugada syndrome (also known by some investigators as idiopathic ventricular fibrillation), a disease associated with an electrocardiographic (ECG) abnormality of right bundle branch block (RBBB) with ST elevation in the right precordial leads (V_1 through V_3), was added to the list of possible causes of sudden death in otherwise healthy young individuals. The purpose of this chapter is to describe the clinical disorder and the genetics of this disease.

Clinical Aspects of Brugada Syndrome

The first identification of the ECG pattern of RBBB with ST elevation in leads V_1 through V_3 was reported by Osher and Wolff,[3] who noted this finding in three apparently healthy males. Shortly thereafter, Edeiken[4] identified persistent ST elevation without RBBB in another 10 asymptomatic males, and Levine et al[5] described ST elevation in the right chest leads and conduction block in the right ventricle in patients

From: Quan L, Franklin WH (eds). *Ventricular Fibrillation: A Pediatric Problem.* Armonk, NY: Futura Publishing Company, Inc.; ©2000.

Dr. Towbin is funded by NIH grants from the National Heart, Lung, and Blood Institute (NHLBI R01–HL33843–06; R01–HL51618–06) and the Texas Children's Hospital Foundation Chair in Pediatric Cardiac Research.

with severe hyperkalemia. Although multiple other reports of patients with variations of this ECG pattern exist,[6–10] this ECG abnormality was largely ignored as being associated with sudden death until Martini et al[11] and Aihara et al[12] focused attention on the possible link. This association was further confirmed in 1991 by Pedro and Josep Brugada,[13] who described four patients with sudden and aborted sudden death with ECGs demonstrating RBBB and persistent ST elevation in leads V_1 through V_3. In 1992, these authors characterized what they believed to be a distinct clinical and ECG syndrome.[14]

ST elevation in the right chest leads has been observed in a variety of clinical and experimental settings and is not unique or diagnostic of Brugada syndrome by itself. Situations in which these ECG findings occur include electrolyte or metabolic disorders, pulmonary or inflammatory diseases, and abnormalities of the central or peripheral nervous system. In the absence of these abnormalities, the term idiopathic ST elevation is often used and may identify patients with Brugada syndrome. The prevalence of idiopathic ST elevation varies from 2.1% to 2.65%,[15] with elevation of the ST segment that is limited to the right precordial leads occurring in less than 1% of all cases of ST elevation.[8]

The ECG findings and associated sudden and unexpected death have been reported as a common problem in Japan and Southeast Asia, where it most commonly affects men during sleep.[16] This disorder, known as sudden and unexpected death syndrome (SUDS) or sudden, unexpected nocturnal death syndrome, has many names in Southeast Asia, including bangungut (to rise and moan in sleep) in the Philippines, non-laitai (sleep-death) in Laos, lai-tai (died during sleep) in Thailand, and pokkuri (sudden and unexpectedly ceased phenomena) in Japan. Generally, victims of SUDS include young, healthy males in whom death occurs suddenly with a groan, usually during sleep late at night. No precipitating factors are identified, and autopsy findings are generally negative.[17] Life-threatening ventricular tachyarrhythmias as a primary cause of SUDS have been demonstrated, with ventricular fibrillation (VF) occurring in most cases.[18]

Brugada Syndrome and Arrhythmogenic Right Ventricular Dysplasia

Controversy exists concerning the possible association of Brugada syndrome and arrhythmogenic right ventricular dysplasia (ARVD); some investigators argue that these are the same disorder or that at least one is a forme-fruste of the other.[19–24] However, the classic echocardiographic, angiographic, and magnetic resonance imaging findings of ARVD are not seen in Brugada syndrome patients. In addition, Brugada syndrome patients typically are without the histopathologic findings of ARVD. Further, the morphology of ventricular tachycardia (VT)/VF differs.[25]

Clinical Genetics of Brugada Syndrome

Like those with ARVD, most of the families thus far identified with Brugada syndrome have apparent autosomal dominant inheritance.[21,25–27] In these families, approximately 50% of offspring of affected patients develop the disease. Although the number of families reported has been small, it is likely that this is due to under-recognition as well as premature and unexpected death.[28]

Molecular Genetics of Brugada Syndrome

In order in identify the gene(s) responsible for Brugada syndrome, moderately sized or large families and excellent clinical surveillance are required for gene mapping studies to proceed with subsequent positional cloning or positional candidate gene cloning. In the latter case, genes previously cloned and mapped to a region of interest (ie, a linked locus) can be screened for mutations to prove that they are responsible for the disease. In cases where excellent electrophysiological hypotheses exist, candidate genes can also be screened randomly for mutations in small families or in sporadic cases.

In Brugada syndrome, several good candidate genes exist. In animal studies, blockade of the calcium-independent 4-aminopyridine-sensitive transient outward potassium current (I_{to}) results in surface ECG findings of elevated, downsloping ST segments[29] due to greater prolongation in the epicardial action potential compared with the endocardium (which lacks a plateau phase).[30] Loss of the action potential plateau (or dome) in the epicardium but not in the endocardium would be expected to cause ST segment elevation and, because loss of the dome is caused by an outward shift in the balance of currents active at the end of phase 1 of the action potential (principally I_{to} and I_{Ca}), autonomic neurotransmitters such as acetylcholine facilitate loss of the action potential dome by suppressing calcium current and augmenting potassium current, whereas β-adrenergic agonists (ie, isoproterenol, dobutamine) restore the dome by augmenting I_{Ca}.[31–33] Sodium channel blockers also facilitate loss of the canine right ventricular action potential dome as a result of a negative shift in the voltage at which phase 1 begins.[34,35] Hence, I_{to}, I_{Ca}, and I_{Na} would be good candidate genes to study. Since I_{Na} (*SCN5A*) has been shown to cause

VT/VF in humans (in the long QT syndrome),[36–38] this gene certainly is worthy of study.

Recently, we reported the findings in six families and in several sporadic cases of Brugada syndrome.[27] The families were initially studied by linkage analysis using markers to the known ARVD loci on chromosome 1[39] and 14,[40,41] and linkage was excluded. More recently, seven other families have also excluded linkage to these loci, thus suggesting that the families recruited with Brugada syndrome to date may indeed be an entity distinct from ARVD. Candidate gene screening using the mutation analysis approach of single-strand conformation polymorphism analysis and deoxyribonucleic acid sequencing was performed and *SCN5A* was chosen for study. In three families, mutations in *SCN5A* were identified,[27] including 1) a missense mutation (C-to-T base substitution) causing a substitution of a highly conserved threonine by methionine at codon 1620 (T1620M) in the extracellular loop between transmembrane segments S3 and S4 of domain IV (DIVS3–DIVS4), an area important for coupling of channel activation to fast inactivation; 2) a two-nucleotide insertion (AA), which disrupts the splice-donor sequence of intron 7 of *SCN5A*; and 3) a single nucleotide deletion (A) at codon 1397, which results in an in-frame stop codon that eliminates DI-IIS6, DIVS1-DIVS6, and the carboxy-terminus of *SCN5A*.

Biophysical analysis of the mutants in *Xenopus* oocytes demonstrated a reduction in the number of functional sodium channels in both the splicing mutation and one-nucleotide deletion mutation, which should promote development of reentrant arrhythmias. In the missense mutation, sodium channels recover from inactivation more rapidly than normal. In this case, the presence of both normal and mutant channels in the same tissue would promote heterogeneity of the refractory period, a well established mechanism of arrhythmogenesis. Inhibition of the sodium channel I_{Na} current causes heterogeneous loss of the action potential dome in the right ventricular epicardium, leading to a marked dispersion of depolarization and refractoriness, an ideal substrate for development of reentrant arrhythmias. Phase 2 reentry produced by the same substrate is believed to provide the premature beat necessary for initiation of the VT and VF responsible for symptoms in these patients.

Conclusion

Brugada syndrome is a clinically heterogeneous disease characterized by ECG abnormalities including ST segment elevation in leads V_1 through V_3, RBBB in some cases, and episodic ventricular arrhythmias including VT/VF. The first genetic abnormality causing Brugada syndrome was recently identified by our group as mutations in the ion channel gene *SCN5A*, which encodes the cardiac sodium channel. Mutations in this gene result in a loss in function of the channels or rapid recovery from inactivation. *SCN5A* was previously shown to be the cause of *LQT3*, a form of Romano-Ward long QT syndrome.[36–38,42–44] The differences in the clinical findings between *LQT3* and Brugada syndrome occur due to the different biophysical results based on the position of the mutations within this gene. Unlike Brugada syndrome, *LQT3* occurs due to a gain of function in *SCN5A*, where persistence of inactivation is seen.

Despite the differences between long QT syndrome and Brugada syndrome, important similarities should be noted. In particular, both of these disorders, in which life-threatening ventricular tachyarrhythmias occur, are due to mutations in genes encoding ion channels. This similarity is somewhat akin to that which has previously been described in familial hypertrophic cardiomyopathy, in which mutations in genes encoding for sarcomeric proteins have been identified.[44–49] Here, seven genes (β-myosin heavy chain,[44] α-tropomyosin,[45] cardiac troponin T,[45] myosin-binding protein-C,[46,47] myosin essential light chain,[48] myosin regulatory light chain,[48] and troponin I[49]), all encoding members of the sarcomeric unit, have been found mutated in patients with familial hypertrophic cardiomyopathy. The clinical phenotype, including outcome, appears to differ based on the gene that is mutated and the specific mutation.[50,51] Similar findings are emerging in familial dilated cardiomyopathy as well.[52] Thus, it appears that if a particular cascade at any point within the final common pathway leading to a specific cardiac function (ie, contractile apparatus resulting in cardiac function, ion channels resulting in cardiac rhythm, cytoskeletal proteins resulting in cardiac structural support) is affected, a spectrum of similar disease (ie, contractile apparatus mutations causes hypertrophic cardiomyopathy, ion channel mutations result in long QT syndrome and Brugada syndrome, mutations in cytoskeletal protein genes result in familial dilated cardiomyopathy) results. This "final common pathway" hypothesis[52] is being used in Brugada syndrome to identify the remaining genes responsible for this disorder.

Summary

Brugada syndrome appears to be a disorder that is genetically distinct from ARVD that results from mutations in the cardiac sodium channel gene *SCN5A*. These mutant channels differ in biophysical profile from the mutations in this gene, which causes the long QT syndrome (*LQT3*); *LQT3* is due to a gain of function and abnormalities of inactivation. It is likely that genetic heterogeneity exists in Brugada syndrome and, based on the "final common pathway" hypothesis, which predicts that all primary ventricular arrhythmias will be due to abnormalities in similar proteins, it is reasonable to expect other ion channel gene mutations in patients with Brugada syndrome.

References

1. Myerburg RJ, Kessler KM, Castellanos A. Sudden cardiac death: Structure, function and time-dependence of risk. *Circulation* 1992;85:I2-I10.
2. Myerburg RJ. Sudden cardiac death in persons with normal (or near normal) heart. *Am J Cardiol* 1997;79(6A):3–9.
3. Osher HL, Wolff L. Electrocardiographic pattern simulating acute myocardial injury. *Am J Med Sci* 1953;226:541–545.
4. Edeiken J. Elevation of RS-T segment, apparent or real in right precordial leads as probable normal variant. *Am Heart J* 1954;48:331–339.
5. Levine HD, Wanzer SH, Merrill JP. Dialyzable currents of injury in potassium intoxication resembling acute myocardial infarction or pericarditis. *Circulation* 1956;13:29–36.
6. Roesler H. An electrocardiographic study of high take-off of the R(R)-T segment in right precordial leads. Altered repolarization. *Am J Cardiol* 1960;6:920–928.
7. Calo AA. The triad secondary R wave, RS-T segment elevation and T waves inversion in right precordial leads: A normal electrocardiographic variant. *G Ital Cardiol* 1975;5:955–960.
8. Parisi AF, Beckmann CH, Lancaster MC. The spectrum of ST elevation in the electrocardiograms of healthy adult men. *J Electrocardiol* 1971;4:137–144.
9. Wasserburger RH, Alt WJ, Lloyd CJ. The normal RS-T segment elevation variant. *Am J Cardiol* 1961;8:184–192.
10. Goldman MJ. RS-T segment elevation in mid- and left precordial leads as a normal variant. *Am Heart J* 1953;46:817–820.
11. Martini B, Nava A, Thiene G, et al. Ventricular fibrillation without apparent heart disease. Description of six cases. *Am Heart J* 1989;118:1203–1209.
12. Aihara N, Ohe T, Kamakura S, et al. Clinical and electrophysiologic characteristics of idiopathic ventricular fibrillation. *Shinzo* 1990;22(suppl 2): 80–86.
13. Brugada P, Brugada J. A distinct clinical and electrocardiographic syndrome: Right bundle-branch block, persistent ST segment elevation with normal QT interval and sudden cardiac death. *PACE* 1991;14:746. Abstract.
14. Brugada P, Brugada J. Right bundle-branch block, persistent ST segment elevation and sudden cardiac death: A distinct clinical and electrocardiographic syndrome. A multicenter report. *J Am Coll Cardiol* 1992;20:1391–1386.
15. Sumita S, Yoshida K, Ishikawa T, et al. ST level in healthy subjects with right bundle branch block in relation to Brugada syndrome. *Eur J Cardiac Pacing Electrophysiol* 1996;6:270.
16. Nademanee K, Veerakul G, Nimmannit S, et al. Arrhythmogenic marker for the sudden unexplained death syndrome in Thai men. *Circulation* 1997;96:2595–2600.

17. Gotoh K. A histopathological study on the conduction system of the so-called Pokkuri disease (sudden unexpected cardiac death of unknown origin in Japan). *Jpn Circ J* 1976;40:753–768.
18. Hayashi M, Murata M, Satoh M, et al. Sudden nocturnal death in young males from ventricular flutter. *Jpn Heart J* 1985;26:585–591.
19. Naccarella F. Malignant ventricular arrhythmias in patients with a right bundle-branch block and persistent ST segment elevation in V1–V3: A probable arrhythmogenic cardiomyopathy of the right ventricle [editorial comment]. *G Ital Cardiol* 1993;23:1219–1222.
20. Fontaine G. Familial cardiomyopathy associated with right bundle branch block, ST segment elevation and sudden death [letter]. *J Am Coll Cardiol* 1996;28:540.
21. Corrado D, Nava A, Buja G, et al. Familial cardiomyopathy underlies syndrome of right bundle branch block, ST segment elevation and sudden death. *J Am Coll Cardiol* 1996;27:443–448.
22. Scheinman MM. Is Brugada syndrome a distinct clinical entity? *J Cardiovasc Electrophysiol* 1997;8:332–336.
23. Ohe T. Idiopathic ventricular fibrillation of the Brugada type—an atypical form of arrhythmogenic right ventricular cardiomyopathy [editorial]. *Intern Med* 1996;35:595.
24. Fontaine G, Piot O, Sohal P, et al. Right precordial leads and sudden death. Relation with arrhythmogenic right ventricular dysplasia. *Arch Mal Coeur Vaiss* 1996;89:1323–1329.
25. Brugada J, Brugada P. Further characterization of the syndrome of right bundle branch block, ST segment elevation, and sudden death. *J Cardiovasc Electrophysiol* 1997;8:325–331.
26. Kobayashi T, Shintani U, Yamamoto T, et al. Familial occurrence of electrocardiographic abnormalities of the Brugada-type. *Intern Med* 1996;35:637–640.
27. Chen Q, Kirsch GE, Zhang D, et al. Genetic basis and molecular mechanism for idiopathic ventricular fibrillation. *Nature* 1998;392:293–296.
28. Gussak I, Antzelevitch C, Bjerregaard P, et al. The Brugada syndrome: Clinical electrophysiologic, and genetic aspects. *J Am Coll Cardiol* 1999;33:5–15.
29. Clark RB, Bouchard RA, Salinas-Stefanon E, et al. Heterogeneity of action potential waveforms and potassium currents in rat ventricle. *Cardiovasc Res* 1993;27:1795–1799.
30. Suzuki J, Tsubone H, Sugano S. Characteristics of ventricular activation and recovery patterns in the rat. *J Vet Med Sci* 1992;54(4):711–716.
31. Lukas A, Antzelevitch C. Differences in the electrophysiological response of canine ventricular epicardium and endocardium to ischemia: Role of the transient outward current. *Circulation* 1993;88:2903–2915.
32. Antzelevitch C, Sicouri S, Lukas A, et al. Clinical implications of electrical heterogeneity in the heart: The electrophysiology and pharmacology of epicardial, M and endocardial cells. In Podrid PJ, Kowey PR (eds): *Cardiac Arrhythmia: Mechanism, Diagnosis and Management.* Baltimore, MD: William & Wilkins; 1995:88–107.
33. Litovsky SH, Antzelevitch C. Differences in the electrophysiological response of canine ventricular subendocardium and subepicardium to acetylcholine and isoproterenol. A direct effect of acetylcholine in ventricular myocardium. *Circ Res* 1990;67:615–627.
34. Krishnan SC, Antzelevitch C. Flecainide-induced arrhythmia in canine ventricular epicardium: Phase 2 Reentry? *Circulation* 1993;87:562–572.

35. Krishnan SC, Antzelevitch C. Sodium channel blockade produces opposite electrophysiologic effects in canine ventricular epicardium and endocardium. *Circ Res* 1991;69:277–291.
36. Wang Q, Shen J, Splawski I, et al. SCN5A mutations associated with an inherited cardiac arrhythmia, long QT syndrome. *Cell* 1995;80:805–811.
37. Bennett PB, Yazawa K, Makita N, et al. Molecular mechanism for an inherited cardiac arrhythmia. *Nature* 1995;376:683–685.
38. Dumaine R, Wang Q, Keating MT, et al. Multiple mechanisms of sodium channel-linked long QT syndrome. *Circ Res* 1996;78:916–924.
39. Rampazzo A, Nava A, Danieli GA, et al. The gene for arrhythmogenic right ventricular cardiomyopathy maps to chromosome 14q23–q24. *Hum Mol Genet* 1994;3:959–962.
40. Rampazzo A, Nava A, Erne P, et al. A new locus for arrhythmogenic right ventricular cardiomyopathy (ARVD2) maps to chromosome 1q42–q43. *Hum Mol Genet* 1995;4:2151–2154.
41. Severini GM, Krajinovic M, Pinamonti B, et al. A new locus for arrhythmogenic right ventricular dysplasia on the long arm of chromosome 14. *Genomics* 1996;31:193–200.
42. Wang DW, Yazawa K, George AL Jr, et al. Characterization of human cardiac Na+ channel mutations in the congenital long QT syndrome. *Proc Natl Acad Sci U S A* 1996;93:13200–13205.
43. Wang Q, Li Z, Shen J, et al. Genomic organization of the human SCN5A gene encoding the cardiac sodium channel. *Genomics* 1996;34:9–16.
44. Geisterfer-Lowrance AAT, Kass A, Tanigawa G, et al. A molecular basis for familial hypertrophic cardiomyopathy: A β-cardiac myosin heavy chain gene missense mutation. *Cell* 1990;62:999–1006.
45. Thierfelder L, Watkins H, MacRae C, et al. α-tropomyosin and cardiac troponin T mutations cause familial hypertrophic cardiomyopathy: A disease of the sarcomere. *Cell* 1994;77:701–712.
46. Bonne G, Carrier L, Bercovici J, et al. Cardiac myosin binding protein-C gene splice acceptor site mutation is associated with familial hypertrophic cardiomyopathy. *Nat Genet* 1995;11:438–440.
47. Watkins H, Conner D, Thierfelder L, et al. Mutations in the cardiac myosin binding protein-C gene on chromosome 11 cause familial hypertrophic cardiomyopathy. *Nat Genet* 1995;11:434–437.
48. Poetter K, Jiang H, Hassanzadeh S, et al. Mutations in either the essential or regulatory light chains of myosin are associated with a rare myopathy in human heart and skeletal muscle. *Nat Genet* 1996;13:63–69.
49. Kimura A, Harada H, Park JE, et al. Mutations in the cardiac troponin I gene associated with hypertrophic cardiomyopathy. *Nat Genet* 1997;16:379–382.
50. Watkins H, Rosenzweig A, Hwang DS, et al. Characteristics and prognostic implications of myosin missense mutations in familial hypertrophic cardiomyopathy. *N Engl J Med* 1992;326:1108–1114.
51. Watkins H, McKenna WJ, Theirfelder L, et al. Mutations in the genes for cardiac troponin T and α-tropomyosin in hypertrophic cardiomyopathy. *N Engl J Med* 1995;332:1058–1064.
52. Towbin JA. The role of cytoskeletal proteins in cardiomyopathies. *Curr Opin Cell Biol* 1998;10:131–139.

Chapter 24

Syncope, Sudden Death, and Sensible Screening

David J. Driscoll, MD

Sudden Death in Children and Adolescents

Sudden death in children and adolescents can be categorized into sudden infant death syndrome, sudden death in patients with known heart disease, or sudden death in presumably healthy children and adolescents exclusive of sudden infant death syndrome. The discussion in this chapter is limited to sudden death in presumably healthy children and adolescents greater than 1 year of age (ie, exclusive of sudden infant death syndrome). This is reasonable because "screening" implies that one is dealing with a population not known to have the problem of interest.

As compared with sudden, unexpected death in adults, sudden, unexpected death in presumably healthy children and adolescents is relatively uncommon. Between 1950 and 1982, there were 515 deaths in Olmsted County, MN, in patients ages 1 to 22 years.[1] Sudden, unexpected death occurred in 12 (2.3%). This represents an incidence of 1.3 sudden, unexpected deaths per 100,000 patient years. Kennedy et al[2,3] studied patients in St. Louis County, MO, and reported an incidence of sudden, unexpected death for children 1 to 9 years of age of 2.5 and 8.5 per 100,000 patient years during 1981 and 1982, respectively. In patients aged 10 to 19 years, the incidences were 2.4 and 5.3 for 1981 and 1982, respectively. Investigators studying sudden deaths in Allegheny County, PA, reported 207 cases of sudden, unexpected death among a total of 948 nontraumatic deaths in patients between 1 and 21 years of age for an incidence of 4.6 per 100,000 patient years.[4] The difference in the incidence rates among these studies may be accounted for by the

From: Quan L, Franklin WH (eds). *Ventricular Fibrillation: A Pediatric Problem.* Armonk, NY: Futura Publishing Company, Inc.; ©2000.

different demographics of the populations studied and by differences in interpretation of the definition of sudden, unexpected death. In the first study, deaths from infectious disease identified prior to death that could be associated with death (eg, meningitis, epiglottis) were not included, whereas these were included in the last study. Hence the "real" incidence of sudden, unexpected death in this age group is somewhere between 1.3 and 4.6 per 100,000 patient years.

In addition to these two studies of the incidence of sudden, unexpected death, there have been numerous non-population-based studies in which causes of sudden, unexpected death have been catalogued. A number of these studies involved sudden deaths that occurred on the athletic field. The list of causes includes, among others, hypertrophic cardiomyopathy, idiopathic dilated cardiomyopathy, myocarditis, anomalous origin of the left coronary artery or its branches from the right sinus of Valsalva, pulmonary vascular obstructive disease, fibrotic coronary artery occlusion, aortic stenosis, Marfan syndrome, mitral valve prolapse, arrhythmic right ventricular dysplasia, tunneled left anterior coronary artery, atherosclerosis, and subarachnoid hemorrhage. In addition, in a significant number of cases, no apparent cause of death was found. One must suspect that in these cases an arrhythmia may have caused the death and, for example, the patient may have had prolonged QT interval syndrome, Wolf-Parkinson-White syndrome (WPW), or other underlying potentially fatal arrhythmias.

Syncope and Sudden Death

Does syncope identify a subset of patients at increased risk for sudden death? Certainly some of the conditions listed above, such as hypertrophic cardiomyopathy, prolonged QT interval syndrome, and pulmonary hypertension, are known to be associated with both syncope and sudden death. This, however, cannot be interpreted to imply that syncope in a general population is, necessarily, a precursor of sudden death.

McHarg et al[5] studied 108 children between the ages of 2 and 19 years who were referred to a pediatric neurologist or cardiologist for evaluation of syncope. They found that 75% of the patients had vasovagal syncope, 11% had migraine, 8% had seizures, and 6% had cardiac arrhythmias. Of the 6 patients with cardiac arrhythmias, 2 had long QT interval syndrome, 1 had atrial flutter, 2 had ventricular tachycardia (1 with associated endocardial fibroelastosis), and 1 had WPW. Only one patient died, and that patient had ventricular tachycardia. This was not a population-based study, and it had inherent ascertainment bias.

Driscoll et al[6] reported the results of a population-based study of syncope in 192 patients 1 to 21 years of age. The long-term survival of these patients was no different than that of the normal population. One patient had prolonged QT interval syndrome. One patient died suddenly and unexpectedly. Exertional syncope occurred in six patients, and the patient who had sudden death and the patient with prolonged QT interval syndrome were among these six.

Screening of Athletes

There have been several reports of the utility of screening athletes with particular emphasis on identifying disorders that could be associated with sudden death. Five studies included echocardiography screening.[7–11] A total of 6684 high school, college, and Olympic athletes were screened. The following conditions were identified: mitral valve prolapse (113 cases), bicuspid aortic valve (14 cases), small ventricular septal defect or aneurysm (5 cases), increased left ventricular septal or wall thickness (but insufficient criteria for diagnosis for hypertrophic cardiomyopathy, 4 cases), aortic root dilation (but insufficient criteria for diagnosis of Marfan syndrome; 4 cases), and others (6 cases). In none of the patients was it thought that the abnormality found put the patient at increased risk for sudden death.

A task force of the American Heart Association recently issued a statement regarding preparticipation screening of athletes.[12] This expert panel concluded that$ext

> a complete and careful personal and family history and physical examination designed to identify those cardiovascular lesions known to cause sudden death or disease progression in young athletes is the best available and most practical approach to screening populations of competitive sports participants, regardless of age.————
>
> The cardiovascular history should include key questions designed to determine (1) prior occurrence of exertional chest pain/discomfort or syncope/near-syncope as well as excessive, unexpected, and unexplained shortness of breath or fatigue associated with exercise; (2) past detection of a heart murmur or increased systemic blood pressure; and (3) family history of premature death (sudden or otherwise), or significant disability from cardiovascular disease in close relatives younger than 50 years old or specific knowledge of the occurrence of certain conditions (e.g., hypertrophic cardiomyopathy, dilated cardiomyopathy, long QT syndrome, Marfan syndrome, or clinically important arrhythmias).[12]

This task force did not recommend incorporating echocardiography or stress testing into a screening program.

One may not be able to extrapolate these findings to a general population. Since the subjects were athletes, one might presume that, in general, they were healthy and also had undergone prior preparticipation evaluations.

Electrocardiographic Screening of Children

There have been studies in Japan of the utility of routine electrocardiographic screening of school children. Aihoshi et al[13] screened 14,227 school children and found 9 cases of prolonged QT interval. In another study (J. Fukushige, written communication, January, 1998), 17,361 school children were screened and 8 cases of left ventricular hypertrophy and 24 cases of WPW were found.

Summary and Recommendations

When considering screening for any problem, several issues must be considered, including 1) the size of the population to be screened; 2) the prevalence of the problem; 3) false-positive results; 4) false-negative results; 5) cost; and 6) legal issues.

There are approximately 77,071,000 children in the United States between the ages of 1 and 19 years. The incidence of sudden, unexpected death in this population is between 1 and 4 per 100,000 patient years. Thus, one could expect from 770 to 3082 sudden, unexpected deaths in presumably healthy children each year.

The potential screening modalities include history, physical examination, chest x-ray, electrocardiogram, stress electrocardiogram, echocardiogram, and, perhaps in the future, genetic screening using a blood specimen or other easily obtainable tissue.

The most common conditions that cause sudden death in this population are cardiomyopathies and coronary artery anomalies. These account for approximately 73% of sudden deaths in athletes. Primary arrhythmias potentially account for 11% of the deaths.[12] Thus, to detect the 73% of cases of cardiomyopathy and coronary anomalies, screening would require some sort of cardiac imaging such as echocardiography. In addition, electrocardiography would be needed to identify patients with long QT interval syndrome. Assuming that echocardiography costs $200.00 per study (a conservative estimate) and electrocardiography costs $25 per study, it would cost $17,340,975,000 to screen US children on one occasion. Because the phenotype of hypertrophic cardiomyopathy may not be expressed at a young age, screening may have to be repeated. However, assuming that there is only one screening encounter, it would cost from $5,626,533 to $22,520,746 per case of potential sudden death. This cost does not include the additional monetary, legal, and emotional cost of dealing with false-positive and false-negative tests.

One could consider routine electrocardiographic screening of children to detect potentially lethal cases of long QT syndrome and WPW. In athletes, this may account for 11% of the cases of sudden death on the athletic field. Based on the data from Aihoshi et al,[13] 0.06% of patients screened had long QT interval. Fukushige's data suggest that 0.04% of children screened had WPW.

Considering all of these issues, the most prudent approach to screening a presumably healthy population of children and adolescents would be to incorporate the recommendations of the American Heart Association Task Force on Cardiovascular Preparticipation Screening of Competitive Athletes into the usual health maintenance evaluation of children and adolescents. Specifically, at each health maintenance visit the following specific issues must be assessed. The examination should include measurement of the brachial artery blood pressure. Cardiac murmurs should be assessed with the patient standing in addition to the patient sitting or supine. Specific historical items to ascertain include those recommended by the task force of the American Heart Association, listed earlier in this chapter.[12]

Currently, in the United States, echocardiographic screening of large populations does not appear cost-effective or medically sound. Routine electrocardiographic screening could be performed, but there are insufficient data available to justify this.

The Future

The key to screening in the future will be genetic testing. This author believes that in the future a blood or saliva specimen will be machine-analyzed and all diseases known to result from gene defects will be identified. To me, this is no more mind boggling than current methods of hemoglobin measurement, white blood cell measurement, and differential and chemistry values would have been to physicians in 1898.

References

1. Driscoll D, Edwards W. Sudden unexpected death in children and adolescents. *J Am Coll Cardiol* 1985,5:118B–121B.
2. Kennedy H, Whitlock J. Sudden death in young persons—an urban study. *J Am Coll Cardiol* 1984,3:485. Abstract.
3. Kennedy H, Whitlock J, Buckingham T. Cardiovascular sudden death in young persons. *J Am Coll Cardiol* 1984,3:485. Abstract.

4. Neuspiel D, Kuller L. Sudden and unexpected natural death in childhood and adolescence. *JAMA* 1985;254:1321–1325.
5. McHarg M, Shinnar S, Rascoff H, Walsh C. Syncope in childhood. *Pediatr Cardiol* 1997;18:367–371.
6. Driscoll D, Jacobsen S, Porter C, Wollan P. Syncope in children and adolescents. *J Am Coll Cardiol* 1997;29:1039–1045.
7. Feinstein R, Colvin E, Kim O. Echocardiographic screening as part of a preparticipation examination. *Clin J Sport Med* 1993;3:149–152.
8. Murray P, Cantwell J, Heath D, Shoop J. The role of limited echocardiography in screening athletes. *Am J Cardiol* 1995;76:849–850.
9. Weidenbener E, Krauss M, Waller B, Taliercio C. Incorporation of screening in echocardiography in the preparticipation exam. *Clin J Sport Med* 1995;5:86–89.
10. Maron B, Bodison S, Wesley Y, et al. Results of screening a large group of intercollegiate competitive athletes for cardiovascular disease. *Am J Cardiol* 1987;10:1214–1221.
11. Spirito P, Pelliccia A, Proschan M, et al. Morphology of the "athlete's heart" assessed by echocardiography in 947 elite athletes representing 27 sports. *Am J Cardiol* 1994;74:802–806.
12. Maron B, Thompson P, Puffer J, et al. Cardiovascular preparticipation screening of competitive athletes. *Circulation* 1996;94:850–865.
13. Aihoshi S, Yoshinaga M, Nakamura M, et al. Screening for QT prolongation using a new exponential formula. *Jpn Circ J* 1995;59:185–189.

Section X

Summary:
Where Do We Go From Here?

Chapter 25

Ventricular Defibrillation in Pediatrics:
Research Imperatives

Leon Chameides, MD

It has been estimated that approximately 400,000 adults experience sudden cardiac death each year and that the overwhelming majority are in ventricular fibrillation (VF) and therefore potentially treatable, if rapidly defibrillated. This potential has been realized under controlled circumstances[1,2] such as the electrophysiology laboratory, rehabilitation program, coronary care unit, and cardiac catheterization laboratory, as well as in the field. The largest number of neurologically intact survivors from cardiac arrest results when the arrest is witnessed, Cardiopulmonary resuscitation (CPR) is started immediately, and the victim is in VF and is rapidly defibrillated.[3,4] This has led the Emergency Cardiac Care Committee of the American Heart Association to develop the concept of the "chain of survival" and to recommend that, for adult victims, the rescuer should "call first" so that a defibrillator and rescuers trained in its use might arrive rapidly.[5,6] For pediatric victims, the recommendation has remained to "call fast" but not "first," in the belief that primary VF is uncommon in this age group and that survival is more likely if the victim is rapidly assessed and CPR is given.

This chapter reviews the issues involved in ventricular defibrillation, especially as they apply to infants and children, and highlights the many areas that remain unknown and might prove fertile ground for further investigation.

Incidence

Before any rational decisions can be made about treatment, the true incidence of VF in infants and children must be ascertained. Most

From: Quan L, Franklin WH (eds). *Ventricular Fibrillation: A Pediatric Problem.* Armonk, NY: Futura Publishing Company, Inc.; ©2000.

studies have concluded that asystole is the most common terminal rhythm in the pediatric age group and that VF occurs in fewer than 10% of infants and children who experience a cardiac arrest.[7–10] Two studies suggest a higher incidence of 19%[11] and 22%[12]; however, as has been pointed out,[13] both of these studies involve selected populations. Victims of sudden infant death syndrome are excluded, and one of the studies[12] includes only patients who were subsequently admitted to a pediatric emergency department.

Weaknesses of all studies on the incidence of VF in pediatrics include the fact that they are retrospective, that a rhythm assessment was not performed early in a large number of victims, and that the total numbers in each study are modest. The true incidence will remain unknown until a prospective, multi-institutional study is performed with agreement on definitions of events according to the pediatric Utstein definitions,[14] and in which rhythms are evaluated early in the resuscitation. The increasingly common availability of automated external defibrillators (AEDs) should make it easier to record and evaluate the initial rhythm.

Are All VFs Equal?

The recommendation for rapid defibrillation of adult victims of sudden cardiac death is based on the fact that such therapy results in the largest number of neurologically intact survivors. This is presumably due to the fact that their cardiac disease and subsequent sudden VF occur at a time when other organs are relatively healthy and defibrillation takes place in a timely fashion before end organs have been irreparably damaged by ischemia. Would that hold true for pediatric victims?

In the most optimistic study of pediatric VF,[11] the total survival was only 9%, and only 4% survived with a good neurologic outcome. It is true that survival in victims with VF was 17% in comparison to 2% survival in those with asystole, but when these figures are more closely examined, it appears that the most common diagnosis in those with VF was cardiac (41%), and the second most common was in those with an overdose (14%). We are not told whether the overdose was with a dysrhythmogenic substance. Three of the five survivors with a good neurologic outcome had an underlying cardiac problem or overdose. Losek et al[8] report a 36% survival rate in children with VF in contrast to 5% in those with asystole. Of the 4 survivors, two were 15 and 17 years of age and, according to current recommendations, should therefore have been treated according to adult criteria. It is interesting to note that of the 4 survivors, 1 had a tricyclic ingestion, 1 suffered from myocarditis, and 1 sustained blunt chest trauma. Three of the 4 survivors in this study presumably had a reversible primary cardiac dysrhythmia. These studies suggest that the children who have a good outcome from defibrillation may be a subset and involve only a small group of infants and children with a cardiac or conduction system problem.

In adults, VF as a result of acute myocardial ischemia is associated with the best chance for survival.[15,16] Patients in secondary VF, ie, those whose VF is not due to acute myocardial ischemia but due to conditions such as cardiac tamponade, tension pneumothorax, pulmonary embolism, congestive heart failure, hypothermia, hypovolemia, hypoxemia, acidosis, electrolyte imbalance, and drug toxicity, appear to have a lower defibrillation success rate.[17] In other words, in those adult victims whose cause of arrest is more comparable to that of infants and children, survival is more likely associated with an ability to recognize and reverse the underlying problem[18,19] than with defibrillation.

Before any major changes are recommended in the resuscitation of infants and children, we must not only define the true incidence of VF in that age group but we should also bear the burden of proving that early defibrillation of these victims will result in better neurologic outcome than with current resuscitation measures.

Energy Determinants of Defibrillation

Current flow (amperes) across the myocardium depolarizes the myocardial membrane and defibrillates the heart. Self-sustaining VF requires a critical mass of myocardium and is more easily supported in larger hearts.[20,21] Garrey[22] demonstrated that when pieces of ventricular muscle with a surface area of less than 4 cm^2 were shaved from the wall of the fibrillating left ventricle, they stopped fibrillating. The remaining portion of the ventricle continued fibrillating until three quarters of the ventricular mass had been removed. This has been verified in an elegant series of experiments by Zipes et al,[23] who also concluded that the critical mass necessary for VF to continue in 13 dogs was 28% of the ventricular myocardium. This may be an important reason for the apparently lower frequency of VF in infants.

In the same series of experiments, Zipes et al,[23] showed that it is not necessary that every myocardial cell be depolarized for successful defibrillation; a critical mass of myocardium must, however, be depolarized. That critical mass is directly related to the mass of the heart; significantly more current is required to terminate VF in heavier hearts.

Use of this information to determine the *safest* electrical energy dose for transthoracic ventricular defibrillation in the clinical setting is complicated by the fact that in a given patient we know neither the *weight* of the heart nor the *amount of current* delivered across the myocardium.

Safety of Electrical Energy

Emphasis on the *safest* electrical energy dose is necessary because the potential ill effects of electrical energy on the myocardium have been well documented. Serum creatine phosphokinase (CPK) increases as a result of electrical defibrillation. Although the majority of this enzyme is in the MM fraction released from skeletal muscles of the thorax,[24,25] Jakobsson et al[26] found a rise in the CPK-MB fraction that was directly related to the total amount of energy delivered and, therefore, most likely due to myocardial damage. Defibrillation has been documented to impair left ventricular function,[27] to cause cellular damage directly related to the energy level,[28] and to cause myocardial necrosis in humans[29] and animals subjected to repeated high-energy defibrillation.[30] The incidence and severity of postdefibrillation dysrhythmias are also directly related to the energy level.[31–35]

Energy Dose/Weight Relationship

A clear direct relationship has been established experimentally between the mass of the heart and the amount of current required for its defibrillation.[23] There has, however, been significant controversy about translating this into practical, clinical terms for adult victims. In 1974, Tacker et al[36–38] suggested that a relationship exists between the energy required for defibrillation of the heart and the victim's weight by noting that rabbits weighing 2.3 kg required much less energy than horses weighing 340 kg although there was a wide species variation. On this basis, they recommended a per-kilogram energy dose and suggested that maximal energy delivered by commercially available defibrillators might be insufficient to defibrillate heavy persons. This has been vigorously disputed by data based on clinical experience and clinical studies.[16,17,39–43] Interestingly, none of the papers disputing the energy dose/body weight relationship point out that there are no adult data that establish a relationship between heart weight and body weight.

The objections raised for the absence of an energy dose/body weight relationship for adults may not necessarily apply to children. Figure 1 shows the relationship between the weight of the heart[44] and age in males and females. Figures 2 and 3 show the excellent relationship ($r^2=0.98$ to 0.99) that exists between the weight of the heart and that of the body (50th percentile) at various ages. The weight of the

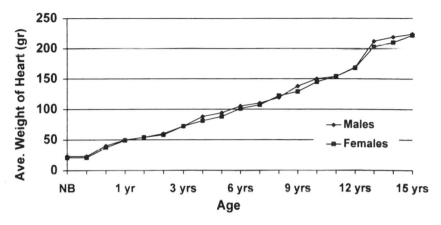

Figure 1. Relationship between the average weight of the heart[44] and age.

body at various ages is taken from a standard growth curve, since the study on the weight of the heart[44] does not provide body weights. This excellent relationship also holds true for the 10th and 90th percentiles. The relationship is almost as good ($r^2=0.95$) for heart weight and body length (Figure 3). Length is easier in an emergency to obtain than weight and has previously been shown to be a useful way of rapidly estimating drug dosages.[45,46] Figures 4 and 5 show that these relationships appear not to carry over into adulthood.

Since there is a paucity of clinical data, it is not known whether the heart/body weight relationship in infants and children is translatable

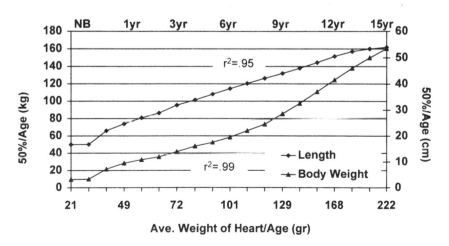

Figure 2. Relationship between the average weight of the heart[44] and the 50th% of body weight and length for girls at various ages.

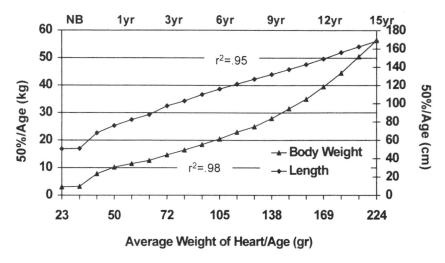

Figure 3. Relationship between the average weight of the heart[44] and the 50th% of body weight and length for boys at various ages.

into clinical practice. A single retrospective study[47] of 71 defibrillation attempts in 27 children showed that an energy dose of 2 J/kg, a dose subsequently recommended by the American Heart Association,[48] was effective in terminating 85% of the episodes of VF. This must be verified in a prospective, multi-institutional study, using Utstein pediatric criteria, to determine the lowest, safest electrical energy required to defibrillate the largest number of infants and children.

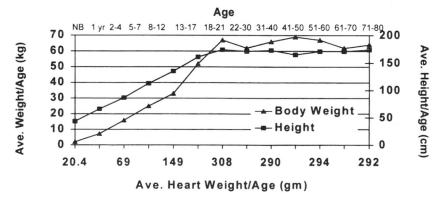

Figure 4. Relationship between the average weight of the heart and body weight by age in males.[66]

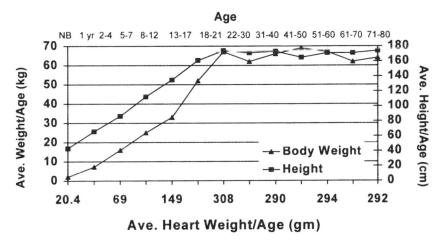

Figure 5. Relationship between the average weight of the heart and body weight by age in females.[66]

Transmyocardial Current

In transthoracic defibrillation, the amount of current ultimately delivered to the myocardium is determined by the energy level (as discussed above), the resistance interfaces that energy encounters, each of which has the potential for decreasing the delivered energy level, and the amount of electrical energy dissipated to other intrathoracic structures.

The major resistance interfaces are the electrode–skin interface and the chest tissue interface, which is more variable and important. The electrode–skin interpose resistance can be minimized by using the appropriate paddle size, location, force, and coupling agent. Small-sized paddles cause a concentrated density of current to be delivered which can cause myocardial injury[49] and depolarize too little myocardial tissue, while paddles that are too large cause more current shunting to the thorax and result in lower current flow through the heart.[50] In a study[51] measuring transthoracic impedance in a group of healthy infants and children, it was demonstrated that the use of adult paddles significantly lowers transthoracic impedance and that adult paddles will fit over the entire surface on chests of infants weighing approximately 10 kg ($\approx$1 year of age). The effect of paddle size on shunting current to other intrathoracic tissues has not been studied in pediatric models or patients. It is therefore not known at this time which effect of large paddles is the more important in clinical situations, their lowered transthoracic impedance or their potential for a lower current flow through the heart.

Transthoracic impedance is determined primarily by tissues of the thorax. When measured in 47 healthy infants and children,[51] transthoracic impedance was found to be not much lower than in adults,[52] and to be significantly but weakly related to body weight and body surface area. Hemodynamic and metabolic effects of cardiac arrest can, however, alter transthoracic impedance. It has been documented experimentally that myocardial tissue resistance is increased by hypoxia[53] and by ischemia[54] and that resistance of blood is inversely related to its velocity.[55]

Dissipated Electrical Energy

Defibrillation occurs when a transcardiac current threshold causes myocardial current density to reach a critical level. In dogs it has been found that 82% of the transthoracic current is shunted by the thoracic cage, and 14% by the lungs. Thus only 4% of the current delivered to the chest passes through the heart.[56] This has subsequently been verified in human adults undergoing cardiac surgery.[57] It is unknown what percentage of transthoracic current is shunted away from the heart in infants and children and what factors might change that percentage. This is critical information inasmuch as it might influence the defibrillation energy dose.

Technological Innovations

Current-Based Defibrillator

The current-based defibrillator measures the patient's transthoracic resistance, which has a fairly large patient-to-patient variability, especially in pathologic states, and adjusts the energy level to deliver a preset amount of current.[58–60] This eliminates one of the variables in the amount of current reaching the heart. Initial experience in adults[61] suggests that this device has the same success rate as conventional defibrillators, but at a lower energy setting. This should result in less myocardial damage and fewer postdefibrillation complications. Kerber et al[62] found that delivering 30 to 37 amperes as the initial shock defibrillates 80% of adult patients and that myocardial damage can occur when shocks of greater than 40 amperes are delivered. There has been no experience with current-based defibrillation in pediatric patients, and the safe current dose is unknown. In animal experiments, peak current dose has been found to be virtually independent of the species at 1 A/kg.[38]

Automated External Defibrillation

The development of the AED[63] has added a new dimension to rapid resuscitation from sudden cardiac death because it has made rapid defibrillation possible by minimally trained personnel. Miniaturization and decrease in cost will make it even more available and accessible in the future. AEDs are not recommended for use in infants and children because their accuracy in the interpretation of pediatric rhythms is unknown and their energy level, currently set at 200 to 360 J, is too high. Before any recommendations are made to change this, several issues will need to be addressed:

1. What is the incidence of VF in infants and children (less than 8 years of age), and is their outcome improved by rapid defibrillation?

2. Are currently used algorithms for rhythm interpretation accurate in infants and young children? Their accuracy in a small number of adolescents has been shown to be comparable to that of adults,[64] but their accuracy in interpreting the rhythm in younger children is unknown.

3. How can the AED be adapted for infants and children without compromising its greatest virtue—its simplicity? Smaller electrodes for infants can easily be added. The appropriate energy level is a more challenging issue that could be solved in several ways. If the length/energy level were verified, then by switching to a pediatric mode, a measuring device could be activated that would determine the energy level. An alternative would be to add settings for 25, 50, and 100 J, which would probably safely satisfy pediatric needs.

At our current level of knowledge, this author's recommendation is that we should encourage the use of AEDs in diagnosing rhythms in infants and children but not adapt them for pediatric use until more information is available.

Low-Energy Biphasic Waveform Defibrillation

There have been attempts to find more effective waveforms, such as biphasic waveforms[65] and waveforms in which the speed at which the wave returns to zero has been altered, that will defibrillate the heart using lower, and therefore safer, energy levels. Whereas these alternatives will be followed with interest as research and experience with them continues, there are no data applicable to children and the American Heart Association has not yet developed guidelines or recommendations even for adults.

Research Imperatives

This chapter has attempted to review the issues involved in ventricular defibrillation, especially as they apply to infants and children, and has highlighted the following areas in which our knowledge is deficient and which might be fruitful research endeavors. Because of the relative infrequency of VF in pediatrics, clinical studies will have to be multi-institutional with unified definitions according to the pediatric Utstein criteria:

- To define the incidence of VF in infants and children via a prospective study with early rhythm evaluations.
- To prove that early defibrillation of infants and children produces better results than advanced CPR.
- To define the lowest electrical energy required to defibrillate the hearts of infants and children and to determine whether that electrical energy dose can be related to the child's weight or length.
- To quantitate the transchest impedance in infants and children with various pathologic states including shock and cardiac arrest.
- To identify in pediatric animal models and patients how much transthoracic current actually crosses the heart.
- To define the accuracy of algorithms for rhythm interpretation of automated electrical defibrillators in infants and children.
- To encourage the use of AEDs in analyzing rhythms of infants and children if the algorithms are found to be, or are modified to become accurate.

Acknowledgment   I wish to express my gratitude to Georgine S. Burke, PhD, for her assistance with the statistical analysis and graphs on the heart weight/body weight and length relationships

References

1. Fletcher GF, Cantwell JD. Ventricular fibrillation in a medically supervised cardiac exercise program: Clinical, angiographic and surgical correlations. *JAMA* 1977;238:2627–2629.

2. Hossack KF, Hartwig R. Cardiac arrest associated with supervised cardiac rehabilitation. *J Cardiac Rehab* 1982;2:402–408.
3. Eisenberg MS, Bergner L, Hallstrom A. Out-of-hospital cardiac arrest: Improved survival with paramedic services. *Lancet* 1980;2:812–815.
4. Eisenberg MS, Bergner L, Hallstrom A. Paramedic programs and out-of-hospital cardiac arrest. I. Factors associated with successful resuscitation. *Am J Public Health* 1979;69:30–38.
5. American Heart Association. Guidelines for cardiopulmonary resuscitation and emergency cardiac care. *JAMA* 1992;268:2172–2295.
6. Cummins RO, Ornato JP, Thies WH, et al. Improving survival from cardiac arrest: The "chain of survival" concept. *Circulation* 1991;83:1832–1844.
7. Eisenberg M, Bergner L, Hallstrom A. Epidemiology of cardiac arrest and resuscitation in children. *Ann Emerg Med* 1983;12:672–674.
8. Losek JD, Hennes H, Glaeser PW, et al. Prehospital care of the pulseless, nonbreathing pediatric patient. *Am J Emerg Med* 1987;5:370–374.
9. Torphy DE, Minster MG, Thompson BM. Cardiopulmonary arrest and resuscitation in children. *Am J Dis Child* 1984;138:1099–1102.
10. Chandra NL, Krischer JP. The demographics of cardiac arrest support "phone fast" for children. *Circulation* 1993;88(suppl I):I193. Abstract.
11. Mogayzel C, Quan L, Graves JR, et al. Out-of-hospital ventricular fibrillation in children and adolescents: Causes and outcome. *Ann Emerg Med* 1995;25:484–491.
12. Hickey RW, Cohen DM, Strausbaugh S, et al. Pediatric patients requiring CPR in the prehospital setting. *Ann Emerg Med* 1995;25:495–501.
13. Hazinski MF. Is pediatric resuscitation unique? Relative merits of early CPR and ventilation versus early defibrillation for young victims of cardiac arrest. *Ann Emerg Med* 1995;25:540–543.
14. Zaritsky A, Nadkarni V, Hazinski MF, et al. Recommended guidelines for uniform reporting of pediatric advanced life support: The pediatric Utstein style. A statement for health care professionals from a task force of the American Academy of Pediatrics, the American Heart Association, and the European Resuscitation Council. *Circulation* 1995;92:2006–2020.
15. Dalzell GW, Adgey AJ. Determinants of successful transthoracic defibrillation and outcome in ventricular fibrillation. *Br Heart J* 1991;65:311–316.
16. Gascho JA, Crampton RS, Cherwek ML, et al. Determinants of ventricular defibrillation in adults. *Circulation* 1979;60:231–240.
17. Kerber RE, Sarnat W. Factors influencing the success of ventricular defibrillation in man. *Circulation* 1979;60:226–230.
18. Gascho J, Sipes J, Cherwek M, et al. Determinants of ventricular defibrillation. *Circulation* 1978;11(suppl II):II203.
19. Gerst PH, Fleming WH, Malm JR. Increased susceptibility of the heart to ventricular fibrillation during metabolic acidosis. *Circ Res* 1966;19:63–70.
20. McWilliam JA. Fibrillar contraction of the heart. *J Physiol* 1887;8:296–310.
21. Porter WT. On the results of ligation of the coronary arteries. *J Physiol (Lond)* 1894;15:121–138.
22. Garrey WE. The nature of fibrillatory contraction of the heart—its relation to tissue mass and form. *Am J Physiol* 1914;33:397–414.
23. Zipes DP, Fischer J, King RM, et al. Termination of ventricular fibrillation in dogs by depolarizing a critical amount of myocardium. *Am J Cardiol* 1975;36:37–40.
24. Ehsani A, Ewy GA, Sobel BE. Effects of electrical countershock on serum creatine phosphokinase (CPK) isoenzyme activity. *Am J Cardiol* 1976;37:12–18.
25. Mattana J, Singhal PC. Determinants of elevated creatine kinase activity

and creatine kinase MB fraction following cardiopulmonary resuscitation. *Chest* 1992;101:1386–1392.

26. Jakobsson J, Odmansson I, Nordlander R. Enzyme release after elective cardioversion. *Eur Heart J* 1990;11:749–752.
27. Stoddard MF, Labovitz AJ, Stevens LL, et al. Effects of electrophysiologic studies resulting in electrical countershock or burst pacing on left ventricular systolic and diastolic function. *Am Heart J* 1988;116: 364–370.
28. DiCola VC, Freedman GS, Downing SE, et al. Myocardial uptake of technetium-99 m stannous pyrophosphate following direct current transthoracic countershock. *Circulation* 1976;54:980–986.
29. Warner ED, Dahl E, Ewy GA. Myocardial injury from transthoracic defibrillator countershock. *Arch Pathol* 1975;99:559.
30. Adgey AJ, Patton JN, Campbell NP, et al. Ventricular defibrillation: Appropriate energy levels. *Circulation* 1979;60:219–222.
31. Weaver WD, Cobb LA, Copass MK, et al. Ventricular defibrillation: A comparative trial using 175 J and 320 J shocks. *N Engl J Med* 1982;307: 1101–1106.
32. Lown B, Neuman J, Amarosingham R, et al. Comparison of alternating current with direct current electroshock across the closed chest. *Am J Cardiol* 1962;10:223–233.
33. Peleska B. Cardiac arrhythmias following condenser discharges and their dependence upon strength of current and phase of cardiac cycle. *Circ Res* 1963;13:21–32.
34. Gold JH, Schuder JL, Stoeckle H, et al. Transthoracic ventricular defibrillation in the 100 kg calf with unidirectional rectangular pulses. *Circulation* 1977;56:745–750.
35. Resnekov L, McDonald C. Complications in 220 patients with cardiac dysrhythmias treated by phased direct current shock and indications for cardioversion. *Br Heart J* 1967;29:926–936.
36. Tacker WA Jr, Galioto FM Jr, Giuliani E, et al. Energy dosage for human trans-chest electrical ventricular defibrillation. *N Engl J Med* 1974;290: 214–215.
37. Tacker WA Jr, Geddes LA, Cabller PS, et al. Electrical threshold for defibrillation of canine ventricles following myocardial infarction. *Am Heart J* 1974;88:476–481.
38. Geddes LA, Tacker WA Jr, Rosborough JP, et al. Electrical dose for ventricular defibrillation of large and small animals using precordial electrodes. *J Clin Invest* 1974;53:310–319.
39. Pantridge JF, Adgey AAJ, Webb SW, et al. Electrical requirements for ventricular defibrillation. *Br Med J* 1975;2:313–315.
40. Campbell NPS, Webb SW, Adgey AAJ, et al. Transthoracic ventricular defibrillation in adults. *Br Med J* 1977;2:1379–1381.
41. Adgey AAJ, Campbell NP, Webb SW, et al. Transthoracic ventricular defibrillation in the adult. *Med Instrum* 1978;12:17–19.
42. Kerber RE, Sarnat W. Clinical studies on defibrillation dose: Effects of body weight and heart weight. *Med Instrum* 1978;12:55. Abstract.
43. DeSilva RA, Lown B. Energy requirements for defibrillation of a markedly overweight patient. *Circulation* 1978;57:827–830.
44. Schultz DM, Giordano DA. Hearts of infants and children. *Arch Pathol* 1962;74:464–471.
45. Lubitz D, Seidel JS, Chameides L, et al. Rapid estimation of body weight

and resuscitation. Drug dosages from length. *Am J Dis Child* 1988;142:403. Abstract.

46. Lubitz D, Seidel JS, Chameides L, et al. A rapid method for estimating weight and resuscitation. Drug dosages from length in the pediatric age group. *Ann Emerg Med* 1988;17:576–581.

47. Gutgesell HP, Tacker HA, Geddes LA, et al. Energy dose for ventricular defibrillation of children. *Pediatrics* 1976;58:898–901.

48. Chameides L, Brown GE, Raye J Jr, et al. Guidelines for defibrillation in infants and children. *Circulation* 1977;56:502A–503A.

49. Dahl CF, Ewy GA, Warner ED, et al. Myocardial necrosis from direct current countershock. *Circulation* 1974;50:956–960.

50. Karlon WJ, Eisenberg SR, Lehr JL. Effects of paddle placement and size on defibrillation current distribution: A three dimensional finite element model. *IEEE Trans Biomed Eng* 1993;40:246–255.

51. Atkins DL, Sirna S, Kieso R, et al. Pediatric defibrillation: Importance of paddle size in determining transthoracic impedance. *Pediatrics* 1988;82:914–918.

52. Kerber RE, Jensen SR, Gascho JA, et al. Determinants of defibrillation: Prospective analysis of 183 patients. *Am J Cardiol* 1983;52:739–745.

53. Wojczak J. Contractures and increase in internal longitudinal resistance of cow ventricular muscle induced by hypoxia. *Circ Res* 1979;44:88–95.

54. Childers RW, Cope T, Lyon R, et al. Tissue resistance in ventricular ischemia. *Circulation* 1979;59 & 60(suppl II):II110. Abstract.

55. Geddes LA, Baker LE. The specific resistance of biological material—a compendium of data for the biomedical engineer and physiologist. *Med Biol Eng* 1967;5:271–293.

56. Deale GO, Lerman BB. Intrathoracic current flow during transthoracic defibrillation in dogs. Transthoracic current fraction. *Circ Res* 1990;67:1405–1419.

57. Lerman BB, Deale OC. Relation between transcardiac and transthoracic current during defibrillation in humans. *Circ Res* 1990;67:1420–1426.

58. Dalzell GW, Cunningham SR, Anderson J, et al. Initial experience with a microprocessor controlled current based defibrillator. *Br Heart J* 1989;61:502–505.

59. Geddes LA, Tacker WA, Schoenlein W, et al. The prediction of the impedance of the thorax to defibrillating current. *Med Instrum* 1976;10:159–162.

60. Kerber RE, McPherson D, Charbonier F, et al. Automated impedance based energy adjustment for defibrillation: Experimental studies. *Circulation* 1985;71:136–140.

61. Lerman BB, Di Marco JP, Haines DE, et al. Current based defibrillation: A prospective study. *Circulation* 1988;78(suppl II):II45.

62. Kerber RE, Martins JB, Kienzle MG, et al. Energy, current, and success in defibrillation and cardioversion: Clinical studies using an automated impedance-based method of energy adjustment. *Circulation* 1988;77:1038–1046.

63. Weisfeldt M, Kerber R, McGoldrick R, et al. American Heart Association report on the public access defibrillation conference. *Circulation* 1995;92:2740–2747.

64. Atkins DL, Hartley LL, York DK. Accurate recognition and effective treatment of ventricular fibrillation by automated external defibrillation in adolescents. *Pediatrics* 1998;101:393–397.

65. Cummins RO, Hazinski MF, Kerber RE, et al. Low-energy biphasic wave-

form defibrillation: Evidence-based review applied to emergency cardio-vascular care guidelines. A statement for health-care professionals from the American Heart Association committee on emergency cardiovascular care and the subcommittees on basic life support, advanced life support, and pediatric resuscitation. *Circulation* 1998;97:1654–1667.

66. Smith HL. The relation of the weight of the heart to the weight of the body and of the weight of the heart to age. *Am Heart J* 1928;4:79–93.

Index